Also by Kate Kelly and Peggy Ramundo

The ADDed Dimension:
Everyday Advice for Adults with ADD
(with D. Steven Ledingham)

The ADDed Dimension:
Celebrating the Opportunities, Rewards, and Challenges
of the ADD Experience (with D. Steven Ledingham)

You Mean I'm Not Lazy, Stupid or Crazy?!

The Classic Self-Help Book for Adults with Attention Deficit Disorder

KATE KELLY

AND

PEGGY RAMUNDO

Foreword by Ned Hallowell, M.D.

SCRIBNER
New York   London   Toronto   Sydney

DISCLAIMER

This publication contains the opinions and ideas of its authors. It is intended to provide helpful and informative material on the subjects addressed in the publication. It is sold with the understanding that the authors and publisher are not engaged in rendering medical, health or any other kind of personal professional services in the book. The reader should consult his or her medical, health or other competent professional before adopting any of the suggestions in this book or drawing inferences from it.

The authors and publisher specifically disclaim all responsibility for any liability, loss or risk, personal or otherwise, which is incurred as a consequence, directly or indirectly, of the use and application of any of the contents of this book.

SCRIBNER
1230 Avenue of the Americas
New York, NY 10020

Copyright © 1993, 2006 by Kate Kelly and Peggy Ramundo

First Scribner trade paperback edition 2006

SCRIBNER and design are trademarks of Macmillan Library Reference USA, Inc. used under license by Simon & Schuster, the publisher of this work.

For information about special discounts for bulk purchases, please contact Simon & Schuster Special Sales: 1-800-456-6798 or business@simonandschuster.com

Manufactured in the United States of America

33 35 37 39 40 38 36 34 32

Library of Congress Control Number: 9440538

ISBN-13: 978-0-684-80116-2
ISBN-10: 0-684-80116-7
ISBN-13: 978-0-7432-6448-8 (Pbk)
ISBN-10: 0-7432-6448-7 (Pbk)

This book is dedicated to my partner and soul mate,
Paul Ravenscraft. He is the answer to a prayer for one who
shares my vision of life as a spiritual journey. Namaste, Paul.

Kate Kelly

I dedicate this book to:
Mom and Pop Eliezer, Roger, Nona and Noni,
Uncle Bill, Phil and Julie.
You have left this earthly plane and I miss you. Though I can't see
or touch you anymore, I hold each of you in my heart—your
memory lovingly wrapped and carried forever in my soul.

Peggy Ramundo

Contents

Here for Anyway?" • Toxic Mental Debris: The Vicious Cycle of Shame, Perfectionism and Procrastination

Acknowledgments

Our wholehearted thanks go to all the people who made this book possible. Please forgive any ADD oopses if you have contributed and fail to find your name mentioned here. While our hearts are full of gratitude, our memories have been known to go south from time to time.

First, we wish to acknowledge those people who made substantial contributions to the original, self-published version of the *Lazy Crazy* book. Rob Ramundo tops the list as the person who put his heart and soul into the publishing and promotion of our first, self-published edition in 1993. Without Rob, we would never have been able to create and run Tyrell and Jerem Press. His "don't tell me no" attitude got us major distribution at a time when all the experts were saying that the big guys were not interested in dealing with a one-title publishing house. The book was so successful, in fact, that soon our phones were ringing off the hook with calls from major publishers wanting to buy it. We can't thank you enough, Rob, for your passion, dedication and hard work. You made it all possible.

Next, we wish to thank Tony Magliano, who created all but a few of the cartoons you will see in this second edition. We liked his original artwork so much that we basically recycled most of his cartoons from the original book, using them in various places in the new chapters.

Thank you, Larry Silver, for writing a foreword to endorse our book back in the days when no one had heard of Kate Kelly and Peggy Ramundo, and very few people knew that the adult form of ADD even existed.

We fondly remember Perry, who manned the phones and took orders for our self-published book from his outpost like *Northern Exposure* in upper Michigan. He had a special talent for getting ADDers off that expensive 1-800 line quickly, without making them wrong. He was a genius at customer service.

David Stull gave us the invaluable gift of the perfect title for our book. We promptly threw out the long list of possibilities when he called us with the results of his brilliant brainstorm.

A grateful thanks go to Rita Stull and George Schober who made substantial editorial contributions.

Many thanks to the following people who provided moral and/or practical support:

The original Cincinnati ADD Adult Support Group, the ADD Council of Greater Cincinnati, Dr. Bonnie Green, Rob Allard, Billy Stockton, Marjorie Busching, Marta Donahoe, Angela Field, Suzanne Behle, Liz Wymer, Bunny Hensley, Doug Pentz, Tyrell Pentz and Mary Jane Johnson.

For the Scriber/Simon and Schuster 1995 hardcover and 1996 paperback edition of *You Mean I'm Not Lazy, Stupid or Crazy?!* we thank our agent, Jody Rein, and editor, Maria Guarneschelli. Special thanks to Jody for her ability to rock and roll with all our ups and downs and writer's heebie-jeebies. Thanks also to Phyllis Heller, publicist.

For the current, second edition of this book, the lion's share of gratitude goes to Paul Ravenscraft, Kate's significant other and our project manager. We could not have pulled it together without his heart-centered involvement and considerable skills. We love you, Paul.

Special thanks go to Dave Brattain, who kept ADDed Dimension Coaching on an even keel while the book was in progress. We also thank him for his contribution to the meditation chapter.

We also express our gratitude to Doug Pentz and Tom D' Erminio for sharing their experience treating multitudes of ADD adults at The Affinity Center.

We wish to honor and acknowledge our coaching teacher and mentor, Madelyn Griffith-Haynie.

Thank you, Ned Hallowell, for writing the Foreword and for all that you have done to inspire and encourage adults with ADD.

We are grateful to the following people and organizations, who contributed ideas, knowledge and moral or practical support:

Terry Matlin, Kathy Aker, Claudia Foster, Steven Ledingham, Wendy Richardson, Sari Solden, Pat Quinn, Kathleen Nadeau, Thom Hartmann, Andrea Little, Neil Anderson, Maegdlyn Morris, Lee Schmidt, Janet Robinson, Michelle Sellers, Ursula Stegall, Richard and Antoinette Asimus, Mark Stucker, Lisa Henry, Roland Rotz, Sarah Wright, Louise Lavey, E. L. Kersten, Ph.D., Julie Nichols, our many clients, The ADDed Dimension Coaching Group, The New Thought Unity Center of Cincinnati, the folks from GDT and The Designers workroom and The Affinity Center.

Beth Wareham, our editor for the second edition, deserves a round of applause for her unflagging support and encouragement. She was endlessly patient and never made us wrong when we needed deadline extensions. We honor Beth as a person who leads from the heart.

Peggy expresses a special thank-you to James Richardson—first my daughter's high school friend and then mine. You seem to know when my now empty nest has me feeling particularly sad.

You appear unexpectedly with your ready smile and encouraging hug. That you trust me with your private hurts and disappointments is a gift I treasure. Thank you, James, for your unconditional love—know that you have mine in return.

Last, but far from least, we thank our families. Our children Tyrell, Jeremy and Alison have enriched our lives and touched our souls. Kate is grateful to her mom and dad, Barbara and Charles Kelly, for doing a terrific job raising a difficult child. Peggy sends a special message to her aunt Elizabeth—you have been a rock and anchor in my life. Your loving support is deeply appreciated.

Foreword

The title of this book alone would have made it a classic when it first came out, but that it also was a wonderful resource for people who had attention deficits sealed the deal.

You Mean I'm Not Lazy, Crazy, or Stupid?! now returns for a new run, updated, refurbished, face-lifted and spiffed up. The authors have applied their usual highly imaginative incantations to conjure up this new incarnation of their classic.

All who read this will learn. Many who do not read it will also learn because someone else will read it for them and tell them about the best parts. That will be a difficult decision because there are so many good parts.

What I like best is not any one part, but the attitude and tone of the book. Open, warm, honest and funny, this book welcomes the reader and never seeks to do anything but help and entertain. The authors are the salt of the earth: no baloney here, just real meat. They also have fabulous senses of humor. I guarantee you will laugh when you read this book. As well as learn. And maybe shed a tear or two.

I am happy to open the book with a few words of my own, but the authors do not need any introduction, as the book carries itself like a cork in a hurricane sea. Buoyant, unsinkable and bobbing along no matter what, this cork will continue to float for years to come.

I hope all who read it will come away filled with hope and enthusiasm, as well as knowledge, and strengthened with the resolve to build upon the talents that all people with ADD naturally possess. The only real disabilities are fear, shame and the loss of hope. This book helps to restore hope, dispel fear and extinguish shame.

What a great gift, indeed.

Ned Hallowell, M.D.
Founder of the Hallowell
Center for Cognitive and
Emotional Health
Sudbury, Massachusetts

Introduction

ADD—Now and Then

It has been fifteen years since we began writing the original version of *You Mean I'm Not Lazy, Stupid or Crazy?!* Back then, we were newly diagnosed and fired up with the awareness of the impact of ADD on our lives. It was a profound experience . . . something like a religious conversion, as a matter of fact. Complete with the intense zeal displayed by missionaries. We saw the light. ADD was the root of all our life problems . . . finally they had a name. We saw ADD everywhere and set about trying to convert (or at least enlighten) everyone in our paths. In fact, it took years to develop the finesse necessary to send a message that would actually be heard. Nobody likes the hard sell. ADD enthusiasm is great, but we get better results when we're aware of our energy levels—too much force and the audience is literally propelled in the opposite direction.

In 1990, almost no one had heard of ADD in adulthood. The common wisdom then was that kids outgrew it sometime during puberty. Very few girls were diagnosed, mostly because the female version of ADD tends to be much quieter than that of the classic hyperactive boy. Boys with the inattentive type of ADD were also overlooked.

A year later, with a rough first draft of the book completed, we sent a number of queries to publishing houses, both major and minor. None of them were interested in buying it. Some of the rejection notices were merely form letters . . . thanks, but no

1

thanks. A few contained personal notes. All of them, however, sent the message that they didn't think there was enough of a market for a book on ADD adults. We thought they had to be kidding . . . didn't they see all the ADD around them the way we did? We knew even then that the less than 3 percent number was way off, that the real number of ADD adults was closer to 10 to 20 percent of the population.

We were pioneers, among the first small group of ADDults to realize that we had been in a fog all our lives, and that it didn't have to be that way. ADD is often subtle. Generally it takes personal experience, either with your own ADD or that of close family members, to get it. Most of the professionals who work with ADDult clients were drawn to the field because they have "in the trenches" knowledge of the disorder. We became ADD coaches because we were so passionate about helping others traverse the same territory we had traveled with very little guidance.

Those of us who specialized in adult ADD had to make it up as we went along—in the beginning. When we set out to write the original *Lazy Crazy* book, we did so partly out of our frustration that there was practically nothing written on the subject at the time. A few articles and a book chapter were all that was available specifically on the subject of ADDulthood. You may be wondering how we managed to write such a long and dense book without much in the way of resources. Well, we read the literature on childhood ADD and extrapolated . . . drawing heavily on our personal experiences and those of others in early support groups. As far as the treatment aspects of the book, other than the medication, much of the treatment recommendations section was an educated guess.

To our delight, we have noted during the revision process that the book has held up very well. Most of it is just as useful today as it was when it was first published in 1993. Now, however, there is more research to back up our educated guesses. In addition, people have been busy writing about adult ADD in the past decade and a half. There are now over a hundred books dealing with the subject.

What has changed since we wrote the so-called bible of ADD? Wait a minute! This introduction would not be complete without at least one ADD mental sidetrack. Why, you may ask, did we write such a l-o-n-g book (a number of people have asked). Well, since there was nothing available at the time, we felt compelled to attempt to give our readers a brain transplant . . . similar to our workshop/speaking style in those days. The "Talk as fast as you can so you can cram in all the relevant information in a limited time frame" school of thought. Never mind that the brain can't process all that so fast. Thank God there are now other resources out there . . . we don't have to drive ourselves and others crazy trying to do it all. If you are an ADDult, you know exactly what we are talking about.

Okay, let's get back to the changes we are including in this revision. One of the biggest changes is the growth and development of an entirely new profession dedicated to assisting ADD adults: ADD coaching. A well-trained ADD coach has a working knowledge of ADD medications and neurology, organizational strategies, specific coping tools and much more. He or she can work with you to help you improve your functioning and satisfaction in all areas of life impacted by ADD.

Coaching, acknowledged to be one of the most important factors in ADD recovery, is at the center of our new sections on getting help. In our experience the four most important areas of focus are the M & M & M & M's—medication, meditation, mental hygiene and moving forward. Your coach can be a resource person in all these areas, although he/she doesn't actually prescribe the medication. So, in our treatment chapters, we will put our coaching hats on and speak to you as ADD coaches, walking you through the process of using medication–meditation–mental hygiene–moving forward to facilitate your ADD recovery. We will also include updated information on medication.

Another important area of change is the new information on gender and ADD. Hormones and biology have a powerful impact on the symptom picture, as do the effects of different socialization for males and females. Currently, most of the information on ADD and gender is focused on the female, so we will devote half of a chapter primarily to the issues of women with ADD. The other half of that chapter is about ADD and sexuality. Yes, ADD follows us into all areas of life, including the bedroom.

Finally, we had to do a search-and-destroy mission for language that included the words "should," "must" or "ought." Although we thought we were being very positive and nonjudgmental when we wrote the original book, we found that we had done much growing in the area of self-acceptance and acceptance of others with ADD. Those nasty "shoulds" just jumped out at us. Mention of the "should" problem brings us to our last, and perhaps most important point: The goal of ADD recovery is not perfect functioning, but a comfortable relationship with your very human self, "ADD oopses" and all. When we ease up on the performance pressure, life is a lot more fun. Almost incidentally, a lot more gets done with less effort. It's like magic.

How to Read This Book

We know that many of you, our readers, are not actually readers at all. Of course, you know *how* to read and you *can* read, but for many ADDers, reading is just not that much fun. Perhaps you have dyslexia—it often travels with ADD. Or maybe reading is just not the strongest learning channel for you. We put this book in an easy-to-read font and broke it up with charts, headers and cartoons because we knew that you, our audience, would need a break while reading all that text.

Don't make a chore out of reading this book! There is no right way to do it. You can read it in little chunks during bathroom breaks or even read it backwards! Pick out the chapters that catch your eye and start there. As they say in AA: Take what you like and leave the rest.

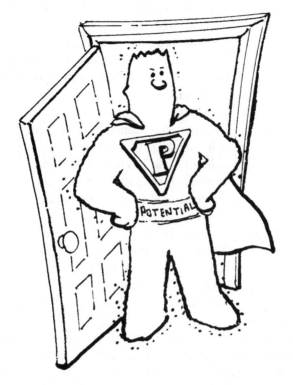

ADD and Your Potential

In the first edition of this book, the Captain Potential cartoon you see on this page was in the final chapter. This time we put him right up front, as a reminder that you really are going somewhere. Honest! When you are slogging through the hard work it takes to get rid of all the baggage associated with undiagnosed ADD, it is easy to get discouraged, to focus so much on the problems that your gifts and strengths recede into the background. We all have enormous potential that can be realized when we discover the operating manual for our unique, quirky selves.

ADD as a "brain style" has a lot to offer. All the "symptoms" of ADD can be worked with to serve us instead of getting in the way. Let's take a different look at the three cardinal symptoms of ADD:

1. Inattention: Did you ever consider that your lack of attention might be telling you that you are not passionate about what you are doing? That the problem is not your inadequacy but a poor fit between your strengths and the task or activity?

2. Impulsivity: This can sometimes be your friend. It can help you take the leap you need to take in order to grow. You may be less likely than your more placid friends to stay in the same routine jobs, relationships and behavior patterns.

3. Hyperactivity: This can be channeled into focused energy. There is nothing wrong with a high activity level per se. Rushing madly in all directions at once is the real problem. We can learn to make high energy work for us, not against us.

We are much more than our ADD. Each of us has a unique profile of strengths that can be used to design and implement a lifestyle that is a good fit for us as individuals. There are many examples of successful ADDers, both historically and in the present. While it is not possible to make a posthumous diagnosis of ADD, what we know about the lives of Thomas Edison, Winston Churchill and Benjamin Franklin, for example, makes us more than a little bit suspicious about their "diagnosability." The CEO of JetBlue Airways, Dustin Hoffman, and Dr. Ned Hallowell are among the many successful people who have come out of the closet about their ADD. And of course, we all wonder about most of the people who do comedy for a living. For every ADD celebrity, there are multitudes of less visible folks who have found a niche for the weird and wonderful brain style known as ADD. Below is a partial list of vocations that can benefit from "diversified thinking":

> *sales*
> *entrepreneurship*

comedy
acting
writing
teaching
parenting
science
design

Actually, anything humans do is enhanced by the capacity to think outside the box. As ADDers, we tend to excel at that kind of thinking. Our task is to tame the chaos and the paper piles enough so that they don't choke the life out of living. We want "good enough" structure and organization, not a straitjacket.

ADD Is a What?

KK: "In the past week, I got a puzzling e-mail from my dad. We had been going back and forth about which political candidate he was supporting. The final e-mail in this particular thread seemed to be a duplicate of the last one I sent him. I chalked it up as an 'oops' and went about my business, keeping the e-mail on the desktop. Some time later, my partner, Paul, drew my attention to the new signature that appeared on the bottom of the e-mail. This was one I had just added after a signature-less couple of months due to a new computer system learning curve. In a pretty font and yummy colors, it read:

Kate Kelly
ADDed Dimension Coaching
addcoaching.com
"ADD—it's not just a disorder, it's an ADDed Dimension"

"Only my dad's version was slightly different. I don't know how he expected my ADD self to pick up on it, but perhaps it was one of those brain teasing tests he delights in administering to the poor unsuspecting soul who is already convinced they are indeed lazy, stupid and crazy. Actually, I think it is just his particular brand of humor, his way of having fun. OK . . . are you ready for my dad's version of the signature? His edited response was:

Kate Kelly
ADDed Dimension Coaching
addcoaching.com
"ADD—it's not just a disorder, it's a bullcrap copout"

"Well! Can you believe he wrote that? In the early days of my own ADD journey I would have shriveled up, curled myself into a little ball on hearing or reading those words. This week I just laughed my head off and sent a message to my dad that publication is the best revenge. I also thanked him for providing the inspiration for part of this introduction."

While these words may seem rude or downright cruel to the ADDer who is struggling to make sense of his or her life, they are just an in-your-face version of the attitudes we deal with on the journey to self-acceptance. We encounter versions of this kind of thinking on talk radio, in books and even in the bosoms of our families. The idea that the kinds of behaviors seen in ADD are the result of a character defect is ingrained in our collective consciousness. Even those of us who have spent our lives slaving to try to control our ADD symptoms without success often wonder if we are just making up excuses for bad behavior.

If anyone tries to tell you that ADD is "all in your head," refuse to take it to heart. You can laugh it off, develop an acute but temporary hearing loss or rephrase the offending words in the privacy of your own mind. You could say, for instance, that "Yes, ADD is in my head—it's a neurobiological condition." Remind yourself that not doing something you are expected to do is not because you won't, but because you can't—at least not without help. Then, of course, there is the tired old phrase "he can do it when he wants to," which is trotted out all too often. This faulty assumption with its ring of truth often results in a lot of self-doubt and recrimination. Remind yourself that it rings true not because you are "guilty as charged" but because ADD is not predictable—somedays we're hot, and somedays we're not.

> *ADD is not an excuse, it's an explanation.*
> *We have been doing our best in very*
> *challenging circumstances.*

If we could sum up the message of this book in a few words (besides the words in the title), we would say that the task in front of you, as you make the journey from diagnosis to self-acceptance, is to:

1. reframe your past experience,

2. forgive yourself,

3. move forward, taking with you the knowledge, tools and strategies that will support your success.

In this book you will find a wealth of information about ADD, as well as practical tips, tools and solutions for living as an ADD adult. We want to say a bit more about reframing here. Imagine a picture frame that you have pulled from the curb on your latest trash-picking expedition. Or one you have stored in your attic or garage for about a century. It is dusty and beat up, perhaps with chipped paint or many layers of ugly paint. Maybe there are some nails missing, so that the frame is coming apart. Even a Van Gogh or a Picasso would not shine as brightly when placed in that sad-looking frame.

That Charlie Brown frame is the one you have been looking through when you view your life. It is constructed from the negative beliefs you collected over the years of living with a hidden disability. The beliefs about not trying hard enough, or just making up excuses, for example. Beliefs are powerful, they affect everything we think, feel, say and do. To change your life, you need to change your thinking, starting with your beliefs. Strip that old frame of the beliefs that don't serve you and are not even true. The ones that say you have not been working hard enough or don't care enough about others. When you re-finish the frame, remember to include the following:

1. You have been working your heart out just trying to navigate life with an unpredictable brain.

2. You have strengths that shine through the disability.

3. None of us is perfect—and all of us are valuable.

As you read this book, keep the image of Captain Potential firmly fixed in your mind's eye. There is indeed a gem buried under all those symptoms and past traumas. We know that you can find it, because we have, and our own lives have been any-thing but tidy. Above all, enjoy the journey.

Warmly,
Kate Kelly & Peggy Ramundo

CHAPTER 1

Understanding the Disorder That Makes Us Feel Lazy, Stupid or Crazy

It's difficult to grow up with the hidden handicap of ADD. Many of us feel that we've spent our lives disappointing everyone—parents, siblings, teachers, friends and ourselves. When we were children, our teachers repeatedly told us we could do our work but chose not to. Our report cards were continual reminders that we weren't very bright. Those Cs, Ds and Fs didn't lie. They defined our self-perception as kids who were lazy. Sometimes we felt smart. We came up with wonderful inventions and imaginative play. We often amazed ourselves, our teachers and our parents with our wealth of knowledge and creative ideas.

We didn't want to cause trouble. We didn't start our days with a plan to drive everyone crazy. We didn't leave our rooms in total chaos to make our parents wring their hands in frustration. We didn't count the thumbtacks on the bulletin board because we enjoyed watching the veins pop out of a teacher's neck when he yelled at us to get to work. We didn't yawn and stretch and sprawl across our desktops, totally exhausted, just to make the other kids laugh. We didn't beg for more toys, bigger bikes or better birthday parties because we wanted our moms and dads to feel terrible for depriving us of these things.

We did these things because we had ADD. But unfortunately, most of us didn't know that. Most of our parents, siblings, teachers and friends didn't know that either. So most of us grew up with negative feelings that developed around behaviors everyone misunderstood.

Pay attention.
Stop fooling around.
If you would just try, you could do it.
You're lazy.
Settle down.
You can do it when you want to.
Why are you acting this way?
You're too smart to get such terrible grades.
Why do you always make things so hard for yourself?
Your room is always a mess.
You just have to buckle down.
Stop bothering other children.
Are you trying to drive me crazy?
Why can't you act like your brother/sister?
Why are you so irresponsible?
You aren't grateful for anything.

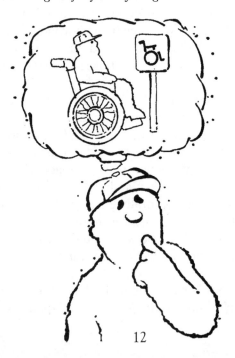

Have you ever heard any of these comments? If you're a parent, have you ever said any of them? Our bet is that your answer to both questions is a resounding "Yes!"

It's unlikely that anyone would tell a child in a wheelchair that he could get up and walk if he tried harder. His handicap is obvious and everyone understands his limitations. Unfortunately, not many people understand the hidden handicap of an ADD child.

PR: "I have sometimes wished that my son had a physical handicap instead of ADD. Of course, I don't really wish he had a physical disability. If he did, though, it would be easier to explain his challenges to people who don't understand. It would be easier for me to understand."

For most of us the misunderstandings and faulty assumptions continued into our adolescent years. Since we were old enough to know better, our behaviors were tolerated even less. By the time we became adults, many of us were convinced that we indeed were—and still are—lazy, stupid or crazy.

Understanding Through Education

As we move through this book, we'll offer many suggestions and strategies for dealing with ADD. But the first and most important one is to repeat at least a hundred times:

"I am not lazy, stupid or crazy!"

If you aren't convinced yet, we hope you will be by the end of this book. We hope you'll be able to formulate a new, positive self-perception to replace the old one. Reframing your self-perceptions is your first job. To accomplish this, you'll need an in-depth understanding of ADD.

To understand your symptoms and take appropriate steps to gain control over them, you have to learn as much as you can about your disorder. Even if you've already done your homework on ADD, we encourage you to read the following section. You may not discover new information per se, but you may discover a new framework for understanding specific issues of ADD in adults. We will use this framework as we examine the dynamics of ADD in your relationships, your workplace and your home.

About Definitions, Descriptions and Diagnostic Dilemmas: Is It ADD or ADHD?

ADD (or ADHD) is a disorder of the central nervous system (CNS) characterized by disturbances in the areas of attention, impulsiveness and hyperactivity.

Media focus gives the impression that ADD is a new problem. Some subscribe to the theory that ADD might not be new but is being used by increasing numbers of parents to excuse their children's misbehavior. In fact, when we first wrote this book, a local principal was referring to ADD as *just the yuppie disorder of the eighties.*

This observation would come as a surprise to Dr. G. F. Still, a turn-of-the-century researcher who worked with children in a psychiatric hospital. We doubt there were many yuppies in 1902 when Still worked with his hyperactive, impulsive and inattentive patients. Although he used the label "A Defect in Moral Control," he theorized that an organic problem rather than a behavioral one caused the symptoms of his patients. This was a rather revolutionary theory at a time when most people believed that bad manners and improper upbringing caused misbehavior.

In the first half of the twentieth century, other researchers supported Dr. Still's theory. They noted that various kinds of brain damage caused patients to display symptoms of hyperactivity, impulsivity and inattention. World War I soldiers with brain injuries and children with damage from a brain virus both had symptoms similar to those of children who apparently had been born with them.

14

Over the years, many labels have been given to the disorder. The labels have reflected the state of research at the time:

Post-Encephalitic Disorder
Hyperkinesis
Minimal Brain Damage
Minimal Brain Dysfunction
Hyperkinetic Reaction of Childhood
Attention Deficit Disorder with and without Hyperactivity

The focus on structural problems in the brain—holes perhaps, or other abnormalities detected through neurological testing, persisted until the sixties. Then research began to focus primarily on the symptom of hyperactivity in childhood. In 1968, the American Psychiatric Association (APA) responded to this research by revising its diagnostic manual (DSM-II). The revision included the new label: "Hyperkinetic Disorder of Childhood."

During the seventies, research broadened its focus beyond hyperactivity and concluded that subtle cognitive disabilities of memory and attention problems were the cores of the disorder. These conclusions, coupled with the discovery that attention problems could exist without hyperactivity and continue beyond childhood, required a second revision of the diagnostic manual.

In 1980, the APA's revised manual, the DSM-III, created new labels: "ADDH, Attention Deficit Disorder with Hyperactivity"; "Attention Deficit Disorder Without Hyperactivity" and "Residual Type" (for those whose symptoms continued into adulthood).

If your son was diagnosed in 1985 with ADDH, why was your daughter diagnosed in 1988 with ADHD? Are you confused yet? Well, you guessed it. The labels changed again in 1987, with the next version of the DSM, the DSM-III-R.

A number of experts believed that hyperactivity had to be present for an ADD diagnosis. They theorized that the other related

15

symptoms were part of a separate disorder. In 1994, the DSM-IV made its appearance, reflecting this theory with yet another set of labels: ADHD, primarily inattentive type; ADHD, primarily hyperactive type; and ADHD, combined type. The DSM-IV is now in its fourth edition, called the DSM-IV-TR. Thank God, the DSM-V won't be ready until at least 2011!

Is there any reason to remember the DSM label revisions? We suppose you could drop terms like the *Diagnostic and Statistical Manual of the American Psychiatric Association* to impress friends at your next party! The information would be useful if you happen to be studying psychology and need the information for an upcoming exam. Otherwise, the only reason to know about the changing labels is that they reflect an ever-changing understanding of ADD.

The debate will continue about ADD issues—what is it exactly and who should be included in the diagnostic criteria? To provide guidelines for diagnosticians, the APA's manual attempts to label and describe various clusters of symptoms, assigning different groups into distinct categories of disorders.

The problem is that human beings don't cooperate with this attempt to categorize behavior. Behaviors just won't fit into tidy little boxes. If you have ever agonized over naming your business report or the song you just composed, you know the limitations of a title. It's difficult to capture the essence of something in a few words.

In practical terms, this means that relatively few people fit the classic DSM diagnoses. There is also much symptom overlap *between* different disorders, so an individual may have symptoms of multiple disorders. The significance for an ADDer is that he shouldn't expect his symptoms to be exactly like his child's, friend's or spouse's.

For our purposes, we've made the decision to use the generic label "ADD" in this book. First, it's easier to type than

"ADHD"! Second and more important, the ADD label avoids the hyperactivity/no hyperactivity issue.

Specific Symptoms of ADD

As we review specific symptoms, you'll become aware of the imprecision of definitions and descriptions, particularly as they apply to ADD in adults. One reason for this imprecision is the complex nature of the brain and central nervous system. This complexity creates a billion-piece jigsaw puzzle of possible causes and symptoms. Each of us is a puzzle with an assortment of puzzle pieces uniquely different from another ADDer. Adding to the diagnostic dilemma are the rapid behavioral changes that make a precise description of the disorder difficult.

Despite the diagnostic dilemma, it is important to understand the impact ADD symptoms have on your life. You don't have to be a walking encyclopedia of ADD, but you do need sufficient knowledge to capitalize on your strengths and bypass your weaknesses. In the following section, we'll examine the three major symptoms of ADD. In Chapter 2, we'll take a broader look at an ADDer's differences that don't quite fit into the diagnostic criteria.

Inattention

Most people characterize an attention deficit disorder as a problem of a short attention span. They think of ADDers as mental butterflies, flitting from one task or thought to another but never alighting on anything. In reality, attending is more than simply paying attention. And a problem with attending is more than simply not paying attention long enough.

It's more accurate to describe attentional problems as components of the process of attention. This process includes *choosing* the right stimulus to focus on, *sustaining* the focus over time, *dividing* focus between relevant stimuli and *shifting* focus to another stimulus. Impaired functioning can occur in any or all of these areas of attention. The result is a failure to pay attention.

17

Workaholism, single-mindedness, procrastination, boredom—these are common and somewhat surprising manifestations of attentional problems. It might seem paradoxical that a workaholic could have attentional problems. It might seem paradoxical that a high-energy adult could have trouble getting started on his work.

These manifestations are baffling only if ADD is viewed as a short attention span or worse, an excuse. When *all* the dimensions of attention are considered, it becomes easier to understand the diversity of the manifestations of ADD.

The Workaholic might have little difficulty selecting focus or sustaining it but have great difficulty shifting his focus. Unable to shift attention between activities, he can become engrossed in his job to the exclusion of everything else in his life.

Similar behavior can be seen in the person who has trouble sustaining attention. He struggles so intently to shut out the world's distractions that he gets locked in to behavior that continues long after it should stop. It's as if he wears blinders that prevent him from seeing anything but the task at hand. The house might burn down and the kids might run wild but he'll banish that last dust ball from the living room!

The Procrastinator has the opposite problem. He can't selectively focus his attention and might endure frequent accusations about his laziness. In truth, he's so distracted by stimuli that he can't figure out where or how to get started. Sounds, smells, sights and the random wanderings of his thoughts continually vie for his attention.

Unable to select the most important stimulus, he approaches most tasks in a disorganized fashion and has trouble finishing or sometimes even starting anything. If the task is uninteresting, it's even harder for him to sustain focus.

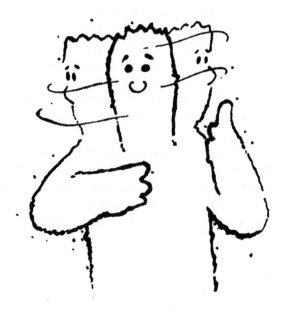

Heightened interest and a belief in one's ultimate success improve the quality of attending. With an inability to maintain focus, many ADDers require intensely stimulating situations to maintain alertness and attentiveness. Without this stimulation, attention wanders, and many of us are told we're unmotivated.

We're not unmotivated! Our problems with selective attention compromise our abilities to stay focused and productive. So it looks as if we don't care and won't try! In reality, we have to exert many times the effort of non-ADDers to maintain adequate levels of motivation.

Impulsivity

Impulsivity is a failure to stop and think. Being impulsive means that many of us act and react with astonishing speed and with little thought about the consequences. Our brains don't control behavior the way they should, so we say and do things rashly.

When we were children, we might have violated classroom rules, insulted our parents or run into the street without looking. As adults, we might blurt out confidential information or share intimate details with relative strangers. We might pull out from our driveways without checking the rearview mirror or leave work two hours early to enjoy a beautiful spring day. Controlling impulses is tough for many ADD adults!

Impulsivity plays out in other, less obvious ways. It can affect the quality of work on the job. The ADDer often rushes through tasks with little preplanning and many careless errors. He might get into debt with impulse buying, discard an important document or ruin a new piece of equipment because it takes too long to read the instructions.

> *"He knows the rules, but breaks them anyway."*
> *"His work is careless because he won't try."*
> *"He's wasting his ability."*

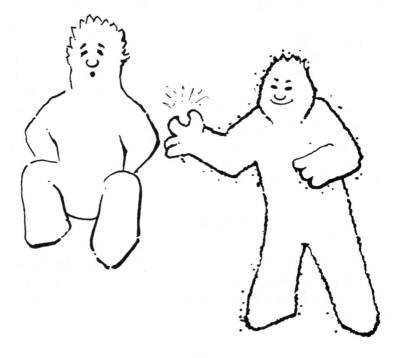

These comments reflect a misunderstanding of the impulsive words and actions of ADDers. Most of us *know* the rules. We *know* our work is neater when we work slowly. We *know* we are capable of more accurate work. Knowing these things, however, doesn't mean we can easily control the impulsive behaviors. People who make faulty assumptions about us don't understand the enormous effort we expend keeping our impulses in check.

Hyperactivity

Hyperactivity is probably the first symptom people think of when they talk about ADD. They might immediately conjure up an image of an overactive child bouncing off the walls and hanging from the light fixtures! Without question, this random, excessive activity can be a primary symptom of ADD. But it describes only one part of a larger activity dysregulation that includes a wide range of behaviors.

Rather than moving too much, some ADDers talk too much! Barely pausing for breath, they talk so much and so fast that no one else has a chance to say anything. The speech has a driven quality to it as if the words have been bottled up for centuries and are desperate to get out!

PR: "At a recent conference, I congratulated myself for sticking to my schedule. Just in time for our break, I shared some information about my own symptoms. I commented that, unlike my son, I wasn't particularly hyperactive.

"A member of my audience stopped me at the coffeepot and shared her observations of my presentation style. She said, 'You might not be hyperactive, but do you know how fast you talk? I have attended lots of workshops, but have *never* learned the quantity of information I just learned! And one more thing. Do you know how many times you took the top of your pen off and put it back on again?' At the end of the workshop, she thanked me profusely for the wealth of material I had shared, so I guess I didn't overwhelm her too much with my nonhyperactivity!"

This anecdote has two messages. First, we can never stop learning about our behavior, even when we think we have a good handle on it. Second, it points out that hyperactivity can manifest itself in more subtle ways than physical overactivity.

These subtle behaviors reflect the generalized restlessness and impatience many of us experience. We may have learned to stop sky diving from the top bunk and snowboarding down the banister, but we might still feel uncomfortable when we have to sit still. So we fidget, tap our fingers or twirl our hair. Relaxing can be impossible, so we might take on numerous hobbies, work second jobs or run marathons on the weekend.

There is a final thing we should mention. Hyperactivity can be either a deficit or an asset, depending on the quality of the behavior. If the activity is purposeful, hyperactivity can help us get more accomplished.

Some researchers have studied hyperactive individuals who don't have any of the other symptoms of ADD. These folk are extremely active but don't seem to have problems with attention, mood swings or any of the other roadblocks that interfere with productivity. The issue for hyperactive ADD adults is that much of their activity is dysregulated, random and unproductive.

But . . . Why??

ADDers are curious folk. They are rarely able to let anything go by without asking, "But why?" You may be asking this question about your symptoms. "I am inattentive, impulsive and hyperactive—*but why* do I have this baffling disorder?" If we could give you a tidy answer to your question, researchers would herald our discovery. Since no one knows for sure what causes ADD, the best we can do is examine possibilities.

To get started, you'll need a crash course in the Neurology of the Brain and the Central Nervous System. Don't close the book yet! We promise to make this as painless as possible. But it's difficult to understand ADD without knowing some of the "whys" of the disorder. Why is your ADD different from each of ours? Why do your symptoms seem to change so much? Why do your symptoms sometimes cause little or no problem? Without some basic knowledge, it's easy to assume that this disorder is your fault. So, here goes.

Research Tools

As knowledge about ADD has grown, research has increasingly focused on the possibility that the ADD brain and central nervous system are somehow *wired* differently. Testing some of the theories is tricky because researchers can't open up an ADDer's skull to study his brain! Even if they could, it would be nearly impossible to isolate and examine a particular chemical or a specific portion of the brain. The human brain is simply too complex, with many interrelated parts.

Instead, scientists are using sophisticated imaging devices to scan the brain. *Brain Imaging* is a promising technique that has provided some information about the differences in ADD brains. MRIs produce clear and detailed pictures of brain structures, while PET scans allow us to observe blood flow or metabolism in any part of the brain when a person is active. The SPECT scan is similar to the PET scan except that the SPECT scan generates images of a person at rest. Generally, these imaging methods are not used as diagnostic tools, although Dr. Daniel Amen has done pioneering work using SPECT in his clinical practice.

Scientists also use drug responses to study brain activity indirectly. They know that certain drugs increase the quantity of neurotransmitters in the brain. A positive drug response suggests an insufficiency of the neurochemical affected by the particular drug.

How does this fit into the theories about the possible causes of ADD? Let's take that crash course in neurology to get a better understanding of the "why's" of your disorder.

The Basics of Neurology

The brain and other parts of the central nervous system (CNS) function as a wonderful and intricate Command Center. This command center coordinates all systems of the human body through a messenger system. It sends messages and receives those sent from various parts of the body and from the outside world. It also regulates and controls behavior.

The messenger system of the CNS consists of millions of nerve cells. These are cell bodies with long, thin projections called *axons* and *dendrites*. Impulses are carried along the length of a nerve cell and jump from one cell to another in much the same way electricity travels through a wire.

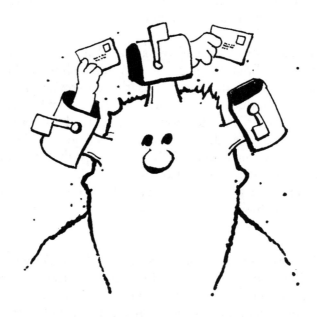

"The Brain's Postal System"

24

Messages are first received by receptors in the nerve cell's dendrite. The message, in the form of an electrical impulse, travels from the dendrite through the cell body and the axon. At the end of the axon is a synapse, a gap between the nerve cells. The electrical impulse, or message, is conducted across the synapse by chemical messengers called *neurotransmitters*. These chemicals carry the message across the gap from one cell's axon to another's dendrite.

You might be familiar with some of these neurotransmitters. *Endorphins* are the pain-relieving neurotransmitters that act as the body's own morphine. An outpouring of endorphins during vigorous exercise causes the marathon runner's "high." This increase protects his body from feeling the pain of stressed muscles and joints—an athlete is often unaware of an injury until he rests. *Epinephrine,* better known as adrenaline, is the neurotransmitter that mobilizes the reaction to danger. This activates the *fight-or-flight* response. The heart beats rapidly and the breathing passages become wider so one can either run or fight an enemy.

That wasn't too bad, was it? Now let's use this information as we consider some theories that have emerged from research.

Current Theories About the Key Players in ADD

Since the command center is so complex, it isn't surprising that there are conflicting theories about the causes of ADD. Although there isn't consensus, many researchers agree that this interrelated system is dysregulated in some fashion. The following discussion examines some of the theories about this dysregulation as well as an assortment of other proposed theories.

Neurotransmitters

Researchers have used indirect drug response research to conclude that an insufficient supply of the neurotransmitter *dopamine* plays an important role in ADD. It is known that the stimulant drugs used to treat ADD increase dopamine levels. Of course, any problem in the brain is far too complex to be the result of a single neurotransmitter malfunction. At the very least, the interaction of multiple neurotransmitters is suspected, with the most likely culprits being dopamine, *norepinephrine* and *serotonin*.

Brain Structures

Using an MRI to scan the brains of children with ADD, researchers found that four brain regions were smaller than those in children without ADD—the *frontal lobes*, the *corpus callosum*, the *basal ganglia* and the cerebellar *vermis*. When we look at the functions of these brain parts, it makes sense that they may play a role in the symptoms of ADD. The frontal lobes are critical to many of the brain's executive functions, including planning, initiative and the ability to regulate behavior. We also know that actual frontal lobe brain damage causes impulsivity, mood swings, disinhibited behavior and sometimes hyperactivity.

The *cerebellum* (the vermis is part of this structure) is responsible for balance and motor coordination. The basal ganglia serves as a connector between the cerebellum and the cerebrum (which includes the frontal lobes). It also helps to regulate moods and control impulsive behavior. The corpus callosum is basically a collection of nerve fibers that connect the left and right frontal lobes, allowing them to communicate.

Is it the actual brain structures or the connections between them that cause our ADD symptoms? Is it the fault of those tiny messengers, the neurotransmitters? Likely, the answer is all of the above. Despite a significant increase in research since we wrote the first edition of this book, scientists are still playing a guessing game when it comes to figuring out how the brain and the nervous system produce the symptoms of ADD.

Primary Sleep Disorder

Some researchers theorize that the core problem in ADD isn't excess activity but rather underarousal. In other words, people with ADD aren't fully awake and alert. These scientists hypothesize that a high activity level might be in part an effort to stay awake. Sleep disturbances are fairly common in ADDers. Many experience irregular patterns of sleeplessness and reawakening. Others sleep so deeply that arousal is difficult.

Research into sleeping and waking patterns suggests to some investigators that the disorder arises from a primary sleep disorder. In other words, the person with ADD sleeps poorly and, as a result, has arousal problems during the day. Other research indicates that deep dream states are necessary to anchor learning in memory. This suggests that some ADD adults may demonstrate associated learning problems because their sleep irregularities interfere with this deep dream state.

Parenting or Heredity?

There are many unanswered questions about ADD, but we know that there is a strong genetic component. Children with ADD are likely to have ADD parents or close relatives. This might not come as a surprise if you are the ADD parent of an ADD child.

Not all family traits result from genetic inheritance. Parents *pass on* characteristics to their children through their behaviors and their child-rearing styles—children imitate their parents and tend to adopt their values. When your son talks to his playmates and sounds like a taped recording of your voice with precisely duplicated words, inflections and pauses, you know the power of modeled behavior.

When it comes to behavior, both nature and nurture play important roles. It is now clear that ADD is a neurobiological condition in most cases. Certainly, a difficult environment will make matters worse, but the root cause is to be found in a dysregulated brain and nervous system.

Theory of Blame

This theory holds that the only reasonable explanation for misbehavior or learning problems is that someone, usually a par-

27

ent, is doing something wrong. If you are a parent, you're probably well acquainted with child-rearing experts who believe in this theory. These folk are the friends, family and teachers who eagerly offer unwanted comments and advice about the correct method for raising your children:

> *"He would never behave like that in my house."*
> *"You are too tough on him."*
> *"You aren't tough enough on him."*
> *"All he needs is grandma's spatula on his bottom."*

Many of us do our own share of blaming, especially before we learn about our disorder. Unaware of the underlying ADD, we often grow up blaming our problems on our upbringing and believing that everything wrong in our lives is caused by our dysfunctional families. Our analysis focuses on the impact of environment, minimizing or excluding consideration of a neurological makeup.

This rather limited view of human behavior may be fostered by the value Western culture places on self-determination. We prefer to feel that we have control over events and can shape destiny by our actions. It's unnerving to think that our children *come as they are* and that we have somewhat limited influence on their behavior.

Pregnancy and Childbirth Complications

No one is sure about the relationship between birth complications, prenatal factors and ADD. In a small percentage of cases, there is evidence that *pre* and *post* birth problems increase the infant's risk of developing symptoms of ADD. The risk factors include poor maternal health, maternal age of twenty or less, long labor, fetal distress or postmaturity.

Most people with ADD don't have a history of these risk factors. Conversely, most children with histories of prenatal and childbirth complications don't develop ADD. It does appear, however, that early damage to the CNS is a factor in a small percentage of ADDers.

Environmental Toxins

There is ongoing debate about an increase in the numbers of children newly diagnosed with ADD. Since definitions of ADD have changed over time, particularly regarding hyperactivity, it's difficult to analyze this increase. Some argue that the incidence hasn't increased but that improved diagnostic methods have identified children with more subtle forms of the disorder.

Others speculate that environmental toxins play a role. It is undoubtedly true that environmental hazards are threatening our health. One-third of children with lead poisoning have symptoms of ADD. The role of other pollutants in causing or exacerbating ADD is a big question mark. It's reasonable to suspect that they might play a part, as other substances do, in various patterns of neurological damage.

Food Stuff

Have you seen the cartoon illustrating a mother in the grocery store with her hyperactive child? While he runs up and down the aisles, she reads the label on a box that promises: "This cereal will take the hyperactivity right out of them!" If only that were true.

Scientific studies have not backed up the claim that sugar causes hyperactivity. This may be a puzzling statement for parents who directly observe the unfortunate results of their child's sugar binge. Scientific studies aside, if sugar seems to make your symptoms worse, it makes sense to eliminate it from your diet. Pediatrician and allergist Dr. Benjamin Feingold developed a special diet to eliminate food additives and salicylates. This diet did seem to relieve the symptoms in about 5 percent of ADD children. It is likely that there is a subgroup of ADDers who are sensitive to certain food substances.

Other Medical Issues

Some medical conditions create symptoms that look very much like ADD. A few examples are thyroid conditions, fibromyalgia and allergies. To make matters even more complicated, ADDers can have both ADD *and* one or more other problems that muddy the diagnostic picture. Fibromyalgia, for example, seems to travel along with ADD in many cases. It produces a syndrome that includes muscle pain as well as mental fogginess. Allergies can also interfere with mental functioning. A person with an overactive thyroid can be hard to distinguish from the hyperactive ADDult.

The question to ask in these cases is not which one of the issues is causing the problem, but how to work with both in a way that maximizes functioning. For some people, taking care of the thyroid imbalance, for example, may be all the treatment that is needed.

Information Explosion
Some believe that the psychological hazards of our increasingly complex society contribute to the higher incidence of ADD. In his book *Future Shock*, Alvin Toffler predicted that dire psychological consequences would result from the rapid changes in modern society.

The theory of information explosion has validity. Many people regarded as entirely *normal* in a simpler society could become overwhelmed by the demands of a fast-paced, complex one. This doesn't mean that the psychological hazards cause ADD. It does seem logical, however, that they could make the symptoms more noticeable and disabling.

Just a Bad Apple
We doubt that anyone is doing research on this popular, unscientific theory! It goes like this: *The erratic behavior of ADD children and adults is intentional, maliciously planned misbehavior.*

This variation on the theory of blame is based on the assumption that an ADDer can control his behavior but *chooses* not to. Of course, these theorists don't have ADD and don't have a clue as to what it's like to live with the disorder.

As an ADD adult, you didn't ask to be born this way, but you do need to work hard to shoot holes in this theory. Using your disorder as an excuse for irresponsible behavior doesn't help your personal growth and gives the Bad Apple theorists ammunition. All of us need to develop strategies to manage our symptoms, but we need to do it with self-acceptance and forgiveness. Every person with a disability has to make the best of the cards he's been dealt.

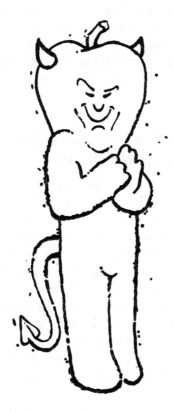

How Common Is ADD?

How many of us are there? Is ADD common? We have to say, somewhat apologetically, that we don't have the answer to these questions! But here are some *guesstimates*.

31

The prevalence figures reported in professional literature vary widely from 1 to 20 percent of the population. Studies that include individuals without hyperactivity cite 20 percent prevalence. The estimate accepted by many professionals is a conservative 3 to 5 percent. Your question "But why?" may be on the tip of your tongue. Why is there so little consensus?

First, there is a lack of agreement about symptoms. Some research studies include individuals without hyperactivity and some don't. Second, most research has focused on children and hasn't included adolescent and adult subjects. The lack of consensus about diagnostic criteria and a somewhat limited number of studies with ADD adults has resulted in statistics that vary from study to study.

"ADD Is a Childhood Disorder That Occurs Primarily in Boys"

We hate to break this news to the *old-school of thought* experts, but authors Kelly and Ramundo are ADDers who are neither boys nor children! The assumption that many more boys than girls have ADD is being challenged as increasing numbers of adult women are newly diagnosed. Historically, six times more boys than girls have been diagnosed with the disorder. The ratio approaches one to one if ADD without hyperactivity is included. These statistics suggest that the learning and adjustment problems of many ADD girls are too subtle to be identified. This apparent underidentification of girls and nonhyperactive boys is a serious problem. These children—and adults—have special needs that are too often overlooked.

We have considered several questions that don't have easy answers. Although most of us are uncomfortable with ambiguity, we need to focus our attention on those issues that do have answers:

> *"How has this disorder had an impact on my life?"*
> *"How do my differences play out in my daily life?"*
> *"How can I help myself?"*

In the next two chapters, we'll look at the impact ADD has had on our lives and at the ways each of us is uniquely different from our non-ADD peers. We'll devote the remainder of the book to the third question and share lots of suggestions for managing symptoms and discovering your ADDed Dimension.

CHAPTER 2

How Are We Different?
How Are We Different?
How Are We Different?

If you have ADD, your disorder makes you different. There's no doubt about it. You come into the world with differences that are part of the wiring of your brain. Not only are you different from others who don't have ADD, you are also different from others who do.

Different Doesn't Mean Defective

Yes, each of us is different, but different doesn't equal defective. It's foolish to ignore our differences or pretend they don't exist. It's equally foolish to focus exclusively on the debit side of those differences. Although our lives would probably be easier without ADD, they wouldn't be more valuable.

In the first chapter we examined the three broad categories of ADD symptoms. Now we'll enlarge the discussion to consider the impact these symptoms have on your daily life. You'll learn about your disabilities. You'll also learn about your abilities—abilities that are sometimes hidden by the challenges you face as a result of your particular ADD symptoms.

So How Do the Differences Affect ADD Adults?

Although we talk of ADD as a distinct disorder, it makes more sense to think of it as a syndrome: a group of symptoms that tend to occur together. The concept of a syndrome seems an appropriate way of thinking about a central nervous system that doesn't work quite right. As previously noted, while researchers disagree about the specific origins of ADD, most agree that the regulatory function of the CNS is somehow erratic and inefficient. With an impaired regulatory system, an ADDer may have wildly fluctuating behaviors from day to day or even minute to minute. He may also have academic problems caused by erratic attention and information processing.

The Wandering Mind Syndrome

Most of us have minds that wander hither and yon. We daydream and drift among loosely and tenuously connected thoughts. As our own thoughts intrude, we change the subject and interrupt with irrelevant comments.

Regardless of the "why" of distractibility, the behaviors associated with it are often mistaken for rudeness or eccentricity. The wandering mind syndrome, like all ADD differences, has its pluses and minuses.

On the minus side, an ADDer might engage in mental free flight when he should be working. Bosses regard his partially finished reports and unreturned phone calls as evidence of incompetence or a poor attitude. In conversations he may listen with one ear but continue on some level to follow his own train of thought. It's obvious to his boss or friend that he isn't *all there*. His seeming uninterest doesn't win friends or influence people!

On the plus side, he can use his wandering mind to notice things others miss and make new and interesting connections between ideas. His creative mind can roam beyond convention into imagination and possibilities.

If an ADDer can learn to control his wandering thoughts and capitalize on their richness, he can discover a valuable asset. Think about the stereotype of the absentminded professor or the talented artist who has incredible gifts but stumbles along trying to manage the practical details of life. We don't believe this stereotype is merely a myth. If we were to survey individuals in creative professions, we feel sure we would find a disproportionate number of ADD adults.

One-Channel Operational System
Most of us are equal opportunity attenders. We give everything and anything the opportunity to grab our attention! An ineffective filtering system makes us vulnerable to distracting stimuli in the environment and in our minds and bodies.

It's hard to get things done when you keep thinking about and responding to so many different things. The quality of the work you do manage to accomplish is often marginal because your focus is interrupted so much. Although some ADDers are able to juggle several things at once, many find this difficult, if not impossible.

To accomplish anything, many of us have to operate on only one channel. Let's use the metaphor of channels on a radio to understand the dynamics of one-channel operation.

During a drive through the mountains, you may have to simultaneously listen to several stations as they fade in and out. You may spend a lot of time hitting the scan button, which is supposed to bring in the strongest channel. No sooner do you happily start singing along with your favorite song than it fades out as a stronger signal takes over your radio.

The normal brain doesn't seem to have trouble with channel selection. When a non-ADDer prepares dinner, he selects the *food* channel. He can attend to this strong signal and cook the food without burning it. At the same time, his brain scans and locates other strong signals that bring in important information. He monitors the *children* channel and switches to it when a sibling argument arises.

An ability to tune in several channels simultaneously is useful and essential. The radio in the ADD brain, however, seems to have a malfunctioning scan button that won't let him switch channels efficiently. Rather than pulling in the strong signal, it pulls in every channel within a thousand-mile radius! He keeps losing track of the channel he's listening to.

For many of us, the solution is to turn off the scan button. It's the only way to prevent the weak channels from interfering with our attention to the one we're trying to listen to. So we stay tuned in to only one channel. If we dare switch to the children channel, the pork chops become dried-out, hardened objects permanently attached to the pan we cooked them in!

We think the one-channel phenomenon has implications for kitchen designers. They really should take a crash course in ADD. If they were aware of this phenomenon, they would never design kitchens with large, open spaces for preparing dinner and chatting with guests at the same time. It may be a great concept for non-ADDers. For one-channel folk, however, this kitchen design results in lousy food or lousy conversation. Handling both at the same time is virtually *Mission Impossible!*

This difference causes undesirable behaviors in a one-channel ADDer. Demands to switch channels are cruel intrusions. He snaps at the interrupting party, snarls at the person on the phone or loses track of what he's doing. He may tune out the interruption, not even noting it or reacting v-e-r-y slowly to it as he undertakes the arduous task of switching gears.

KK: "When I worked on a psychiatric unit, I shared the responsibility for answering the telephone. I had trouble switching gears fast enough to pick up the phone after a few rings. Often, I never heard it ring at all. Other staff members resented my failure to do my share of this job. They mistakenly assumed I thought I was 'too good' to do this mundane task."

An ADDer can be at a disadvantage in the workplace when he has to tune in to many channels. The *phone, boss* and *coworker* channels all compete for his attention. Many workers complain that numerous interruptions force them to bring most of their work home. They can't get anything done at the office.

The Locking-In and Blocking-Out Phenomena

An interesting correlate to the one-channel phenomenon is over-persistence. When an ADDer becomes locked in to a task, he can't stop. His overpersistence can make switching gears very difficult. It can also cause a friend, colleague or spouse to leap to erroneous conclusions: (1) "It's obvious he can pay attention when he wants to." (2) "He's so rude! He completely ignores me."

Erratic focus and the general dysregulation that cause problems with concentration and stick-to-itiveness seem incompatible with overpersistence. Aren't unfinished tasks and short attention spans characteristic of ADDers? Well, the paradoxical answer is yes . . . and no!

Much of ADD behavior is paradoxical. Overpersistence could be just another difference that is at odds with a "short attention span." But we submit that it's more than that. An ADDer expends great energy and effort to shut out the distractions of other channels. With an unfiltered sensory world rushing into his brain, he has to develop some rather powerful defenses to survive. Overpersistence may be one of them.

An ADD adult may deliberately use this locking-in ability to shut out the rest of the world. It can insulate him from the wear and tear of handling the flood of incoming information. A one-channel ADDer may use his overpersistence as a compensatory strategy in a society that values the ability to bounce many balls at one time.

There may be another reason for overpersistence: Comorbid Obsessive-Compulsive Disorder (OCD). It is not uncommon for the ADD adult to have symptoms of OCD as well. Even in the absence of the compulsive, ritualistic behavioral component of OCD, obsessive thought patterns may be at work, causing excessive rumination. The inner experience is of having thoughts seemingly captured on a short loop of a tape recording—one that replays itself over and over on a recorder that has no Stop function.

Overpersistence is definitely a double-edged sword. Spouses and friends marvel at the ability to sit at a computer and write for hours, oblivious of everything else. Envy of this self-absorption turns to annoyance, however, when rain pours unnoticed through open windows or the tornado siren evokes not even a blink!

The good news is that this disability/ability difference can be used to good advantage. The bad news is that locking-in can be inappropriate, counterproductive or downright dangerous in certain situations. Remember the tornado siren—locking in to the computer instead of racing for the basement could have disastrous consequences!

The "I Hate Details" Dynamic

Many of us have an aversion to details. An inability to scan and switch channels plays into this aversion. To scan for details, we have to attend to numerous pieces of data. We find that our brains are uncooperative when we try to absorb many details simultaneously. We may forget much of what we see or hear. When we try to remember sequential details, we can lose the first step before we can assimilate the second. Our preference for the gestalt (the big picture) over miscellaneous details may in part result from this difficulty with data processing.

The "Don't Do Today What You Can Put Off Till Tomorrow" Dynamic

Many people live by this creed. Requesting several extensions on a federal income tax filing can put off this onerous task as long as possible. But we're not talking about a conscious decision to procrastinate. We're talking about the frustration many of us feel every time we try to get started on anything.

What appears to be stalling or an apparent unwillingness to do something is often a sign of the superhuman effort required to begin concentrating on a new task. Refocusing is painful. It takes a lot of blood, sweat and tears. Although an ADDer may do well after he gets going, he has to work hard to shut out the rest of the world and turn off the other channels. It's possible to become more efficient at self-starting but it takes time and self-discipline to learn this skill.

A Defective Filter

Another brain function that goes awry in ADD is the filtering mechanism. A brain that is working at peak efficiency can select what it needs to concentrate on and filter out extraneous distractions. It works much like the oil filter in a car. It filters out the dirty, useless particles so the engine can operate efficiently with clean oil. Coffee filters perform a similar function, preventing the bitter grounds from getting mixed in with the liquid.

A defective filter permits the "grounds to get mixed up with the coffee." An ADDer experiences the world as a barrage to his senses—noises, sights and smells rush in without barriers or protection. Normal noise levels can interfere with his ability to hear conversations or maintain a train of thought.

Even in a relatively quiet restaurant, background noises compete for attention and interfere with the ability to listen to the server. During a telephone call, the ADDer may snap at a spouse who makes the slightest noise in the room. Unfiltered visual distractions can make shopping a nightmare. The process of scanning the contents of a large department store can be agonizing. The quantity of choices is overwhelming and often creates feelings of intense anxiety and irritation.

Touchy Touchability

An ADDer can be very touchy about being touched! His sense of touch is as vulnerable to overstimulation as the rest of his sensory channels. An intolerance of touch or close physical proximity is a fairly common difference noted by ADD adults. The term "tactile defensiveness," found in occupational therapy literature, captures the essence of this difference. Similar to most ADD symptoms, it waxes and wanes. At times the need for physical space is acute, and an ADDer simply can't tolerate being around other people.

It's ironic that with his poor sense of physical boundaries, he may bump into someone else's physical space while he fiercely protects his own. One ADDer ruefully observed: "People like me—other ADDers—can drive me crazy. I hate to be touched, and they keep bumping into me." Others say they don't like living with animals because pets don't have respect for physical boundaries!

Roller-Coaster Emotions

ADDers Live on Emotional Roller Coasters

We're not exactly sure what causes the problems with mood and emotion in ADD. We do know that ADDers often say they live on emotional roller coasters. Feeling states fluctuate, with extreme alterations in the highs and lows over hours or even minutes.

Maintaining emotions on an even keel is an intricate process involving fine adjustments by different parts of the brain and nervous system. For an ADDer, this process seems to be dysregulated. He walks precariously on his high wire never knowing how he'll feel at a given moment. The people in his life may tiptoe around him, fearing his next bad mood.

Intense INTENSITY

People often describe ADD adults as *intense*. Feelings are amplified and blasted out with little restraint. When an ADDer is angry, he might yell or throw things. When he's happy, he often captivates people with dazzling displays of positive energy.

41

Low moods feel like the end of the world. Many of us have passionate natures, artistic temperaments that react quickly and to an extreme. Our tendency to boast and exaggerate may result from experiencing the world so intensely. If we always see the world in vivid living color, we'll describe it that way to others. It isn't a planned exaggeration but a valid reflection of our perceptions.

A Short Fuse

When something pushes an ADD adult's temperamental buttons, impulsivity often kicks in. It may take little to set off his explosive temper or turn him into an irritable grouch. The outburst that results can be as baffling to him as it is frightening to the people around him. After the explosion that seems to come from nowhere, he often feels ashamed. He can't understand why he made such a big deal out of nothing.

His anger usually disappears as quickly as it appeared, but the anger he elicits in other people doesn't go away quite as fast. They shake their heads at his childish reaction to a burned piece of toast. He could just get another piece. Instead, he fusses and fumes. Since setbacks throw him off balance so easily, he starts complaining when he should be trying to solve the problem.

The IDP Dynamic—Irritability, Dissatisfaction or Pessimism

The moodiness in ADD can be expressed as generalized irritability. There may not be dramatic explosions of temper but rather a continual grumpiness. Unfortunately, the irritable ADDer misses out on the highs, instead experiencing chronic dissatisfaction. He seldom expresses positive thoughts or feelings and travels through life exuding an aura of pessimism. Through no fault of his own, he views his world through gray-colored glasses.

Another manifestation of this generalized irritability has less to do with pessimism than with a feeling of being constantly annoyed by other people and events. The ADDer may be sarcastic, rude or abrupt with others because they have overstimulated him or interrupted his train of thought.

Affective Disorders?

The symptoms of affective disorders (such as bipolar disorder, dysthymia and depression) and those of ADD can be remarkably similar. Mental health professionals sometimes have difficulty distinguishing among these disorders.

Sometimes the various affective disorders and ADD occur together in the same individual. Dysregulated emotions can also appear to be symptoms of, say, depression when they're not. The symptoms can mask underlying attentional problems. It isn't uncommon for a mental health professional to make a diagnosis of depression and totally miss the ADD.

The depressionlike symptoms of ADD adults might be part of the neurological dysregulation that causes the disorder. They might be part of an emotional response to repeated failure. Likely, the moodiness of many ADDers is a little of both. Differentiating ADD from other affective disorders can be difficult but very important. The emotional piece of ADD is often just the tip of the iceberg of other problems that must be addressed.

Bottomless Pit of Needs and Desires

"I want . . . I need . . . I must have . . ."

On any given day, parents everywhere hear these immortal words! In the grocery store checkout, the begging can be for a pack of gum or candy; at the toy store it's for the latest, greatest water pistol. Although it isn't easy for children to learn that they can't have everything, they usually grudgingly learn to accept the deprivation. For many ADDers, the intense feelings of need continue forever. It's part of the dysregulation of ADD.

An insatiable ADD adult experiences ongoing problems with his appetite for many things—sex, alcohol, excitement, etcetera. He is a bottomless pit of needs, always looking ahead and never feeling satisfied. The simpler pleasures of life are too mild. Intense experiences must match his voracious appetite.

This insatiability can manifest itself in varied ways. Inside, it feels like an overwhelming craving. The craving is often non-specific—it's for *something* but not for anything in particular. An ADDer might use food, sex, liquor or shopping sprees to appease the greedy Needs Monster. Unfortunately, feeding the monster makes him grow larger and more insistent, so the ADDer sets a vicious cycle in motion. He can exhaust friends and lovers with demands for attention and affection because *no amount is ever enough.*

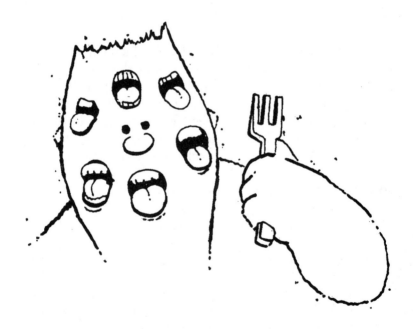

Some ADDers develop patterns of behavior that include habitual overeating or binge drinking. It is likely that a significant percentage of the members in the Anonymous groups—for alcoholism, codependency, sex addictions and others—also have ADD. For a wealth of information about the connections between ADD and addictive behavior, read Wendy Richardson's excellent book *When Too Much Isn't Enough.*

With hard work, an insatiable ADD adult can learn to say "No" to the nonstop "I want, I need, I must have" message of his Needs Monster. He might quiet his restless cravings by dabbling in sports car racing or bungee jumping. He might assuage his need to shop till you drop through a strategy an acquaintance of ours has designed. She goes on periodic shopping binges, frantically charging hundreds of dollars' worth of merchandise. Having happily fed her Needs Monster with all her packages, she heads home. But wait a minute. Doesn't that make him grow even larger? In her case, it doesn't because there's a second part of her strategy. The key is that she has taught herself to bring the packages home and *never open them.* She has learned that within a few hours or days, the cravings for her purchases will have subsided. Then she goes on another shopping trip to return everything she bought!

Of course, what the Needs Monster is really looking for is more brain juice. Enough stimulation to wake it up in order to simply feel *alive.* Food, sex, shopping, substance abuse, etcetera are ways that ADDults attempt to self-medicate a sleepy mind.

Activity Levels in Flux

> *Some ADDers are hyperactive, though not all the time.*
> *Some ADDers are hypoactive.*
> *Most ADDers are hyperactive and hypoactive.*

Literature frequently refers to ADDers as *hyperactives*—a reference to excessive activity levels. This reflects a viewpoint that is both controversial and somewhat outdated. Although some professionals still focus on high activity levels in diagnosing ADD, we prefer to consider the issue of hyperactivity as one piece of a more generalized *dysregulated activity level*. This dysregulation can include *too much* action (hyperactivity), *too little* action (hypo-activity) and *fluctuations* between the two extremes.

Some ADDers know something that many professionals don't understand: Hypoactivity can be a troubling part of ADD. A hypoactive ADDer moves in slow motion and often hears "Get moving." If only he could. It would take a bonfire beneath him to cause any movement at all! He may envy his hyperactive counterpart.

A hyperactive ADDer's differences are most noticeable when he has to sit still. That's when he starts swinging his leg or gnawing on his pencil. If his job permits physical activity, the hyperactive adult can be indistinguishable from his non-ADD colleagues.

Traveling salespeople cope with restlessness by staying on the road and on the move. Nurses joke about needing roller skates to get from one end of the shift to the other. Likewise, the con-struction worker has a job that lets him expend physical energy. The level of activity required in these jobs can provide a needed outlet for hyperactivity.

Many ADDers are both hyperactive and hypoactive. It seems that activity levels fluctuate between extremes, much like the other dysregulated symptoms of ADD. Sometimes the ADDer moves and talks at mega-speed, only to flip to a state of inactiv-ity that makes him appear nearly comatose.

Some ADDers report that on a given day, their activity levels seem to build from morning to evening. They are slow-moving and thinking in the morning, functioning well only if they can carry out routines without interruption. Early morning conversations with family members can consist of grunts and one-word answers. These ADD adults describe themselves as operating on "auto-pilot," capable of little more than routine, automatic functions.

Nothing helps to speed up this process. These folk begin to gain alertness by midmorning, which is a problem when they work standard daytime hours. By noon, they're going full tilt, using their energy to talk nonstop to coworkers over lunch. With energy reserves drained by midafternoon, the big slump often hits with a fight to stay awake. The cycle often continues with a late afternoon shot of newly found energy when they start revving up again. For many, the evening hours are the most productive—late afternoon or evening shifts enable them to work at peak efficiency.

This pattern is certainly not unique to ADDers. After eating, in particular, many people suffer from a slow down as their bodies mobilize for food digestion. The practice of the siesta in many countries is related to this normal physiological cycle.

An ADDer's cycles, however, seem to have more intense peaks and slumps. As a group, ADD adults tend to be night owls. Many have trouble getting started in the morning and display irregular patterns of hyperactivity and lethargy throughout the day.

Although many experts regard hyperactivity as a primary symptom of ADD, others hypothesize that it's an attempt to compensate for underarousal. Likely, both theories hold parcels of truth. At times, the ADDer seems to be frantically trying to keep himself going by being physically active. Instead of taking Ritalin to maintain focus and regulation, he might use strenuous exercise to boost his flagging energy and attention level. At other times, he seems frantically driven by his hyperactivity, a force over which he has limited control.

People with high energy levels can accomplish many things in a short time. While others complain that a twenty-four-hour day isn't long enough to get everything done, an ADDer might search for extra things to fill up the unused hours. Hyperactivity can be helpful. Unfortunately, many ADD adults energetically spin their wheels, go in circles and get nowhere. The goal of treatment or self-help can't be just to slow the ADDer down, but to help him learn to use and direct his energy more efficiently.

Thrill Seeking

Lack of restraint can cause an ADDer to risk life and limb in pursuit of excitement. As a group, we tend to be thrill seekers, minimizing inherent risk and danger. As children, we fell out of trees and dove from great heights. We have made frequent trips to the emergency room to have our bruised and battered bodies patched up. As adults, we're on our own without anyone to remind us of the dangers. We may still be making emergency room visits for far more serious injuries. Instead of climbing trees, we are climbing mountains or skydiving.

An ADDer isn't the only adult who enjoys activities with a high element of risk. But he may approach these activities without sufficient planning. His behavior can be more risky because he engages in thrill seeking without recognizing the inherent risks involved. He fails to pay sufficient attention to register them. Since he doesn't register or process the information about risks, he doesn't really believe in them. Fuzziness about the external world makes him feel invincible and gives him a false sense of safety.

The Intractable Time Tyrant

Time is an elusive entity to many of us. Sometimes we feel as if we've entered a time warp—a twilight zone where we tread water, get nowhere and accomplish nothing. Our sense of time is elastic, and we characteristically underestimate the time it will take to do anything.

As children, we're late for school, stay out beyond our curfews and miss homework deadlines. As adults, we might be late for work and have trouble completing projects on time. Teachers, bosses and coworkers often misinterpret the tardiness as laziness or an indifference to their needs. In reality, our behaviors can result from an altered time sense and an inability to plan.

An unscientific diagnostic tool could be to count the items on a person's "to do" list for a given day. In Chapter 11, we'll offer a "test" we've developed to diagnose ADD as a measure of disorganization! The daily list of an ADDer usually includes far more than any human could accomplish in three or four days. A professor friend planned to write three articles, a book and two grants over the summer months. His unrealistic goals were quite typical for an ADDer!

Perhaps there is a brain function called "Time" that doesn't operate efficiently in an ADDer's brain. More likely, his time troubles are caused by various deficits and his failure to factor in their impacts on his life. He figures that it shouldn't take more than two hours to prepare a small dinner for friends. So he decides to add a few extra things to his afternoon plans. Regrettably, he fails to plan for the inevitable distractions that will derail him. Preparing the meal always takes much longer than he thinks it will.

Time troubles play out in other ways as well, with time passing both more quickly and more slowly than it should. When an ADDer is lost in his own compelling thoughts, the hours fly by in an instant, whereas routine work hours inch along at an excruciatingly slow pace.

Sometimes even unpleasant tasks can grab the ADD adult. Most people don't think of housework as their favorite activity. Then why does an ADDer who hates housework spend hours "spit-shining" his house while other chores remain unfinished? The answer lies in overpersistence. It's not uncommon for him to become locked in, obsessively attacking tiny specks of dirt. The day evaporates as he scrubs a small portion of a room into antiseptic perfection. This would be okay if he had the time or inclination to spend his life pursuing the elusive dream of a spotless home. Of course, his time is limited and must be divided among a variety of chores.

The time he never accounted for is eaten up by lists that are too long: Another day is gone . . . It's three o'clock in the morning . . . The alarm will go off in three hours . . . Doesn't the Time Monster ever sleep???

Space Struggles

An ADD adult can also have a distorted sense of space and problems with directionality. As an adult, he might still rely on the visual clue of his wristwatch to identify right and left. He might have difficulty following a road map or understanding the compass settings of north, south, east and west.

He can also have a distorted sense of how his body moves in space in relationship to other objects. As a consequence, he bumps into people or furniture. He might be unable to gauge the speed and direction of a ball in tennis or baseball games. Sports that demand finely tuned spatial abilities can be particularly difficult for him.

Similar to a distorted sense of time, an altered sense of space might be related to excessive speed and deficient planning. It can also result from the impaired information processing of a specific learning disability.

Spatial problems aren't limited to sports activities and directionality. They also have an impact on organization. An ADD adult often lives with a daunting amount of clutter and disorganization. Even when he slows down to take the time to tidy up, he faces a nightmarish task of figuring out what to do with his chaotic surroundings. He may dream of having enough money to hire the right person to organize all the *stuff* in his life so he can get on with the business of living.

The ADD brain seems to have trouble *sorting and filing*. We ADDers tend to focus on all the exceptions to the orderly rules of the world. We play a perpetual game of "But what about . . . ?" It's difficult to organize either space or a filing system without an ability to decide which things belong together.

Memory also plays a role in an ADDer's space troubles. Before he can organize his belongings, he has to remember where they are. After he finds them he still has to figure out what to do with them!

Some of us dismiss the effect of clutter on our lives, assuring ourselves that tidiness is simply a waste of time. Others become obsessed with putting things in order and have time for little else. Although neither course of action is particularly helpful, problems with spatial organization are common for many of us with ADD.

The ADDer's environment is a confusing one over which he constantly struggles to gain a semblance of control. A certain degree of order is important for emotional well-being. Preventing the overwhelming feelings of confusion that result from untamed piles of junk is an important goal.

Information Processing
Some of the differences of ADDers can be understood within the context of information processing. How do we think about and act on the information we receive from the environment? Do we have unique ADD thinking and acting styles? To answer these questions and examine other differences in ADD adults, we'll use the theory of systems as a working model of the brain's functions.

Systems consist of assorted parts organized into a whole to serve a function or reach a goal. Every system uses energy and resources from the environment as its input. It transforms, or processes, the input into an alternative form called output and sends it back to the environment.

A computer system takes input from humans by way of the keyboard. It processes it and produces new information as output on a printout. Similarly, the human brain receives input from the outside world through the senses, processes it and produces output in the form of words or actions.

If a computer malfunctions, we look at the three parts of the system to find out what's wrong. Human error can interfere with input if information is keyed incorrectly. A problem in the information processing of the computer itself may also exist. Finally, the output function can be flawed if there is a mechanical problem with the printer.

Breaking down the workings of the brain into these three components can help us better understand what's happening when things go wrong. A significant problem for many of us with ADD is mismatched input, information processing and output capacities.

An ADDer can often process internal information rapidly but has a less efficient capacity for the input and output functions. Problems with selective attention and filtering compromise the quality of input—getting information into his brain. Difficulties with impulsivity, activity levels, memory retrieval, motor control and rambling speech compromise the quality of output—effectively communicating or acting on the processed information. Let's take a look at how input/output weaknesses and internal processing strengths create some unique ADD differences.

Action and Inaction Imbalance

We know that as ADD adults, we have problems with attention. That's why our disorder is called an Attention Deficit Disorder. We have trouble with *selective attention*—focusing on one part of the vast array of information that bombards our senses. This is just the first step in processing information, however.

We also have trouble with the second step, *selective intention*—selecting one response from a variety of possible action choices. Melvin D. Levine, M.D., examines the interplay of selective intention and selective attention in his book *Developmental Variation and Learning Disorders*. He makes the point that it's rare to find a person who has difficulty with attention without also having difficulty with intention, or action.

When your teacher complained that you weren't paying attention, was he observing the neurological process in your brain? Of course not! He was observing behavior. Your action—

looking out the window rather than at your math book—resulted from listening to the blue jay instead of your teacher.

The action part of attention depends on balancing the forces of action, *facilitation,* and inaction, *inhibition.* The brain needs to facilitate, or support, helpful actions while it inhibits, or blocks, the harmful ones. Many of the differences unique to an ADDer result from an imbalance in this area. When he should be in his inaction mode, he blurts out a hasty, sloppy response he should have inhibited. When he should be in his action mode, he fails to answer a question he should have facilitated.

In tennis, facilitation helps him react quickly to return a shot and inhibition prevents him from reacting too quickly and moving when he should be waiting. A bad game of tennis is one thing, but social errors pack a bigger punch.

Disinhibition causes many of the social problems an ADDer experiences. He says things he shouldn't say, interrupts conversations and intrudes on a friend's personal space. Because he has trouble slowing down enough to stop and think, he may not even realize his mistake. Sometimes he may realize it but is too embarrassed to apologize.

Failure to restrain or inhibit can cause problems far more serious than a social faux pas. An ADDer tends to react quickly and intensely to his impulses. He may strike out at his children or let loose a stream of verbal abuse. Arguments with his spouse can quickly get out of hand as he says things in the heat of the moment only to regret them later.

He doesn't mean to lash out and is ashamed of his behavior. The hasty words or actions were neither planned nor intended.

> *If behavior is judged by intentions, we ADDers are blameless—we didn't mean it!*

While it's true that we're not calculating criminals, we need to look beyond good intentions. These impulsive words or actions can impact relationships and psyches. We have to consider the impact of our behavior on other people, especially our loved ones.

A failure to inhibit one's words isn't always a negative quality—an ability to say just about anything can come in handy. Talking about personal experiences and problems can open doors for others to share confidences. Most people are enormously relieved to discover that others share their fears and insecurities. The mushrooming number of support groups is evidence of this need to share and be intimate. Many people seem to be starved for connections to others.

People laugh when the truth is exaggerated, twisted or expanded to the level of absurdity. An ADDer who doesn't inhibit the flow of his thoughts can dream up outrageously funny things to say—things that others wouldn't dare to utter! If he can learn to monitor himself sufficiently to keep from stepping over the line into offensiveness, he can contribute a sparkling sense of humor.

The Supersonic Brain
Stated simply, the ADD brain goes fast! Although we've listed it separately, the supersonic brain is closely related to the action/inaction balance.

An ADDer's *altered cognitive tempo* can translate into unmonitored rapid-fire speech. Without pausing for breath, he may prevent someone else from getting a word in edgewise. Handwriting and other aspects of task performance can also suffer as he fails to slow down enough to balance his internal processing and physical capabilities (output). As a result, he makes careless errors and has trouble with motor tasks. The authors, for instance, have had a long-standing love/hate relationship with tennis that has resulted in part from the supersonic brain phenomenon.

PR: "Kate and I should have our names listed on a plaque of notable accomplishments, a kind of *Guinness Book of Records*. We merit inclusion on the basis of our record-setting number of years in beginner and advanced beginner tennis lessons! Regardless of how hard we worked at our game, we never seemed to make much progress. After we both started taking Ritalin, we experienced a startling improvement in our skills on the tennis court.

"Lest struggling athletes read this and race to their pharmacies for their physical skill pills, I need to emphasize that the improvement we experienced was one of *mental* skill. We were playing better because we were thinking better, or at least more slowly and with better planning.

"Taming our runaway thinking tempos gave us a more accurate sense of time. Our abilities to strategize and s-l-o-w d-o-w-n improved our game. With relief and a sense of accomplishment, we finally graduated from our beginner lessons."

Applying the brakes to our supersonic brains often gets easier by the time we become adults. Many of us manage to achieve some degree of balance and an ability to stop and think—at least more often than we did as children. Unfortunately, as soon as we start feeling complacent, something invariably goes wrong.

KK: "I'm certainly no whiz at higher mathematics, but I can accurately add long columns of figures. I prefer doing my addition without a calculator so I don't have to worry about pushing the wrong buttons.

"Years ago, however, I made the mistake of rapidly calculating our household budget to figure out if my former husband and I could afford a major renovation. I didn't recheck my figures before assuring him that the project was financially do-able. I swept away his natural caution with my enthusiasm and energy and implied that he was a stick-in-the-mud for raising questions and objections. After we had committed to the project and were up to our ears in plaster dust, I found a glaring omission in my figures. I had neglected to add the mortgage payment to our monthly budget!

"My grandmother bailed us out. If she hadn't given me a portion of an inheritance we might still be in debtors' prison—assuming such places still exist!"

This anecdote is illustrative of an important balancing act for many of us with ADD. We have to put the brakes on our racing thoughts gradually enough that we don't come to screeching halts, paralyzed by fears of making impulsive mistakes. Alternately, we don't always apply the brakes when we should, especially when we're working on something easy or familiar. When we're feeling overconfident we may "put the pedal to the metal" and send our racing thoughts careening out of control!

Paralysis of the Will

The balance can also tip in the other direction, with a failure to act at all—something like a paralysis of the will. The output function totally stops working. When this happens, the ADDer may find himself in a frozen state, unable to take appropriate action. He may watch the softball whiz by as if he were a spectator instead of the player responsible for intercepting it. When it's time to answer someone's question, he may stand back feeling stupid, because he can't think of a response. Input problems probably also play a part in this paralysis of the will. If he hasn't input the information he needs to properly respond, the quality of his output will be impaired.

Did you know that this little section on the paralysis of the will sparked a thread on about.com that ran to over four hundred postings? Obviously, it struck a nerve with many ADDers. As of the writing of this second edition, you can still find that thread on add.about.com. You might want to go there to check out what others have said about paralysis of the will.

Reaction Time Irregularity

Our discussion of the fast-thinking brain may seem puzzling. You may be thinking, "That's crazy! My brain moves with the speed of a glacier and it makes me feel pretty stupid." This is another of the ADD paradoxes. Your brain moves both very slowly and very rapidly, depending on the task.

If an ADDer is free to direct his own thoughts and actions, the rapid freewheeling aspect of his brain takes over. When he has to fit into someone else's agenda either with words or actions, he finds it more difficult to function well. In other words, *it's easier to act than react.* Reacting depends on the problematic input and output functions of an ADD brain. If you can rely on your ability to process information internally, you can often take swift and decisive action.

Fluent self-expression is independent of the ability to respond to questions. A person with the gift of gab who ignores you when you ask direct questions, might not be rude or uninterested. He might simply have trouble retrieving things from memory in a demand situation.

PR: "I have a particular gift for speaking and conduct workshops without missing a beat. When I get ready to share information with an audience, I become energized and focused. I thoroughly enjoy this work and am never at a loss for words. But informal gatherings are a totally different matter. Even in a group of friends, I often find myself groping for things to say in response to questions.

"This baffling behavior confused me until I understood my ADD. Now it makes perfect sense. I am in charge of my thoughts and the direction of my work during my conferences. I rely on the wealth of my knowledge and my excellent long-term memory to orchestrate these sessions. The question-and-answer period isn't a problem either, because the focus is something I know well. But at the social gathering, I have to react and respond to conversation generated by other people. My brain often doesn't work fast enough to find what I need to say. On the way home from these gatherings, I usually think of many things I could have said."

Clearly, most people function best when the task or subject is something they know well. You don't have to have ADD to be at a loss for words. But ADDers seem to experience this phenomenon on a regular basis. It results from a significant imbalance in action and reaction capabilities.

Connections to the world are generally slow and inefficient while internal connections work with lightning rapidity. Output can be difficult because the ADDer has to synchronize his mental speed with his slower output. An inability to respond quickly to requests seems to be stubborn or noncompliant behavior. In reality, these behaviors can be manifestations of irregular reaction capabilities. His mouth, brain and body just don't cooperate very well in demand situations.

As many of us struggle with mismatched input/output capabilities, we feel out of control. We live in a world of paradoxes, a world that seems to toss us about by inexplicable forces. Our need for control doesn't come from a desire to be one up on others. It is often a desperate attempt to manage a situation so we can function with a degree of competence. Otherwise, it's so easy to look and feel stupid.

ADD children may not work well in the group setting of a classroom but perform well with a tutor. An ADD adult can have difficulty working as a committee member yet perform admirably as the chairperson. He may stand around the kitchen of a friend preparing a dinner party, unable to figure out how to assist. But he may successfully orchestrate a social activity of his own design.

These behaviors can make you feel lazy and bad about yourself. It's important to remember that this is another piece of ADD. These contradictory behaviors can reflect your genuine inability to react quickly and efficiently to situations.

The Minuscule Mental Fuel Tank
Unless you happen to be in excellent aerobic health, a frenzied hour-long chase through the park after your escaping Great

Dane would probably do you in for the afternoon. If a nap wasn't warranted, a *kick back, put your feet up and read a book* break probably would be. You are exhausted!

This scenario is similar to the daily experiences of an ADDer. Though his body might not dash madly around a park, his thoughts can race around his head. He is mentally tired. A rapidly working brain expends much energy and quickly uses up its daily allotment.

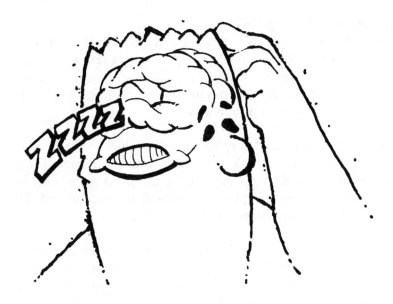

ADDers tend to process information at a mind-boggling pace and burn out just as quickly. An eight-hour workday can be torturous for someone whose mental energy and productive times simply don't last long enough. Some have sufficient energy to get through the day but run out of steam when they get home. Families can't believe that the slug in front of the TV could ever be of any use on the job. For years, they have never seen him move off his couch!

Many of us think faster and fatigue more quickly than our non-ADD peers. Each of us needs to be aware of the impact of cognitive fatigue on our work tempo. Some adults conserve their resources by coasting at work, particularly if their jobs aren't too demanding. This strategy can backfire. Without a high level of motivation, the ADDer's job performance can really suffer. Conversely, the mental fatigue caused by a demanding job can overload his brain's capacity to function well. The challenge is to conserve his mental energy by working at his own pace and rhythm.

Shutdown Susceptibility

What happens when the brain's capacity to process information is exceeded? *It shuts down.* Many of us live in terror that we'll shut down at a critical moment and become useless in a crisis. We may freeze in response to loud noises or unexpected events and feel that we're in slow motion.

An ADDer's overloaded system can make him so tired he can barely move, talk or think. It is as if he is in a temporary coma. He experiences attempts at communication as assaults on his very being. He either ignores the assault or snaps an irritable reply—taking any action is an impossibility.

An overloaded brain is similar to an overloaded computer system. If you load up the working memory of a computer with excessive data, it might crash, losing data or the functions of the software. Your program will be temporarily useless. With excessive sensory information, the brain can also suffer from overload.

Even the most efficient, resilient person can become disorganized under certain conditions. Discoveries in the brains of individuals suffering from *Post-Traumatic Stress Disorder* are good examples.

Post-traumatic stress disorder (PTSD) is a syndrome that can occur following frightening trauma such as war, sexual abuse or natural disaster. The symptoms include nightmares, flashbacks, substance abuse and an exaggerated startle response. Previously well adjusted people aren't immune to the disorder—the symptoms can occur in anyone who has experienced severe trauma.

PTSD is not just a psychological problem. Psychobiological researchers have discovered actual biochemical changes in the brains of people with PTSD. It appears that the massive overload experienced in extreme situations can actually alter the brain.

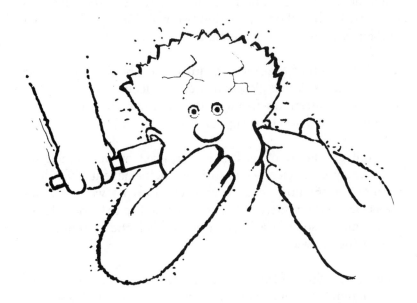

Although no one can explain the biochemistry that causes shutdown, we know from experience that it's troubling for many ADDers. Of course, we aren't the only people who shut down under demanding situations. The difference is a matter of degree. It takes a fairly low level of stress for the ADD brain to yell "uncle." And when it happens, it's definitely not fun!

This baffling coma of shutdown is troubling but essential for our continued well-being. It is as if our brains must stop the onslaught so we can heal ourselves and renew our depleted reserves of mental energy. Rather than fighting it, we need to give in to it and accept the self-imposed rest time. Our brains must recharge. Each of us has to find the best way to facilitate this renewal.

Undependable Memory and Learning Systems

If you look at a picture of the brain, you won't find an area labeled The Memory. Memory is a process rather than an identifiable part of the brain. The function of memory is a system with multiple parts scattered throughout the brain. Some of the differences ADDers experience are related to problems with memory. In the following section, we will examine the impact of ADD symptoms on the memory process.

The First Step of Memory: Acquisition. The first step in the process, acquisition, is closely related to selective attention. Besides paying attention to incoming information, it involves a preliminary decision to accept and store it.

As ADDers, many of us feel embarrassed by how much we don't know. Our selective attention deficits make it difficult to acquire information that never even finds its way into our memories! The positive side is that an ability to notice things others miss results in a fascinating and eclectic storehouse of interesting knowledge!

The Second Step of Memory: Registration. We have to register information before it can become part of memory. In this second step of the memory process, we consciously make an effort to secure the information in our memories for subsequent recall. If we superficially register the data, we'll have difficulty retrieving it later. Problems of arousal or alertness often impair adequate registration. We may only partially understand conversations, phone messages or directions and jump the gun on new tasks.

Coding and *rehearsal* are two important parts of registration. Every time you use a file cabinet, you are using a system of coding. You decide whether to file the piece of paper by subject, writer's name or type of required action. As you may recall from the discussion of spatial organization, this is no small task for some ADDers.

Registering information involves essentially the same kind of sorting and filing. We decide to code, or file, incoming information as a visual image, a word or a sound. For example, we can code the name "Tom Thumb" in several ways. The code can be a "picture" of Tom, the midget with an enormous thumb (visual); a word, "finger" (verbal) or a sound, "Tom Thumb is a bum" (auditory).

Rehearsal is what children used to do in their one-room schoolhouses—memorizing by reciting their lessons aloud. We use rehearsal to practice and repeat information until we anchor it in our memories. To be effective, rehearsal must be more than rote memorization. It must include *elaboration* of information. If you have ever memorized a word list by singing a silly song you created from the words, you have used rehearsal elaboration.

Rehearsal is another problem for an ADDer because it's tedious and requires patience. These are usually not his best qualities! He is creative, though, and can be quite inventive with the sometimes off-the-wall coding methods he designs.

The Third Step of Memory: Storage. The third step involves storage of the processed information. There are four storage systems: *instant recall; active working memory; short-term memory;* and *long-term memory.* These storage systems aren't characterized by their size but by their duration, or how long information is stored in each.

Instant recall has the shortest duration. Seeing the flash of lightning in your mind's eye is an example of instant recall. Touch-typing also uses this kind of memory. The typist holds the key's location in his mind only long enough to press on it.

Active working memory functions much like the working memory of a computer. While you work, the words on the screen are held in the computer's temporary storage. If the power goes out, you lose your work forever unless you have saved it to permanent disk storage.

RAM memory capacity varies from one computer to another. If you try to run memory-intensive software, your computer might respond to the overload with a shutdown and loss of data. If you're lucky, it might give you a chance to close files or change software by alerting you to its low memory.

Similar to RAM memory, your active working memory can shut down if you try to overload it. It's too bad your brain doesn't give clearer messages of impending shutdown—maybe something like, "This is your brain. I am preparing to self-destruct!" Complexity of detail seems to shrink the storage capacity. An ADDer often has a remarkably unreliable temporary memory that regularly loses power and data. He begins the first step in solving a complex problem only to lose it as he undertakes the second step. The jigsaw pieces keep falling off the table before he can put the whole puzzle together.

Short-Term Memory also functions as temporary storage. Its capacity is quite limited with a maximum of five seconds or seven items (plus or minus two). Its unique limitations make it vulnerable to a variety of interferences. Distractibility wreaks havoc with short-term memory. It doesn't take more than a brief mind trip for a person to lose data that he wasn't mentally present to register.

An imaginative thinking style can also interfere with short-term memory storage. Elaboration and association of old and new data is a great anchor for long-term storage. But it can compromise the quality of short-term storage that requires focus on specific details.

Long-Term Memory is the permanent, seemingly unlimited storehouse of facts, experiences, values, routines and general knowledge. You can think of it as a huge bank vault that contains numerous safe-deposit boxes. Memories you need to store forever are in a separate box deep inside the cavernous vault. The ones you need to remember while you complete your errands are in your safe-deposit box right inside the vault's steel door.

The data in this bank vault is *consolidated,* or translated into a permanent code. The code determines which box will store the information. When you identify a Honda, Buick and Ford as automobiles, you are using consolidation. From experience and learning, you form associations by elaborating on the characteristics of each car and cross-referencing them to other vehicles.

A rich imagination enhances these associations and is an asset for long-term memory storage. Since an ADDer tends to be a conceptualizer rather than a rote learner, his consolidation skills can be superb. He may possess a wealth of information in his bank vault but routinely forget where he put his car keys!

Fourth Step of Memory: Access. Access is the process of recalling stored information through recognition or retrieval memory. Recognition relies on *familiarity* to refresh the memories of superficially learned data. For example, you use recognition memory to take a multiple-choice test or find your way to a location by noting landmarks along the way.

On the other hand, *retrieval* requires precise, accurate recall on demand. When you take an essay exam, you have to retrieve information as an accurate whole. Finding a specific word in your memory banks is another retrieval task.

Retrieval relies on data you have firmly fixed in memory. To anchor data in memory, you have to use specific strategies. Precise recall is only as good as the strategies you used to store the information. That's why rote recitation is a less effective strategy than memorizing by principle. Rote learning results in isolated details rather than general ideas and abstractions.

An ADDer's unique abilities and disabilities cause great variability in his ability to access information. Accurate retrieval is a combination of attention to the details of what he needs to memorize, planned strategies for storage and fast information processing.

With an aversion to details, an ADDer tends to approach memory chores in a rapid, superficial and haphazard manner. This compromises his ability to develop strategies for registration. His limited reserves of mental energy impair his ability to maintain sufficient effort to memorize something. As he quickly burns out, he often rushes to get the memory chore finished.

His divergent retrieval is usually much faster and more accurate than his convergent retrieval. Remember the dynamics of reaction time? An ADD adult functions better when he *acts* (divergent retrieval) on his own ideas than when he *reacts* (convergent retrieval) to a direct question. He often impresses his friends and himself (!) with the fluency of thoughts structured around his knowledge base. Everything is great until someone interrupts with a question or even worse, changes the subject. He suddenly feels anxious and annoyed that he has to switch to his faulty convergent retrieval.

Fifth Step of Memory: Transfer. Transfer is a complex process of rearranging individual pieces of data to form new knowledge. It can include combining fragmented pieces into a larger whole. It can include applying data from one application to another. It can also include generalizations of the common threads between seemingly unrelated ideas or events.

A precise memory for facts is invaluable in answering questions about a specific subject. It is less valuable in information transfer that depends on associations. For instance, children and adults with mental retardation have difficulty transferring skills from one setting to another. They need to learn skills in each of the settings they will use them.

Transfer of knowledge depends on the creative and flexible use of a knowledge base. If data is stored in separately labeled boxes, transfer of knowledge is impossible. Mixing the contents of the boxes or combining them in new ways is unthinkable!

An ADDer tends to be a creative, divergent thinker with an ability to put knowledge and ideas together. He resists putting things in boxes with neat labels. Although this can be a disadvantage when he needs precise memory, it is a decided advantage for transferring knowledge. He can wander through his safe-deposit boxes, finding information to use in new and interesting ways. He can apply knowledge and solve problems in ways undreamed of by more orderly thinkers.

━━━━━━━━━━━━━━━━━━━━━━━━━━

ADD adults don't have faulty memories, but their unique symptoms create gaps in the memory process. Although each of us has a unique memory profile, we share some fairly consistent patterns. Recognition memory is usually good. That's why many of us performed well in classroom discussions about the historic implications of world events but failed miserably on tests that required one-word answers.

It makes sense that your memory would be good for a specific subject or task that comes easily to you. But what about that tough physics class in high school? Why did you do so well in a difficult subject that required *on demand* memory retrieval? Your teacher might have wondered the same thing. He might have pointedly used this as evidence of your ability to do it *when you wanted to.*

Your teacher was partially correct in his assessment. Your ability to excel was related to motivation but not in the way he thought—your lack of motivation wasn't the result of your poor attitude. It was the result of an ADDer's need for intensely compelling motivation to grab the dysregulated selective attention. It also had a lot to do with individual teaching styles.

Everyone has his own unique learning style. The visual learner learns by seeing, the auditory learner by hearing and the kinesthetic learner by doing/experiencing. If you are a visual learner and the course in question was taught with many charts, diagrams and other visual aids, your brain received the optimal kind of stimuli. Your memory was given just what it needed to function efficiently.

Recognizing individual learning styles can be very helpful in bypassing weak areas and focusing on strengths. The memory of an ADDer can compromise his attempts to learn, converse and carry out instructions. Understanding the process goes a long way toward helping him readjust his self-assessments.

We ADDer's aren't stupid or oppositional. We just need to learn, and to demonstrate what we've learned, differently than others do. We'll examine these differences in greater depth later in the book.

Social Skills' Impaired Control Center
ADD has a profound impact on all areas of life, including social adjustment. Symptoms of the disorder can affect interpersonal relationships in a variety of ways.

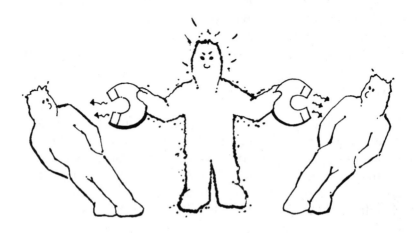

Some people seem to be born with social gifts and skills of intuition that they use to "read" other people. Perhaps they have highly developed Social Skills' Control Centers in their brains! With little effort, they seem to interact admirably in social situations. Many of us with ADD, however, really have to work hard at learning and using social skills.

We learn manners and other forms of social rules in childhood, but successful relationships require more than memorized rules. The rules are somewhat flexible and can change from situation to situation. The development of social skills is more an art than a science because we must learn to read the ever-changing reactions of others. If deficient selective attention gets in the way, an ADDer's perceptions may be flawed by inaccurate or incomplete information.

If we are unsure of the rules in a given situation, we watch other people for clues and gauge their reactions to our behaviors. An inability to process information efficiently can result in a failure to assimilate the new rules quickly enough. Combined with impulsivity, this deficit can lead to numerous social mistakes.

Developing friendships can be difficult for an ADDer whose restlessness interferes with the process. Building lasting friendships requires slow, careful planning and nurturing. Many of us simply can't wait around long enough for this process to take its course. So we try to speed it up and come on like gangbusters, pushing ourselves into others' lives.

"I know you said that you would call me, but I figured I'd just drop over and see what you were doing. Yeah, I know it's two a.m. Yeah, I know I already called three times today."

An ADD adult may have brief conversations with many people but be unable to focus long enough on a given relationship to make a connection. It's just too difficult to hang in there for the duration. Intimacy, with its demands for careful attention to another person, may elude him. He works so hard at following the rules and not looking foolish that he may have insufficient energy left to focus on someone else.

If you are an ADD adult who has grown up feeling like a social reject, don't despair! It's never too late to develop a social network. You may have unrealistic expectations for yourself, believing that you should have friends dropping in all the time. It can be healthier for your soul to recognize that this lifestyle may be unnecessary and undesirable. Using your energy to develop one or two positive relationships can be a much better way to go.

Some of the eccentric traits that caused an ADDer's childhood peers to label him "weird" often become admirable traits in adulthood. Weird becomes unique, special or interesting. Creativity, a special talent, a sense of humor or an enthusiastic zest can be a social magnet, drawing other people to him.

By this point in your reading, we hope you have a better understanding about what ADD is and the impact it has had on your life. We hope you have begun to forgive yourself for the failures and shortcomings you may have blamed on your lack of character. We hope you know that your ADD isn't your fault.

In the next chapter, we'll look at some additional dynamics of ADD. Our focus will be the unproductive ways many of us have learned to cope with our disorder. Growing up different affects the way each of us interacts with our individual world and the people in it.

By understanding your disorder you've already begun the process of dismantling your self-defeating assumptions. To continue this important process, you need to consider both the adaptive and maladaptive strategies you've been using to cope with being different. With this knowledge, you can make decisions about your behaviors and modify those that are getting in the way of your recovery.

The Not So Fine Art of Coping

"I won't think about that today . . .
I'll think about it tomorrow."

Scarlett O'Hara used this classic line several times in the movie *Gone With the Wind*. She had mastered the art of dealing with the problems in her life by avoiding them—she put them out of her mind. Scarlett may have been a fictional character, but she did what *all* human beings do: She developed coping strategies, defense mechanisms, to defend herself against psychological and emotional pain.

Defense mechanisms are the survival techniques we learn through our life experiences. Scarlett learned to protect herself against feeling guilty for her less than admirable behaviors with her "I'll put it out of my mind" defense. Defense mechanisms become armors that shield all of us from hurts and disappointments.

Because of our differences, we ADDers endure more than our fair share of disappointments, rejections and feelings of inadequacy. By the time we reach adulthood, many of us have erected elaborate defense systems to hide our differences or distract others from seeing them. *We don't want to be different* and will jump through hoops to fit in and gain acceptance. So we build shields to defend ourselves against emotional harm.

Defense mechanisms can be psychologically beneficial. They can be adaptive, positive coping mechanisms. They can also be psychologically harmful, maladaptive coping mechanisms that undermine growth. Scarlett sometimes used her denial defense—"If I don't think about the problem, it doesn't exist"—as an adaptive coping mechanism. When she killed a man in self-defense, her refusal to think about the devastating circumstances enabled her to survive its horror.

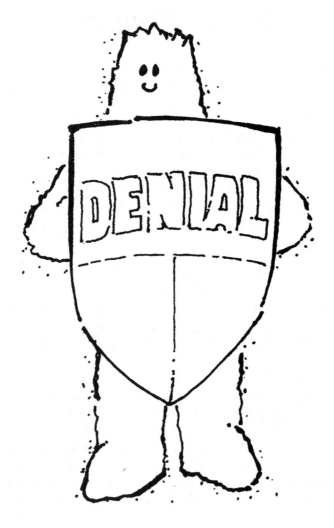

Unfortunately, Scarlett overused the defense. She used it not only to cope with extreme circumstances but also to insulate herself from ever thinking about the possible consequences of her actions. Because she didn't allow herself to consider the impact of her behavior, she realized too late that she was destroying her marriage. Even in the final scene when Rhett Butler leaves with his declaration that their relationship is over, Scarlett refuses to confront reality. Again she invokes her standard refrain, "I won't think about that now, I'll think about it tomorrow."

The defense mechanisms that ADDers use are sometimes helpful and sometimes harmful, creating more problems than they solve. It's important for each of us to recognize the maladaptive behaviors that get us in trouble. In later chapters about recovery, we'll examine some adaptive coping strategies we can substitute for the harmful ones.

We've compiled some character sketches of real people struggling to cope with their differences. Each uses a maladaptive coping strategy. If you recognize yourself in any of their descriptions, you will already have taken an important step in your recovery. If you can analyze your maladaptive defenses, you can begin to substitute emotionally healthier ones.

Bad Is Better than Stupid

Susan is fifteen years old. Just a few years ago her classmates thought she was weird. They teased her for being in the "ozone" during class. She was puzzled and hurt that no one wanted to befriend her. Now at long last she has found a group of kids who embrace her.

Susan and her new friends wear extreme hairstyles and clothing. They have a doomsday mentality. Since they're sure the world is going to hell no matter what they do, they think it's useless to work hard at school or try to excel at anything. They are smart kids. They use their collective intelligence to write nihilistic poetry and make darkly humorous jokes. They flirt with death as they take drugs and have sex without safeguards.

Although the group isn't overtly violent, each of the kids has a hostile, sarcastic and tough manner. Their peers are afraid of them. Sometimes Susan is scared too by the talk of suicide and the use of IV drugs. But at least she feels accepted by a group of her peers. The other kids don't dare make fun of her now, and she is off the hook as far as schoolwork goes.

Elementary school was always difficult for Susan, but junior high and high school have been nightmares. Many ADDers can empathize with her. She has always felt incompetent, stupid and rejected. Slow and awkward in learning new sports and mastering the art of conversation, she hasn't fared any better in physical prowess or in her social life.

She has, however, learned one thing very well: Adolescents admire kids who are cool and in control. Driven by the adolescent's intense need to fit in, Susan has learned that rebellious behavior is more acceptable than the uncertain fumblings of someone struggling with disabilities. She has decided that Being Bad is better than Being Stupid.

Faced with reality as she experiences it, Susan chooses inclusion in the gang over humiliation and alienation. She has a third choice. She can learn new ways of dealing with her differences. She doesn't consider this option because she is driven to save face. She's always in trouble with her parents and teachers but is willing to pay this high price for acceptance.

The defense mechanism Susan has learned is common in adolescence. A defiant and *smart* reply to a teacher's questions can get a few laughs and perhaps some admiration from other kids. It's a way to avoid answering a question without looking stupid. The stint in detention hall that follows can be a reasonable price to pay for maintaining one's image. And anyway, getting plenty of detentions is cool.

TOUGHNESS creates a smoke screen
to mask VULNERABILITY.

74

If you separate Susan and her friends from their group and manage to dig beneath the tough shells, you find troubled, uncertain kids. Many vulnerable ADD adolescents continue to wear their shields of toughness into adulthood. They usually manage to keep themselves and their tough facades within the bounds of society's rules and don't become major-league criminals or radicals. A hostile attitude, however, intimidates other people and prevents anyone from getting too close. This defense mechanism does double duty as a cover for problems and an insulator from other people. Unfortunately, Susan and her counterparts may pay a high price, indeed.

The Perfectionist

Unlike Susan, who protects herself by rebelling against society's rules, Debra has taken the opposite tack. She has decided that being the best, regardless of the cost, is the only way to hide her deficits. Debra is a perfectionist.

She has ADD, but those who know her would never believe it. Although her poor-conduct grades reflected her restlessness, her behavior wasn't disruptive enough to cause serious discipline problems in school. In general, she followed the rules and did what was asked of her. Before she graduated—in the top 3 percent of her high school class of one thousand—she took part in many extracurricular activities. Everyone counted on her to volunteer for any task that needed to be done.

You might be asking how someone with ADD could function so well. Actually, Debra wasn't really functioning very well despite her carefully constructed facade. She rarely slept more than four or five hours each night. This had nothing to do with insomnia. She didn't sleep much because she didn't have time—she had to study twice as long as everybody else to learn the material. She regularly pulled all-nighters and never had time to relax or hang out.

Sometimes she desperately longed to get off her treadmill but didn't dare risk disclosure. If she failed to do everything, her secret would be out. Everyone would know she wasn't normal.

The hitch was that Debra didn't have a clue about what "normal" was. She had kept her secret so long that she had inflated ideas about what other people could accomplish. She thought that if she said "No" to anything, she would be found out.

Her inability to say "No" got her into serious trouble in all areas of life. Beginning in seventh grade, she had sex with any boy who asked, and pushed the bad feelings about herself to the back of her mind. Even a pregnancy and an abortion didn't change her sexual behavior. Her impaired sense of self, distorted by differences she didn't understand, caused her to do anything that would bring acceptance.

Now thirty-two years old, Debra is married and has a set of twins and a successful business. She still works herself to death, compelled to *do it all*. It's becoming increasingly more difficult to do it all with so many conflicting demands on her time. Children, husband, volunteer work and clients all vie for her attention. Lately she feels that she's losing control and that at any moment something horrible is going to happen. She can't keep all the pieces together anymore.

While Debra may look good to outsiders, she feels terrible inside. She has to spend all her energy running and hiding behind her facade of perfection. Knowing that she has just about pushed herself beyond her limits, she wonders when she'll totally self-destruct.

There are many Debras around. It's interesting to speculate on the number of *super* men and women who struggle with disability beneath their *in control* exteriors. Readers who are familiar with codependency may recognize similar traits in Debra. She's trying to gain control of her life by taking care of everything and everybody. Recovering codependents could tell her that it doesn't work.

The Blamer
Steve never admits he's made a mistake. When he can't find important papers in the black hole that constitutes his office,

he accuses his secretary of losing them. He terrorizes his wife, kids and employees by flying off the handle and accusing them when anything goes wrong.

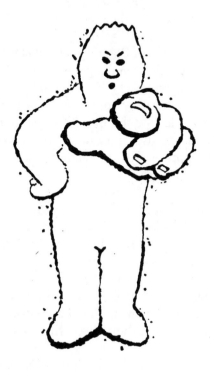

At fifty-four years old, Steve is a chronic blamer. If food falls out when he jerks the refrigerator door open, he yells at his wife for putting the groceries away incorrectly. If his kids don't understand his instructions, he blames it on their stupidity or inattention. It's an impossibility that his instructions were unclear. Enduring his daily accusations and anger, his family begins to believe they are at fault.

Most people who know Steve characterize him as an arrogant SOB. What they don't realize is that beneath his blustery, aggressive exterior is a scared, rejected kid. Steve is shielding himself against feelings of inadequacy by shifting the blame to others. This keeps everyone from looking too closely at his performance. He's terrified that he'll be exposed for the bumbling idiot he thinks he is. Although he's a successful businessman, he still feels like the kid who was regularly ridiculed and punished. Tapes from the past keep playing in his head: "How could you be so stupid! You'll never be worth anything!"

The defense mechanism of Blaming is similar to Being Bad except that the blamer fends off people by actively accusing them of stupidity or wrongdoing. The Bad person keeps others off balance with anger and hostility but not necessarily with criticism. Blamers can never let anything go. To maintain their fragile emotional equilibrium, they must have a scapegoat to blame for everything that happens. For the blamer, accidents don't exist.

"Who Cares?"

Jim is thirty years old and has worked as a waiter or cabdriver most of his adult life. He is intelligent and well-informed. He loves to engage in lively discussions about current events with his friends and anyone else who will listen. He has a good sense of humor about things in general and himself in particular. At his legendary high school graduation (his friends were amazed he ever managed to graduate), he joined in the laughter as his buddies carried him down the aisle on their shoulders.

People enjoy being around Jim because he's likable and easygoing. Nothing seems to bother him, even when bosses and coworkers ask him to work unpopular or extra hours. They know he won't complain.

Jim makes excuses for the people who do him wrong or maintains that the things they do don't bother him. He professes to be content with his life the way it is. Secretly he feels bad that he didn't go to college as his brothers and sisters did. He isn't at peace with himself and has many physical symptoms to prove it: tension headaches, high blood pressure and an ulcer that regularly flares up.

Jim feels he's a failure and masks his feelings of inadequacy with his Who Cares persona. His wide circle of friends and broad knowledge base don't make up for his academic shortcomings. The defense mechanism he uses to protect himself is similar to Susan's. Borrowing from the fox-in-the-sour-grapes fable, both pretend that things out of reach aren't worthwhile, anyway. Susan's arrogance and Jim's indifference are shields of armor to prevent anyone from seeing their disabilities.

Jane presents a slightly different version of the Who Cares defense. Jane, a forty-two-year-old mother of two, is intelligent and creative and has impressive artistic talents. Despite her gifts, Jane's ADD made school a monumental struggle. It took twice the customary time for her to complete college. Before choosing to stay home with her children, she had always held jobs well below her educational level.

Jane is outspoken about the excessive competition and materialism in today's society. She is proud of her skill at budgeting money and has learned to live without the many consumer goods others consider necessities. She doesn't own a VCR or clothes dryer.

Jane's wise use of resources enables her to devote time to her family and have enough left over to pursue her own interests. Her choice of saying "No" to the rat race to live by her own values is admirable. The problem is, Jane isn't entirely comfortable with her decision. She "doth protest too much" when she scoffs at academic and career achievement. There is a distinctively angry, defensive edge to her voice when she rationalizes her life choices. She spends much time explaining herself.

Jim's indifference is passive and Jane's is assertive, but both are carefully designed masks. Jane doesn't feel successful. She uses so much energy on defense that she can't accept herself or honestly evaluate her choices. Perhaps beneath the bristly Who Cares defense is a real desire to accomplish some of the things she rejects. Perhaps the choices she has made are right for her. Regrettably, she works so hard at protecting her fragile sense of self that she has little energy left for living the life she has chosen.

Jim, on the other hand, can't realistically assess himself because he works so hard at pretending nothing bothers him. His "what, me worry?" attitude masks real feelings that probably include anger. He is angry at himself for his shortcomings and at the people who take advantage of him. His armor protects him but also prevents him from grappling with ambitions he's never been able to admit. If he's ever able to let his guard down, he'll need to confront his anger. If he can learn to deal with his feelings up front, he may even find that his physical health improves.

Manipulation

Todd is forty-seven years old and is restless, attractive and charming. He frequently changes relationships, living arrangements and jobs. He uses his disarming, boyish manner as a powerful lure to hook others into willingly taking care of him. He never pulls his weight at work, relying instead on his mastery of manipulation to get others to do the work for him.

Faced with a tedious or difficult task, Todd flatters and cajoles others into bailing him out. Sometimes he acts helpless, getting coworkers to do his job under the guise of teaching him. He says something like, "I never was any good at that. I really admire people who can do it." Sometimes he tells a tale of woe about his boss piling work on him or about emergencies in his life. His manipulative behavior usually works and someone steps in to bail him out. As soon as he feels restless or coworkers get on to him, he simply changes jobs.

Todd usually makes decent money but regularly ends up flat broke because he's careless and impulsive with his spending. To deal with his financial difficulties, he relies on the women in his life to support him. His women do more than simply contribute to his financial support. They are also charged with keeping him out of trouble. They keep track of his checkbook and his household and social responsibilities. Todd manipulates them by using guilt, charm, sex appeal—whatever maneuver will work in a given situation.

Often he manipulates his current woman into keeping him to-gether enough to hold down his job. She gets him up in the morning, monitors his performance and smooths things over with the boss when Todd messes up. More often than not, he ends the relationship when he feels too constrained by the "mothering." His behavior sounds a lot like an alcoholic's but he doesn't drink. He has just learned to manipulate like some-one who does.

Todd might seem like a ruthless, unfeeling user who will stop at nothing to ensure that his needs are met. He isn't pure villain, however. He's an ADD adult who has learned to use manipula-tion as a cover for his underlying problems.

He lives in a constant state of emergency, running scared all the time. He knows he regularly makes mistakes but feels helpless to prevent them. So he survives by using other people to cover for him. It's the only way he knows to survive, although he's aware that it's unacceptable for a grown man to be cared for this way.

Todd simply hasn't figured out an alternative method for satis-fying his needs. His manipulations are neither conscious nor premeditated. He doesn't connect his actions with their impact on others. His impulsivity and lack of attention to detail make him unaware of much of his behavior and its consequences.

Webster defines manipulating as "controlling or playing on oth-ers using unfair means." It may be a dirty word but everyone uses manipulation on occasion. Although we may not like being manipulated as puppets on a string, occasionally we may need to use this defense as a matter of survival.

ADD adults in particular can become masters of the art of ma-nipulation. It's a tough, competitive world out there with dire consequences for those who sink to the bottom of the heap. Many of the newly homeless are hardworking folk who slid over the line into poverty following a setback such as unemployment or illness. If someone starts out in life with a physical handicap, learning disability or ADD, the stakes are higher and riskier. There is a great temptation to use any available means to improve one's odds of survival.

This isn't to say that the majority of people with disabilities become manipulative. Most are rather heroic in their striving to achieve. They generally cope by learning to work harder than nondisabled people. ADD adults, however, have additional risk factors that increase the odds of their becoming masters of manipulation.

Withdrawal

Barb is both unattached and detached. Twenty-five years old, she lives with her parents and works as a file clerk. She has rarely dated, has no close friends and spends most of her free time watching TV. Occasionally she goes out to dinner with a coworker, but that's the extent of her social life. She spends her vacations tagging along with her parents. Although Barb has an above-average IQ, she is a marginal worker on the job. She makes many mistakes and has trouble keeping up with her colleagues.

Barb is different from most of the ADDers you've met in this chapter. She isn't anxious about her performance and doesn't worry about her less than glowing appraisals. After a childhood of academic and social failures, she has decided that giving up is the safest thing she can do. She has chosen to accept mediocrity. The price she pays is a life of boredom, loneliness and depression. Barb is free from the risks she would face if she decided to live her life fully. But is it worth it?

Like that of many ADD adults, Barb's handicap has never been identified. She is neither hyperactive nor impulsive. Everyone has always told her that she is lethargic and spacey. Barb believes this characterization. She has chosen survival through withdrawal.

This defense is a cousin to the Who Cares stance but operates slightly differently. Barb has given up completely and has carefully buried her feelings and doubts. She never gives any thought to the possibility that her life could be different. Jim, on the other hand, maintains nagging doubts about his abilities and lack of achievement. On some level, he continues to think about these issues that trouble him.

Insulated from pain by suppressing feelings of inadequacy, Barb can't make a thoughtful decision about her life. The Barbs of this world haven't made peace with themselves—it's as if they're buried alive.

Chip on the Shoulder

While Barb quietly withdraws, Paula aggressively poises for full-scale battle every moment of her life. She's only nineteen but has developed an especially prickly suit of armor. When her husband asks if she has taken out the trash, she reacts defensively. She offers a long-winded explanation of why she hasn't been able to get around to the chore yet. As she becomes increasingly angry and indignant, she switches to the offensive, attacking her husband for overworking her with his demands.

Paula's husband asked about the trash only because he was going outside and wanted to take it with him if it was still in the house. He wearily retreats from the house, wondering how his good intentions ended up in this ugly scene. Paula retreats to nurse her anger at a world that is always dissatisfied with her efforts.

Paula is a selfish shrew, making her saintly husband's life miserable. She has a colossal chip on the shoulder, responding to innocent comments with a barrage of defensive excuses and explanations. At least this is the way she acts. But appearances aren't always what they seem.

Paula is an ADD adult who spent much of her childhood rebuked for things she forgot to do or didn't finish. Her psyche is raw from all the times she worked her heart out only to be chastised for the one thing she didn't do. Her life has been filled with false accusations of thoughtlessness and laziness that no one knew were symptoms of her subtle disability. She ruminates about the injustices in her life and the unfairness of it all.

Paula's chip on the shoulder is a protective suit of armor designed to shore up her sense of self. She continually defends herself as a matter of reflex even when she isn't being attacked. The intensity of her defensive stance may be out of proportion to the imagined slight, but her life experiences have taught her to expect criticism. She can never let down her defenses. She has to be ready for the next assault on her being.

Paula's defense serves another purpose. It inoculates her against requests for her time or energy. With deficits that interfere with an organized lifestyle, she frantically tries to keep up with demands that are sometimes overwhelming. Her prickly shell fends off at least some of the extra demands as it makes people think twice about approaching her with questions or requests for her involvement.

There isn't anything inherently bad about emotional self-defense in the face of real injustice. In Paula's case, however, her knee-jerk defensiveness is the maladaptive suit she wears every moment of her life. She has suffered so many wounds that she can't differentiate between real and imagined assaults. She focuses exclusively on protection, never allowing herself to find the strengths that would lead to positive growth.

Take Me or Leave Me

You probably know highly effective people whose self-confidence you admire. They are self-assured and comfortable with themselves. They assume a healthy attitude of "What you see is what you get—I'm okay and have nothing to hide." They use this in a positive way. They are unlikely, for example, to waste time on relationships that probably wouldn't work anyway.

Pete is a Take Me or Leave Me man in his midthirties. He is attractive and affable, drawing people to him with his sense of humor and gift of gab. He comes across as honest, straightforward and comfortable with his limitations. He sincerely apologizes when he misses an important deadline at work or forgets to attend his daughter's school play. Pete disarms most people by being the first to admit his weaknesses. He frequently makes himself the butt of his own jokes.

"What you see is what you get" Pete has chosen a positive coping mechanism . . . or has he? What makes Pete different from the self-confident people we described? The difference is that Pete's "take me or leave me" attitude is a carefully fabricated facade behind which he hides.

He is a grown-up class clown who "keeps 'em laughing" so no one will notice the things he can't do. He uses his excellent sense of humor to create a smoke screen to hide difficulties and deflect criticism. Would-be critics find the wind taken out of their sails when Pete beats them to the punch by making a joke about his failings. He leaves them with nothing to say.

It's healthy to take ourselves less seriously. Pete, however, does it to excess. Though he readily admits his weaknesses, he never does anything about them! He retreats behind his self-deprecating facade instead of honestly studying his behavior.

He's busy hiding and is unaware of the increasing frustration and anger of his friends. They continue to forgive his failings but are beginning to have nagging feelings that something is rotten in Denmark. Pete's basically a "good guy," but he's totally undependable. He isn't doing anything to improve himself. His mistakes are getting less funny, and his refusal to take anything seriously is causing increasing resentment.

Pete's coping mechanism does protect him, but it's maladaptive. It prevents the introspection he needs to make positive changes in his life.

It Ain't So

Donna's family of five lurches from crisis to crisis. She always attributes her family's problems to external events and people.

Everything will be fine when the excitement of Christmas is over or when one of the kids gets a new teacher. She spends much of her time waiting for things to return to normal, but they never do.

Donna is forty-five years old and has given up a professional career to stay home with her three children, who are all hyperactive and disobedient. Donna is gentle and spacey, rarely raising her voice to her children or asserting herself with other adults. She works hard at a difficult parenting job, but her children continue to be unruly, and her household remains noisy and disordered. When a crisis erupts, she consults with professionals but promptly disregards their advice. She denies that a real problem exists.

Several years ago Donna was diagnosed with ADD. Her physician prescribed Ritalin and she took it for a short while. She explains that she stopped taking the medicine because it interfered with her sleep, but she never told her doctor about the side effect.

It's obvious to anyone who knows Donna that her ADD has a big impact on the problems she experiences. The chaos created by her unruly children overwhelms her. Her deficits make it nearly impossible to provide the firm discipline and structure her children need so desperately. She continues to delude herself into thinking she can manage everything by herself.

Donna avoids her problems the way Scarlett O'Hara avoided hers. She chooses to deny they exist. Denial is an integral part of grief when a loved one dies. It provides time for mobilizing strength to cope with the realization of the loss. Denial is a healthy, essential step that leads to ultimate acceptance.

The end of a relationship or a job, the loss of a body part or an alteration in self-image can also set the grief process in motion. Donna is grieving the loss of *a perfect, healthy self,* replaced with the label of ADD. She has always known that something was wrong but hasn't found comfort in her diagnosis. Similar to a widow who keeps her long-deceased spouse's belongings as if he were still alive, Donna is stuck in denial. Because she can't acknowledge her limitations, she can't move beyond them toward a stage of acceptance.

Donna uses her It Ain't So defense to run frantically in circles, trying to avoid facing herself. Unable to *own* her ADD, she continues to attribute her problems to something or somebody else. She refuses to take needed medication or avail herself of professional help. She expends considerable energy trying to keep everything together. Her misguided efforts, however, don't yield results. If she can ever face her situation realistically, she'll be able to use her creative mind to find solutions.

Learned Helplessness

Tracy is a modern-day Prissy, the flaky servant girl in the movie *Gone With the Wind* who didn't "know nothin' 'bout birthin' babies." Played by Butterfly McQueen, Prissy affected a simpleminded air that helped her avoid responsibilities.

In the era of slavery this defense was useful. "Stupid like a fox" Prissy used her helplessness as a mechanism for control without risking the severe consequences of outright rebellion. Tracy has learned that helplessness works as effectively for her as it did for Prissy. Approaching her fiftieth birthday, she has spent years learning to play the role to the hilt.

Tracy never worries about failure. Similar to the manipulator, she avoids her responsibilities at work and in her social life by getting others to do everything for her. She smiles charmingly as she appeals to others for help. Her method differs from Todd's. She openly uses helplessness as her ploy. She flatters and boosts the egos of her rescuers, contrasting her poor, *dumb little me* act with their competence.

Women have been frequently characterized as incompetent and helpless. We aren't trying to perpetuate an unfortunate stereotype by casting Tracy in her maladaptive feminine role. Her helplessness is a coping strategy used by many members of oppressed groups such as minorities and women. If you are otherwise powerless as Prissy was, you can use helplessness to survive and exercise some control. Few men use this coping strategy because playing helpless isn't an acceptable male role in our society. Men can't get away with it!

Although Tracy is bright and personable, her ADD has always made her feel unable to cope with the realities of her life. Learned helplessness makes her life easier to handle. She manages to remain unstressed, but also unchallenged. Tracy needs help in affirming her abilities so she can feel comfortable enough to risk failure and find success.

Controlling

You probably know Jack or someone similar. At sixty-two years old, he lives by the adage "He who has the gold, rules." He establishes himself as the undisputed ruler of his kingdoms at home and at work. He has used his intelligence, creativity and high energy level to rise to a high-powered position in a large corporation. Jack has aggressively and relentlessly climbed high on the ladder of success. He seems to have used the symptoms of his ADD to his advantage and should be congratulated for his efforts . . . or should he?

Jack measures his success against external rewards of financial gain. Unfortunately, he has orchestrated his success through his domination of the people in his life. He monopolizes conversations and insists on having the last word. He makes all decisions at home and on the job. He regards his beautiful wife as an earned bonus and treats her as a subject in his kingdom. At work, he always sets the agenda at meetings even when it isn't his responsibility. If someone else chairs a meeting, he subtly undermines the agenda, steering it in a direction that suits his needs.

He makes unilateral decisions, often incurring the wrath of his peers for his failure to consult with them. His resentful colleagues and employees are ready to lynch him. His wife is fed up and is thinking about leaving him. He has made an impressive array of enemies who would like nothing more than to overthrow the king.

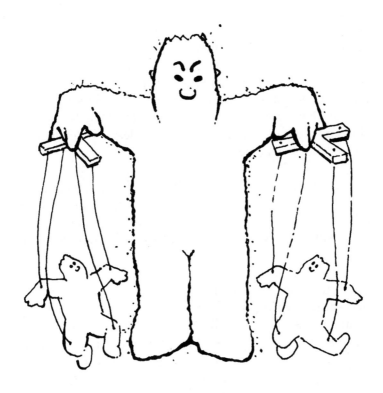

While it isn't readily apparent from his behavior, King Jack lives in perpetual terror of looking stupid. At home, he controls his family's agenda to avoid the risk that his wife will choose an activity that will expose his weaknesses. At work, he commands all discussions because he knows he's effective only when he follows his own train of thought. By not letting anyone else contribute, he avoids the confusion and embarrassment he feels when questions and comments derail him.

Jack's controlling defense mechanism may backfire. One false move and he may maneuver himself out of a job and a family.

Character Sketches of People You May Know

The ADDers you've met use acquired defense mechanisms to protect themselves from public exposure of their deficits. We've examined the rationale for their choices and the ways in which their coping strategies are maladaptive.

Human behavior is too complex to explain within the context of defense mechanisms alone. Beneath the defenses are the individual characteristics we are born with. Maladaptive ADD behaviors are a combination of various learned defensive maneuvers and specific deficits.

In this section, we'll look more closely at behavioral manifestations of specific deficits. These vignettes aren't condemnations of ADDers—we get plenty of them! Rather, we have designed them to illustrate what can happen if ADD symptoms flourish without control or intervention.

The Peter Pan Syndrome: Forty-Eight Going on Twelve

You may be familiar with the Peter Pan syndrome, popularized in a book on the subject. People in our society normally experience some regret at leaving childhood and taking on adult responsibilities. Most of us, however, manage to bite the bullet and make the transition into adulthood. Chris is a Peter Pan who has decided that growing up is simply not worth it.

As Chris approaches his forty-ninth birthday, he continues to live in a state of perpetual childhood. He has a personality that attracts people. Energetic optimism, a wacky sense of humor and a warm acceptance of others make the people around him feel good.

He always has more invitations than he can accept. The ease with which he connects with people promises an intimacy that never materializes. After an initial period of intense connection, would-be lovers and close friends find him an elusive man, impossible to pin down. He refuses to make plans, preferring to live from moment to moment. The notion of commitment to goals or a relationship is incomprehensible to Chris. He just wants to have fun and is mystified when other people feel betrayed by his broken promises.

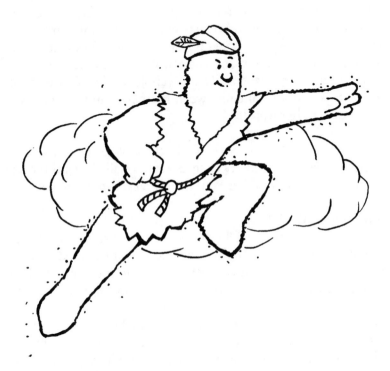

He disappoints bosses and coworkers as well as friends. His high energy level and intelligence generate expectations for superior job performance. After an initial burst of energy, Chris typically becomes bored with a project and loses motivation. His work becomes sloppy and careless. When a job becomes boring or a boss begins pressuring him to get serious, Chris switches to another one.

Lovers get similar treatment. When they begin to make demands for a more committed relationship, they find that Chris has moved on. The women hurt by his "love 'em and leave 'em" lifestyle feel used and abused. Chris believes, however, that he's just operating under a different set of rules. He lives according to the pleasure principle and its primary goal of maximizing pleasure and minimizing pain.

All of us operate on the pleasure principle to a certain extent. When we're born, we're virtual bundles of wants and needs without any sense of people outside ourselves. As we grow and are socialized by family and society, we gain awareness of our responsibilities to others. The psychologically healthy adult learns to strike a balance between her needs and the needs of the people in her world.

Chris is an adult by virtue of his chronological age, but he hasn't developed psychologically or emotionally beyond the age of twelve. Similar to Peter Pan, he just *don't wanna grow up*.

The Space Cadet

It isn't uncommon for ADD adults to say they are spacey. When the mental fog descends, they can become disoriented and forgetful. Some of us, however, settle too comfortably into waking dream states, becoming lifers in the Academy for Space Cadets!

Sean is thirty-seven years old and has joined the academy. He is a gentle soul with a fanciful imagination and a gift for poetry. He spends his days daydreaming, writing and having long philosophical conversations with his cronies. Sean takes little notice of practicalities. He earns meager wages as a writer but doesn't worry because material things are of no consequence to him.

He does his own thing, oblivious of the world around him. When he was single, his lifestyle wasn't a problem. But now he's married and has four children. Sean's wife is exhausted and at her wit's end trying to cope single-handedly with the large family. Sean is always pleasant and soft-spoken with his spouse and children. He tries to do whatever they ask of him—that is, when they manage to capture his attention!

Sadly, Sean makes little effort to tune in to the world around him. Unless someone demands his attention, he's content to spend time drifting on his own mental clouds. He never set out to dump all the responsibility in his wife's lap, but that's effectively what has happened. He plays with the kids when he wakes up long enough to notice them, but his wife rarely leaves him alone with them. She's terrified that the toddler would poison herself right under her daddy's less than watchful eye. Sean isn't callously allowing his wife to work like a dog while he sits and daydreams. *He doesn't even notice.* The varied duties and details of family life totally escape him.

Emotional Incontinence

This behavior doesn't have anything to do with bodily functions! Rather, it is rampant, uncontrolled emotional output. As ADDers, we have a hard time modulating our erratic moods. Staying reasonably calm can be a full-time job! Unless we want other people to write us off as immature or crazy, we have to expend the effort.

At twenty-seven years old, Jeff has a serious case of emotional incontinence. He doesn't make any effort to control his extreme ups and downs. The atmosphere in his house is always thick with the fallout from his latest mood. His family rides the roller coaster along with him, cowering from his rages, sinking into gloom or becoming infected with unreasonable giddiness. The members of his household feel exhausted and tense. They deplete their energy reserves as they try to cope with his moodiness. He has lost more than one job because of his temper and is close to losing his second wife, as well.

Sadly, in social situations beyond his home, Jeff doesn't have any impact at all. Other people size him up quickly and decide not to take him seriously. They view his rages as the pathetic tantrums of a young child.

In Jeff's case, *more is definitely less.* Emotional expression has greater impact as it becomes more intense, but only to a point!

Drama can quickly deteriorate into melodrama, evoking laughter rather than empathy. People like Jeff who don't control their emotional output run the risk of becoming caricatures of themselves.

The Blabber

Mary is Jeff's close relative. She also has a bad case of incontinence, but hers is verbal incontinence. Although her official title is manager of order processing her colleagues have dubbed her Typhoid Mary, Rumor Distribution Manager. They can count on hearing the latest office dirt from Mary, who has assumed responsibility for broadcasting everyone's confidential information.

With her warmth, good listening skills and grandmotherly manner, sixty-year-old Mary easily made friends with coworkers. Her new friends, however, quickly learned to keep their distance when they discovered that Mary talked as much as she listened! Now everyone fears the effects of her loose tongue.

She isn't a vicious backstabber. She truly cares about her colleagues and wants to lend an ear when they have problems. But she fails to reflect on the confidentiality of shared information and indiscriminately and inappropriately distributes rumors.

The angry reactions that greet her news continually surprise her. Since she has no qualms about sharing her own deepest secrets with total strangers, she can't understand why others are upset when she shares their secrets. To Mary, the human race is just one big happy family, and families don't keep secrets from one another, do they?

The Bulldozer

A bulldozer is a well-designed piece of machinery. In short order, it can transform an acre of tree-covered land to a flattened, barren landscape. In similar fashion, some ADDers bulldoze their way through their lives, leaving little untouched or unharmed. This is Richard's style, and it has left him with an empty life.

Richard's mother says he was born with a will of iron and a voice that could shatter glass with a whisper. From his earliest days, he made everyone in the household dance to the tune of his angry cries. Throughout childhood, he went directly for anything he wanted and shoved aside anybody who got in his way. Now that he's a forty-three-year-old adult, he seems ruthless and cold as he continues to bulldoze his way over other people's feelings. He is successful in business but lives in a lonely world. He doesn't understand why people seem to avoid him.

Richard really doesn't get it at all. He's oblivious of the impact of his forceful nature and is honestly puzzled when others keep him at arm's length. As he pushes his way through life, he's aware only of his goals and takes little notice of the people he shoves aside to reach them.

Please remember that the negatives of ADD make up only one dimension of the disorder. ADDers come in an assortment of packages. There are differences in specific symptoms and in the ways each of us manages these differences. Many of us do an amazingly wonderful job of coping with symptoms of the ADD we never even knew we had!

Lacking an understanding of their deficits, many ADDers feel compelled to spend inordinate time and energy trying to *pass* as normal. This is a term we've borrowed from African-American history. With a long history of discrimination in this country, it isn't surprising that some lighter-skinned African Americans managed their lives pretending they were white.

In similar fashion, many of us with ADD can pass as normal (whatever that means). We work hard at hiding our differences. We can identify with the adults in this chapter who have been somewhat successful in their efforts but who have paid dearly for fitting in.

We spend our lives in fear,
feeling like impostors who will be found out at any moment.

A recurring theme throughout the vignettes is the importance of squarely facing one's behaviors and honestly evaluating them. Many of us, along with the people in our lives, have spent lifetimes wondering why we do the things we do. We have never considered our behaviors as symptoms and haven't analyzed our coping strategies as defense mechanisms developed to hide inadequacy. Lacking knowledge about the role ADD plays in our lives, we resign ourselves to the "truth" of the assumptions made about us—we are indeed lazy, stupid or crazy!

If a parent or teacher suspected a problem, she usually attributed it to poor motivation or a dysfunctional family. Even when a diagnosis of hyperactivity was made in childhood, the prescription was for Ritalin and patience. "Take this pill twice a day, Monday through Friday during the school year, and wait until you outgrow your hyperactivity in adolescence." Some of us have been waiting a very long time for this miraculous change to occur!

The fact is, many of our readers have never been evaluated at all. Although there isn't anything magical about a diagnosis, it is a vital, initial step in changing faulty self-perceptions. Even if you feel fairly certain that you have ADD, you owe it to yourself to have a complete evaluation.

In the next chapter we'll look at the process of a diagnostic evaluation and share information that can help you make some decisions about accessing this help. As you may guess, the diagnostic evaluation of ADD adults is less well defined than that of children. So you'll need to proceed with caution in finding the professional you'll work with in this important part of your recovery.

CHAPTER 4

I Know . . . I Think . . . I Have ADD: What Do I Do Now?

The diagnosis and treatment of a garden-variety illness is fairly straightforward. A throat culture uncovers a strep infection and the patient takes a round of antibiotics and goes on his way. A few days later he feels great. He has come to expect that powerful antibiotics will quickly and easily fix his illness. He views his medical care as a relatively simple process:

Symptoms—medical tests—diagnosis—treatment—CURE!

The process of uncovering ADD is considerably more complicated. Often, the process never even begins because the symptoms are behavioral, not physical. Many people view behavior as the *cause,* not the *symptom* of disorder. It usually goes something like this:

Behaviors—faulty assumptions—blame—
punishment—POOR PROGNOSIS!

For many if not most of us, the initial discovery of ADD doesn't come from a professional. It comes from reading an ADDer's life story that could be our autobiography. It comes from talking with a friend whose description of his ADD sounds remarkably similar to our own behaviors. It comes when our children, who are "chips off the old block," are diagnosed with ADD.

Adults in support groups talk of learning about their ADD in all these ways. Most of these adults say they waited a while before seeking professional help to confirm their self-diagnoses. They used this time to read about ADD and to examine their lives to see if the information fit their experiences.

Your Job as a Mental Health Consumer

If you are beginning a similar process of self-discovery, your first responsibility is to thoroughly educate yourself about this disorder. Part of your self-education should include learning about the professional resources in your community. When you're ready to proceed with an evaluation, you shouldn't let your fingers do the walking through the yellow pages of the phone book to find the services you'll need!

We recommend that you contact the nearest chapter of an ADD support group. The group can give you leads on ADD-informed professionals in your area. Make sure you ask for names of professionals who are competent in diagnosing and treating adults. Also ask your local organization to put you in touch with other ADD adults who can tell you about their experiences with professionals on the referral list. You may be fortunate to locate an ADD adult support group that can be an invaluable, informal referral network. For help in locating a group in your area we refer you to the CHADD Web site (chadd.org) and the support group listing in the back of *Delivered from Distraction*, by Edward Hallowell and John Ratey.

Remember that you are the customer and a consumer of mental health services. To be an informed consumer, you need to do your homework before you make your first appointment. You need to proceed carefully, because many good therapists have little knowledge about ADD.

When you first meet with the mental health professional you have chosen, ask as many questions as you want. If you aren't comfortable after your initial meeting, don't hesitate to go on to the next professional on your list. Your mental health is too important to entrust to someone you don't think understands your issues.

After the evaluation is completed, be sure to request a follow-up appointment to discuss the results of your testing. If you don't specifically ask, the professional may just send a highly technical report to you or your psychiatrist.

Who's Who

Practitioners from many different fields are qualified to perform diagnostic testing. If you have limited experience with the mental health profession, you may well find the various titles and professions confusing, including but not limited to:

Ph.D, Psy.D, Ed.D, MSN, MSW, LISC, M.D.
Clinical Psychologist, Neuropsychologist, Cognitive Psychologist, Education Psychologist, Psychiatrist, Mental Health Nurse Practitioner, Developmental Pediatrician, Licensed Social Worker, Master of Social Work

The professional backgrounds listed above can be divided into two main groups, medical and mental health. Any of these professionals are qualified to perform diagnostic testing. The most important question is that of expertise. Is the professional experienced in diagnosing ADD and its comorbid disorders—disorders separate from but frequently coexisting with Attention Deficit Disorder? The various psychologists, for example, are typically skilled at identifying the specific learning disabilities and dyslexia often present in the individual with ADD.

It may seem odd that developmental pediatrician is included on the list. Interestingly, with extensive experience working with ADD children, the practices of many pediatricians have evolved naturally into treating the parents, many of whom have ADD as well. The advantage of working with a medical professional is that additional testing can be done should a specific medical condition be suspected as a contributing factor in an individual's symptoms. Also, if medication is indicated following an ADD diagnosis, you can continue working with the same person for this part of your treatment.

Consider working with a specialty ADD group practice if one is available in your area. The benefit is *one-stop shopping,* since both medical and mental health professionals are part of the team.

The Diagnostic Evaluation

There is no medical or psychological "test" that will tell you absolutely that you have ADD. The best diagnostic tool currently available is an experienced professional who takes the time to listen to your story. A diagnosis of ADD is generally made on the basis of your retrospective history. They will want to know about your ADD symptoms and how they impacted your life in the past and present. For more detailed information about the process of making an ADD diagnosis, we refer you to Chapter 11 of *Delivered from Distraction.*

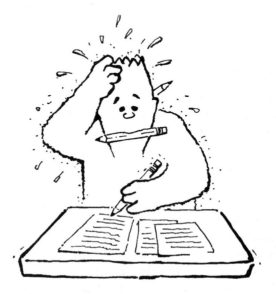

Tests—aren't those the things we always failed??

While there is no generally accepted test for ADD, researchers are doing the work that may lead to some useful biological tools for identifying it. Stay tuned for further developments. One medical diagnostic test that seems promising is the QEEG, which measures brain waves. Doctors Hallowell and Ratey, acknowledged ADD experts, have begun to use this diagnostic tool in their work with ADDers. Another interesting possibility is the SPECT scan, used at this point primarily by ADD pioneer Dr. Daniel Amen. Bear in mind that you are not likely to find these cutting-edge technologies in your backyard.

Of course, ADD doesn't generally travel alone. ADDers often *also* have learning disabilities and comorbid conditions—that is, other disorders that may complicate your ADD, such as depression, obsessive-compulsive disorder and other issues. If learning disabilities are suspected, the person in charge of your diagnosis may recommend some neuropsychological tests to be done by a psychologist.

KK: "It may not matter that the point of these tests is to 'fail' them. When I took my neuropsychological tests years ago, I was aware of having an intense anxiety about going too slowly on the written tests. I tried to beat the clock, even though I was taking the test to get a diagnosis so I could get some *help*! It's just not that easy to confront your weaknesses head-on."

Understanding Your Diagnosis
Your follow-up appointment should be a detailed fact-finding mission. You should ask questions about why certain tests were used, what they measured and how you compared with the normal range for a particular test. When your psychologist explains your results, ask for clarification of terms you don't understand.

No two ADD people are alike. You should use your follow-up meeting to learn as much as you can about your unique neuropsychological profile. If you leave this meeting armed only with your checklist of deficits, you'll have only half the information you need. You must also have a clear understanding of your unique strengths and the positive compensatory strategies you already use.

You can't expect to leave this meeting with all the tools you'll need to manage your ADD. You can expect to leave with specific information about your individual strengths and weaknesses and a framework of treatment options.

After the Diagnosis—Your Role in Treatment
The homework you did in locating your mental health professional will pay dividends as you begin treatment. It is important to become an active participant in your treatment, working with the professionals on your team to problem-solve. Since information about adult ADD is limited, a flexible, experimental approach to treatment is usually necessary.

If you're going to use medicine in your treatment, it's essential that you establish a partnership with your physician. Finding the right medication and dosage is generally a trial-and-error process. There isn't any magic formula the physician can use to determine in advance the medicine that will work best for you.

If your mental health professional becomes defensive or pats you on the head when you ask questions or offer ideas, find a new one! We've been contacted by adults who can't find informed professionals in their area. Should you end up in a similar situation, you may have to seek out someone who is willing to learn!

The Practical Side of Evaluation and Treatment— What's It Going to Cost?
This discussion wouldn't be complete without a word about cost. The testing process is time-consuming and can rapidly run up a large bill. Before committing to testing or treatment, ask about approximate costs and ways to cut corners if you are uninsured or on a tight budget. You may be able to work out a payment schedule in advance if the bill for testing is too large to pay at one time.

Carefully scrutinize your insurance policy. Some policies don't cover or only partially cover psychological services. Some specifically exclude ADD from coverage. We don't want to discourage you from seeking a diagnosis and treatment. *You are worth the price* even if it means skipping your summer vacation this year. We just want you to be prepared so you can plan and avoid rude financial shocks.

In a later section we'll talk specifically about various treatment options for ADD adults. Although professional help will likely be an important part of your treatment, we want to focus primarily on self-help, which is the guiding principle of this book. We firmly believe that you are capable of helping yourself, and we want to help you learn how to do it.

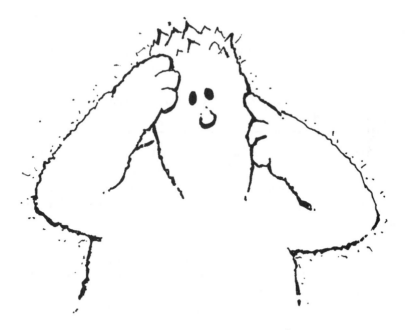

Getting Down to Work

Okay, so you know, or feel fairly certain, that an Attention Deficit Disorder is at the root of your problems. You know you were born with the deficits and grew up with them. You know you're different from someone without ADD. You know you've learned various not-so-great ways of coping with them. SO WHAT DO YOU DO NOW?

What you do now is take a deep breath, find some time for yourself and look squarely at your ADD. It is inseparable from who you are. What you do now is decide that *you are worth all the work it will take to recover.*

Recover:

1. a. to get back (something lost, stolen, etc.)
   b. to regain (health, consciousness, etc.)

2. to compensate for; make up for (to recover losses)

3. a. to get (oneself) back to a state of control, balance, composure, etc.
   b. to catch or save (oneself) from a slip, stumble, betrayal of feeling, etc.

New World Dictionary of the American Language, Simon and Schuster, 1980

To regain, compensate, get back control and balance, save oneself— this is what you do now. The remainder of this book is about this process of recovery. We'll move from the theoretical to the practical and offer specific guidelines and suggestions that can make recovery possible.

We can't emphasize enough that recovery is a process that requires a lot of work. It isn't something that will magically happen after you read this book. You must commit yourself to believing that you are worth all the work it will take to recover.

If you're still reading, we can assume that you've made this important commitment to yourself. You won't be sorry. You have so much to offer and so many talents to discover! Let's get started and take a look at some important issues you'll need to consider.

ADD is inseparable from who you are. We made this observation at the outset, but what does it really mean? ADD is an acronym for Attention Deficit Disorder. *Deficit . . . ? Disorder . . . ?* If ADD is inseparable from who you are, does this mean that disability is your only dimension? Absolutely not!

Your differences are only one part of you. If society has learned anything from the efforts of the physically disabled to gain equal access, it's that we are all people first. If more time and energy were spent developing the unique abilities of all people, we would have a more productive society.

As you learn to help yourself, you must never focus more on your disabilities than the total person you are. It's a mistake, however, to totally ignore your differences. The tricky thing for ADD adults is that many of us grew up never knowing we had a disability. ADD is inseparable from who we are because we forged our senses of self around it, never knowing it was there. Most of us haven't grown up with the benefit of knowing we had a handicap. We grew up thinking we just weren't as smart, competent or valuable as other people.

Now that you know you have ADD, it should be easy to make a recipe to turn out a great person, right? Well, it doesn't quite work that way. You may know intellectually that you have ADD. Grappling with that knowledge on an emotional level, however, is a very different proposition:

It is a task of truly accepting that you aren't perfect.

You must say good-bye to your old self-image, whatever that may have been, and admit that your problems won't go away by changing your job, your friends or your spouse. The vague feeling you've always had that something was wrong has been confirmed and given a name. What a scary place to be—in adult-hood, trying to figure out who you'll be when you grow up.

Your newly acquired self-knowledge may be scary but it's also liberating. It offers a wonderful opportunity to take control of your life by looking squarely at your limits and growing beyond them. This requires courage and time. It requires working through a process of self-acceptance that begins with grieving.

When a loved one dies we can't move on with our lives until we have grieved and moved through the stages of shock, anger, denial, bargaining and depression. Similarly, when we lose a part of our psy-chological selves, including an alteration in our self-concept, we must grieve the lost sense of self before we can work on building a new one. You may not have thought of your ADD in this way, but:

Grieving is the beginning of your self-discovery.

Let's take a look at how the process works. You may already have moved through some of the stages.

Grief—The Shock of Recognition

The diagnosis is often both a punch in the stomach and a vin-dication of years of struggle and feelings of inadequacy. We knew something was wrong and now we have the test results to prove it. We don't have to feel like impostors anymore, living in fear of being found out. What a relief!

KK: "When I went through psychotherapy in my twenties, my constant theme was that I felt different. I always struggled with comparing myself to other people, unable to figure out how they could so easily manage the things I sweated over. I won-dered if they had some secret to which I wasn't privy or if they managed to accomplish a lot at the expense of their families.

"Since I couldn't go to college and do much of anything else at the same time, I assumed that being a student meant giving up everything outside school. I didn't know that it was just easier for other people. I assumed that I was too self-indulgent to accept the challenges.

"When I was diagnosed with ADD, the relief was enormous—I was finally able to make sense of my struggles. Having ADD meant that I wasn't bad, lazy, unmotivated or stubborn. It meant that I could look at my life through different-colored lenses. I could stop filtering my accomplishments through the expectations I based on comparisons to others. I began to marvel at all I had managed to do in spite of a significant disability.

"The midlife crisis I had been working on resolved itself when I shed a positive light on the life I had lived up to that point. Although I had gained positive self-esteem as a result of psychotherapy, it was nothing compared to the boost of my changing view of myself as a heroically struggling adult.

"I began to feel less apologetic for my shortcomings and more deserving of help and understanding. Accompanying the relief was the hope that I could be fixed now that I finally understood the basis for my problems."

PR: "I always struggled silently with my deficits. Neither my grades in school nor any of my relationships ever suffered outwardly. The only person who knew I was a failure was me. It was an incredible burden.

"The people in my life didn't destroy me. I destroyed myself with intense feelings of inadequacy. Perhaps the worst period in my life was when my little brother died. I was fourteen years old and into driving my parents crazy with my adolescent stuff. Roger hit a tree when he was sledding and died the next morning. He was only ten years old and indisputably the perfect child in my family. He was so perfect. I was so imperfect. And he had to die! I knew that it should have been me.

"No one ever knew how I felt. I agonized over screwing this one up by not being the one who died. Learning at thirty-nine that I had ADD didn't miraculously free me from my impaired sense of self, but it offered a peace I had never known before. It was a relief to know, at least in my intellectual self, that my feelings had a basis. My struggles came from deficits over which I had no control. The diagnosis alone didn't undo years of silent pain but gave me a reality I could use to work on readjusting my self-image.

"I wish my brother hadn't died, but I've been able to alter my perspectives of his life and mine. Neither of us had more value than the other. His death just happened, and I finally believe that it's okay that it wasn't me instead."

Grief: Anger—"Why Me?"

The initial stage of relief and euphoria often gives way to a period of anger. The diagnosis that frees us from faulty assumptions begins to feel like an unbearable burden. Facts don't lie. We are imperfect and it just isn't fair!

"Why me? Why did I have to be born this way?"

"Why did everyone—parents, teachers, therapists—blame my difficulties on depression, lack of motivation or poor character?"

"Why didn't somebody believe in me?"

"Why did everybody assume the worst—that I just wasn't trying hard enough?"

"Why was I misunderstood and reprimanded when I was trying my heart out?"

"Why did all those mental health professionals pretend to know more than they really did?"

We may feel furious at the people in our lives who failed to recognize our deficits. We understand that no one knew much about ADD ten or twenty years ago. But somehow we still feel that if only our parents had loved and respected us enough, they would have figured it out. They should have known our problems were real. We often begin to feel helpless and victimized.

Grief: Denial—Not Me!

Remember Donna? She struggles with her inability to move beyond the *intellectual* knowledge of her ADD to the *emotional* knowledge. It's not that she rejects the reality of her disorder. She simply denies its impact on her life.

Denial can take several forms. After an initial sense of anger, we might decide to reject the diagnosis, wondering why we ever wasted our money on the evaluation. We might, as Donna does, announce to friends that we have ADD but then not seek treatment. We might pick up our prescription but never use it. We might take the medication with the mistaken belief that we have found the cure for our problems. We move into this new phase of our lives with rosy fantasies of how, with the help of our local pharmacy, we can conquer the world.

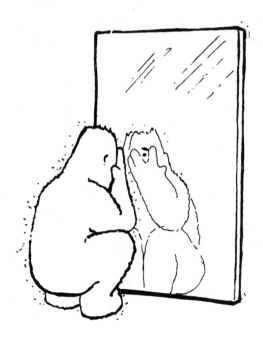

Regardless of the brand of denial we choose during this stage, we aren't dealing yet with the reality of our ADD. We need time to process our new knowledge and confront ourselves with our weaknesses. At this early stage in the process of recovery, we don't recognize the face reflecting back to us in the mirror:

"That isn't the person I used to be,
and I'm not ready to figure out who it really is."

Bargaining—It Can All Be Fixed

As we begin to make sense of everything, we bargain with God or fate to forestall facing the inescapable fact of our disorder. The deal goes something like this: "If I'm really good, you'll give me back what I've lost."

For many ADD adults the bargaining is around medication that often brings at least initially dramatic, positive changes. A whole world opens up as the medication helps us emerge from lifelong fogs. Sights and sounds that had previously drifted by our conscious awareness are noticed for the first time. We are better organized and focused. We feel energized with a new sense of purpose and feel calmer and happier. This new tool is a great bargaining chip.

We promise ourselves to work diligently at pursuing the right dose of medication. When we find it, we know that our symptoms will go away. We'll be able to take responsibility for our behaviors and be like everybody else.

This strategy works for a while until awareness grows that maybe this isn't the answer to our problems. Our improved ability to pay attention makes us increasingly aware of our mistakes. We grudgingly acknowledge that our medicine hasn't cured them. It doesn't make us normal even though we promised to do everything right if only the Ritalin or Adderall would fix us. We begin to notice the drug's uneven symptom control over the course of the day and our decreased functioning when the drug is at a low level.

Our diagnosis vindicates us against the invalid assumptions people have made about us. We've spent our anger railing about the injustice and have taken a step toward dealing with our symptoms. But we aren't fixed. Our bargaining doesn't work but we're still not ready to own our disorder. *We still aren't ready to accept that our ADD is not just going to magically disappear.*

Reality Sinks In—Depression

Our diagnosis is supposed to free, not imprison us. But that's often what happens at some point in our grief process. As adults, we resent having to relive the identity crisis of adolescence. We may not have been doing great before, but at least we thought we knew who we were. At this point depression often sets in. For some ADD adults it returns periodically, threatening to undermine progress.

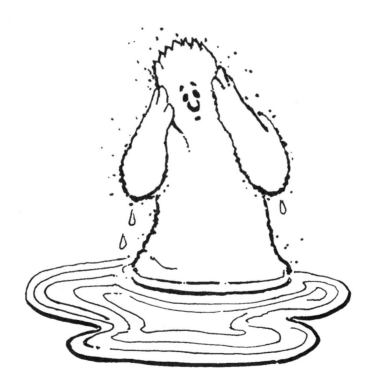

KK: "When depression set in, it was compounded by the growing certainty that my daughter also had ADD. I mixed us up in my mind during that time. Tyrell was my bright hope for the future. I put a lot of energy into carefully nurturing her self-esteem so she wouldn't have to go through what I did as a child. When I realized that ADD was at the root of many of my problems, I was frightened for my daughter.

"In my state of gloom, I began to think that she was doomed as I was. If this problem was inherited and biological, there was no escape. I agonized over Tyrell's fate and my own. I ruminated about all the things I couldn't do and all the times I had failed. I relived each painful and humiliating experience from my past. My positive attributes and accomplishments ceased to exist. There was the triple whammy of feeling helpless as a parent, generally incompetent and without hope for the future. I said good-bye to many of my dreams, both the realistic and the unrealistic ones.

"This stage was marked by extreme fragility. I constantly burst into tears, and innocent remarks set me off. I laugh at it now but just hearing the word 'memory' would bring tears to my eyes because it reminded me of my deficits. I sat in church every Sunday trying to hide the tears streaming down my face."

PR: "The relief I felt after my diagnosis was short-lived. In the months that followed, it was replaced with an assortment of conflicting feelings. Depression was one of them. It was a place I had frequently visited during my life. This time, however, there was no vagueness about my feelings of gloom.

"I had often lived under a cloud of helplessness and hopelessness. The discovery of my ADD, however, brought my negative feelings crashing down around me. I had previously been able to pull myself out of my black fogs by reasoning that things really weren't that bad. My diagnosis brought this reasoning to a crashing halt. Things really were that bad! I would never be okay.

"I had accepted that my then-eight-year-old son's symptoms would never go away. I vividly recall the moment two years earlier when my fantasies about R. Jeremy abruptly ended. I sat in the psychologist's office, mentally checking off all the things he would never be able to do. Four months pregnant with a baby girl conceived after several years of infertility treatments, I felt gut-wrenching terror for both my children.

"Remember my brother Roger? Well, I had given my son his name and I had an intense, frightening feeling of déjà vu. What awful curse had I visited on my son? Would he also come to some terrible end?

"Depression set in with a vengeance. I had previously resolved my issues around Jeremy's disorder and had accepted that he would have lifelong challenges. But here it was again—that damned ADD. This time it was mine. My feelings and fears about both my son and myself converged into some pretty self-destructive thoughts. Just when I was getting a handle on his problems, I was faced with the reality of my own.

"It wasn't easy to move beyond my depression. It didn't happen overnight. But I did it. With persistence and a sense of humor, I climbed out of my deep, black hole again. I decided I didn't like it in there—it was too dark and I'm into bright, open spaces! I figured that with my family of four, I was *two down, with two to go*. I did it twice and if I had to, I could do it again."

Out of the Depths—ACCEPTANCE!

If you keep working on the grief process, you will come to a new and better place in your life. The stages you will go through are often difficult and painful, but *they're essential*. When the going gets rough, don't get discouraged. Visualize where you're going—to a place where you will discover and learn to use your valuable gifts.

PR: "One summer, a terrible thunderstorm rocked our house and terrified my young daughter. When it finally ended there was an incredibly beautiful double rainbow stretching across the sky. Alison was dumbstruck because she had never seen a rainbow. After watching it awhile, she announced that she hoped we'd have another bad storm soon so she could see another rainbow. Her fear disappeared, replaced with a child's optimism.

"I've thought from time to time about that storm since Alison comforted herself with the wonder of the resultant rainbows. It may be a cliché, but my journey through my own personal storm has taught me to believe in the gold at the end of rainbow. It's there. It's real. It's within my grasp.

"Maybe I'll have more storms than rainbows, but that goes with the territory. I know that my journey will be an uphill struggle, but the rewards are worth my efforts. I accept my son and myself as we are. We're all we've got, so we'd better make the most of our lives. Those complex and beautiful rainbows symbolized limitless possibilities. And so do we, my son and I."

KK: "I don't remember exactly when the depression began to lift. I know one sign of my emergence from gloom and doom was regaining the ability to laugh at myself. I joked about starting a new kind of AA group for people like me. I would call it Airheads Anonymous.

"Understanding that I wasn't to blame for the way I was relieved me of the guilt I had lived with for so long. I was a valuable person with a disability. I had deficits but they no longer defined who I was. They took their rightful place as one dimension of a multidimensional person. I began to feel more confident about my parenting skills and became less anxious about my daughter's future. I reasoned that if I could make it without any help during my childhood, Tyrell could do even better with support.

"Coming to terms with my ADD meant spending far less time and energy hiding my deficits. I concentrated on understanding them without being consumed by them. I was finally free to take charge of my life and realistically assess it.

"The months that followed were exciting and productive as I evaluated various career options. It became clear that I had a gift for writing and an ability to understand and connect with people. I was already using my people skills in my teaching and nursing, but I realized that many of the routine details of my work were painfully difficult for me. I decided to use my risk-taking ability to embark on a new venture, although it wasn't readily apparent what it would be!

"I had been intensely interested in ADD since my diagnosis and wanted to specialize in it in some way. I just didn't know what direction to take. I liked the flexibility of teaching and enjoyed mentoring students, but sensed that perhaps this wasn't quite the right niche. I wrestled with the issue of security versus optimally using my interests and talents. With my newfound sense of inner strength, I was sure that I would eventually find what I was looking for.

"When the answer came, everything fell into place. I decided to write this book and asked Peggy to join me in this venture. The project had my name on it! I knew there were millions of people struggling with ADD and that there was limited help available for them. This book would be the perfect work choice for me.

"I had impeccable credentials—who could know ADD better than someone who lived with it? I could use my experiences, varied background in education and mental health and my people and writing skills to work at something in which I was intensely interested. What a perfect job!

"Life still has its ups and downs, but I feel that I'm living it more fully now than I ever could have before this journey. Instead of hiding my weaknesses or working at things that are wrong for me, I can now celebrate my gifts."

In the remaining chapters of this book we will offer a framework you can use to maximize your abilities and minimize your disabilities. The focus will be on what you *can* do rather than what you *can't* do. We want to help you discover your hidden strengths and talents and celebrate the person you are.

We don't presume to have all the answers. We can, however, help you formulate the questions you need to ask as you take responsibility for your recovery. We share your pain and your hope because we are struggling alongside you.

As you continue on your personal journey of recovery, consider the following quote by Cathy Better of Reisertown, Maryland. It appeared in the *Community Times* newspaper and is an empowering affirmation of the possibilities available to you with hard work and a deep commitment to yourself.

Each day that we wake is a new start, another chance.

Why waste it on self-pity, sloth and selfishness?

Roll that day around on your tongue, relish the taste of its freedom.

Breathe deeply of the morning air, savor the fragrance of opportunity.

Run your hands along the spine of those precious 24 hours

and feel the strength in sinew and bone.

Life is raw material. We are artisans.

We can sculpt our existence into something beautiful,

or debase it into ugliness.

It's in our hands.

CHAPTER 5

About Balance, Toyotas, Porsches, Circus High Wires and the Twelve Steps of Alcoholics Anonymous

Did we get your attention? Are you wondering about the connection between balance, cars, high-wire acts, AA, ADD and recovery? Well, there is a connection and it's an important place to start learning how to effectively manage your ADD.

Balance may be something you think about only at the end of the month when your bank statement comes. One of life's little joys is a balanced checkbook. This doesn't happen nearly often enough. How many times do you decide that it isn't worth trying to figure out the discrepancy, that it's easier to accept the balance your bank says you have?

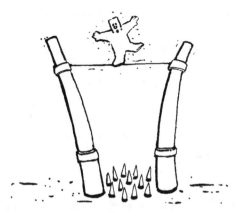

"The ADDer's Precarious High-Wire Act"

As ADDers, achieving balance in our lives is critical and considerably more difficult to achieve than balance in our checkbooks. What is balance? It's a general concept, similar to freedom or success, that each of us defines individually. Let's find out how balance issues have an impact on the lives of ADD adults.

Warning—It's Very Easy for an ADDer to Lose Her Balance!

ADD folk have nervous systems that are erratic and poorly regulated. Rapid thoughts and an excitable nature are at odds with a central nervous system that can't handle too much input. The paradox is of an enthusiastic, creative and impulsive ADD adult who is often driven to get involved in more than she can handle. Since having ADD means that her basic nature is at war with itself, her life can indeed be a high-wire act!

Achievement and Less Tangible Goals: There are many ways for an ADDer to lose the balance in her life. The delicate balance between achievement and other, less tangible goals is a critical balancing act. These days it seems that many people feel they live on fast-moving treadmills that lack Off switches. Careers eat up family time, and escalating demands create pressure-cooker environments.

Unlike people who react to this pressure with mild stress symptoms, ADDers can fall apart completely. Of course, this is often a first, essential step toward recovery. Falling apart can be the equivalent of an alcoholic's hitting "rock bottom." For some alcoholics, rock bottom is getting a DUI citation. For others, it is a string of DUIs, a divorce, unemployment and hitting skid row. As awful as rock bottom may seem at the time for an alcoholic or an ADDer, it's often the starting point for a new and better life. It begins the recovery process because its awfulness forces the person to make some changes.

Structure and Freedom: To keep ourselves from falling off our high wire, many of us also need a proper balance of structure and freedom. We ADDers often balk at the structure we desperately need. A tendency to become easily overstimulated means that chaotic lifestyles can get us into trouble. On the other hand, lives routinized into dullness by too much regimentation don't provide sufficient challenge.

We know that an ADD child needs externally imposed structure to thrive. When she becomes an adult, she continues to need limits but has to provide them for herself. Adults are expected to manage their own lives. The challenge is to establish a balance that offers order without stifling creativity, one of many ADD adults' best attributes.

Ways of Thinking, Activity Levels, Emotions and Needs: ADD brains and nervous systems are often out of balance, with behavior swinging rapidly from one extreme to the other. An ADDer tends to excesses, alternating between bouts of workaholism and sluggish inactivity. Her moods swing up and down and her performance is erratic. The following list outlines some of these balance issues that can cause you to lose your footing on the high wire:

Work vs. Play
Do you tend to get overinvolved in one or the other and have trouble shifting gears?

Your Needs vs. Others'
Are you oblivious to the feelings and points of view of others, or do you always put yourself dead last?

Over- vs. Understimulation
What is your optimal level of stress, noise, work and challenges?

Hyperactivity vs. Hypoactivity
Are you so active that you drive others crazy, or do you vegetate most of the time? This includes sleep and rest patterns as well as daily activity levels.

Detailed vs. Global Thinking

Do you get caught up in too much detail, unable to see the forest for the trees, or do you tend to focus on the gestalt or whole picture? If you focus on big pictures, do you have trouble keeping track of details?

Depression vs. Euphoria

Are your moods out of balance, with too much sadness or excessive happiness? Do you swing between these two extremes?

The Value of Examining Balance Issues

It's easy for your balance in each of these areas to become skewed in either direction at different times. Alternately, you may find yourself regularly swinging erratically from one extreme to the other. The point of examining each of these areas is that imbalance in any of them can cause problems for your mental health or family life.

What's the connection we mentioned between balance, Toyotas and Porsches? In some respects, the ADD adult is designed like a Porsche. She is spirited, dynamic, powerful, exciting and ready to go with the rapid acceleration of an expensive sports car. Her non-ADD peers are more like the family Toyota. Equally well engineered, this Toyota has a more "even temperament." It is designed for comfort, reliability and fuel efficiency. If the ADD adult is to maintain and maximize the high performance of her Porsche, she has to take especially good care of herself.

One of the best ways you can do this is to work on achieving balance in your life. Having a well-balanced lifestyle is akin to taking good care of your car. It subjects the system to less wear and tear. To use the metaphor again, working on balance is similar to continually tinkering with and tuning up your car. If you want to keep your whole system in working order, you'll have to make ongoing adjustments.

With limitations they can't ignore, ADDers who recover may well lead the rest of society to a saner way of life. Competence and levels of achievement have become the societal standard that measures a person's worth and success in life. Those who are "unproductive" owing to age, health or disability have been devalued because they don't "measure up." Society no longer values children or the aged as it previously did. A shocking number of children sink into poverty, while stressed caregivers abuse many senior citizens.

This philosophizing isn't just the wandering of creative minds but relates directly to achieving balanced lives. You have a unique opportunity to redesign your success model and get off the crazy treadmill everyone else is on.

If you pay attention to the messages of your body and soul, you'll realize that you can't be all or do it all. If you work at your recovery, you can use your new self-knowledge to design a life that really works for you. You can be at peace with yourself and your environment while the rest of the world skyrockets out of control.

We've already talked about the connection between balance, cars and high-wire acts. Now let's consider the last part of this chapter's title—Alcoholics Anonymous—as we move from general concepts to practical applications for achieving balance in your life.

How-To's of Achieving Balance

To help you get started, we're going to borrow the invaluable framework of the Twelve Steps of Alcoholics Anonymous. Although this program specifically refers to alcohol and alcoholics, it's possible to substitute virtually any chronic problem or disability. A variety of support groups have adopted this framework, which is a sound program for creating a balanced life.

Briefly, the program is a systematic plan for acknowledging limitations to oneself and others, making amends to others whenever possible and coming to a greater self-acceptance. *Working the program* means making a commitment to follow the steps in daily life.

The Twelve Steps of A.A.

1. We admitted we were powerless over alcohol—that our lives had become unmanageable.

2. Came to believe that a Power greater than ourselves could restore us to sanity.

3. Made a decision to turn our will and our lives over to the care of God as we understood Him.

4. Made a searching and fearless moral inventory of ourselves.

5. Admitted to God, to ourselves and to other human beings the exact nature of our wrongs.

6. Were entirely ready to have God remove all these defects of character.

7. Humbly asked Him to remove our shortcomings.

8. Made a list of all persons we had harmed, and became willing to make amends to them all.

9. Made direct amends to such people wherever possible, except when to do so would injure them or others.

10. Continued to take personal inventory and when we were wrong, promptly admitted it.

11. Sought through prayer and meditation to improve our conscious contact with God as we understood Him,

praying only for knowledge of His will for us and the power
to carry that out.

12. Having had a spiritual awakening as the result of these
Steps, we tried to carry this message to alcoholics, and
to practice these principles in all our affairs.

Using the Twelve Steps for Your Personal Recovery from ADD

The steps are framed around a central concept of spiritual
awareness that has relevance for ADDers. It's the glue that
holds all the steps of the program together so that peace and
self-acceptance can be achieved.

Spiritual awareness isn't specific to organized religion. The
Twelve Steps carefully talk about *"God as we understand him,"*
leaving the specifics to the individual. The word "God" can be
replaced with a more generalized "higher power" that has
meaning for each individual. The higher power could be the
fellowship of other alcoholics (or, in our case, other ADDers)
or the whole of mankind. The idea is to focus on something
greater than ourselves and realize that *we can't go it totally alone.*
The Serenity Prayer sums up this philosophy:

GOD GRANT ME THE SERENITY
TO ACCEPT THE THINGS I CANNOT CHANGE,
TO CHANGE THE THINGS I CAN,
AND THE WISDOM TO KNOW THE DIFFERENCE.

Closely related to spiritual awareness and integral to the program is the issue of morality and wrongdoing. For the alcoholic,
this is a critical part of her recovery. Typically, the alcoholism
has caused havoc in the lives of her friends and family, and she
must assume responsibility for her actions. This includes making amends to each of the people she has directly hurt.

These issues aren't relevant to your recovery from ADD except
as they relate to those aspects of self you can change. For in-

stance, if you've learned to use some maladaptive coping mechanisms that have hurt other people, it is healing to take responsibility for your behaviors and make appropriate amends.

The issue of *powerlessness* detailed in the first three steps, however, has a direct implication for you as an adult with ADD. It means that you are powerless over your ADD in that it isn't anyone's fault and can't be cured.

Applying these steps in your own life means that you need to stop blaming your parents, spouse, children and yourself for the problems caused by your ADD. This doesn't mean that you absolve yourself from all responsibility for your behavior. It means that you acknowledge the reality of your imperfect self. Confronting your powerlessness includes an admission that you can't do it all—you are human and have unique limitations. If you have begun your process of grief, you may already be confronting and working at accepting your limitations.

The fourth principle also has significance for you as an ADD adult. This step instructs the individual to take an inventory. This should be similar to the one you develop for your homeowner's or renter's insurance. Rather than noting the condition and value of possessions you should examine and list your assets, abilities, liabilities or disabilities.

Your inventory is central to your recovery. Since your ADD can't be cured, your goal shouldn't be to *eliminate* your deficits. Instead it should be to *identify, accept* and *manage* them. A failure to confront your limitations can result in damaged emotional and spiritual health and a diminished sense of self. Later in this discussion we'll offer some suggestions about how to compile this important inventory.

Evaluating Balance Issues in Your Life

We talked earlier in this chapter about general balance issues that can be important for you as an ADD adult. Now it's time for you to think about the balance in your own life. The following is a list of questions you can use to get started. You may never have really thought about some of them and may not be able to answer all of them right now. But keep them in mind throughout the discussion in this chapter. If you try some of the things we suggest, you may be able to answer them later.

1. What is your daily/weekly work capacity?

2. How much sleep and rest do you need, including "down time" when there are no demands placed on you?

3. What is your financial bottom line—how much income do you require to maintain an acceptable standard of living?

4. How much time can you devote to family and friends?

5. What must you do to renew yourself spiritually, not just in the sense of religion but regarding anything that gives your life meaning?

6. How much and what kind of recreational activities are critical for your well-being?

7. How long can you work efficiently without a break?

8. What obligations can you fulfill?

9. What things are cluttering your life and could be eliminated?

10. How much time do you spend daily on self-maintenance: grooming, dressing or health care?

Is Your Life in Balance?

You probably know that "all work and no play makes Johnny a dull boy." A balanced life must include time for work, relationships, spiritual renewal, recreation and rest. In today's fast-track, dual-career society, the pressures are such that even calm, well-organized people become frazzled as they attempt to find time for everything.

The juggling act is daunting for you as an ADD adult. If you just go with the flow, you're likely to find yourself drifting in directions that aren't particularly helpful. You can get immersed in work and forget that you have a family, or allow your socializing at work to interfere with the quality of your performance. Since you're distractible and have an elastic sense of time, you can't expect to let balance take care of itself. You need to carefully design it. To work the steps in your personal balance plan most effectively, we recommend that you hire an ADD coach to assist you in the process.

Conduct Your Own One-Rat Study

To answer the questions we posed about the balance in your life, you'll need to conduct your own research experiment. It should include a daily log that tracks your activities for several weeks. Write down everything you do and how much time it takes. Also, keep track of the difficulty of each task or event.

Rate the difficulty on a scale of one to ten. If you have trouble deciding how to rate something, pay attention to stress indicators. What happens when you face too many demands? Some people react to stress with muscle tension or headaches. Others become irritable or start tuning out. What is your pattern of stress indicators?

When your diary is complete, examine it for observable patterns. Did your stress indicators increase after a certain length of time on a task? If so, you have discovered how long you can work without a break or a shift to another activity. In similar fashion, you can begin to estimate your overall daily and weekly work capacity.

By keeping track of stress symptoms and altering the number of hours you work, you can determine how long you can work efficiently. Don't neglect the other areas of your life when you analyze your diary. Does exercise seem to lower your stress level and improve the quality of your work? What about the time you spend with your family?

Make a Personal Schedule

It's time to develop a tentative weekly schedule that includes an estimate of the time it takes to do each activity. As you pencil in time estimates on your schedule, be very careful. Refer to your diary to find out how long it took to complete various tasks, and factor in extra time. Doubling your estimate for everything except sleep will give you a cushion for unexpected events and the distractions that inevitably derail ADDers. Don't forget to include transition time from one activity to the next. Unfortunately, technology is not sufficiently advanced to allow us to "beam up" from one place to another.

We can almost guarantee that after the first week, you'll decide that your schedule is unworkable! You will probably find that everything you needed to do didn't fit into your time frames. We bet that if you did manage to stay on schedule, you were frazzled by the end of the week.

Your life is out of balance because you're trying to fit too much into it! This includes not just the quantity of activities but an accumulation of demands on your capacity for work and stress. After you've recovered from the shock of recognizing the impossibility of doing it all, you'll need to review your schedule with the goal of slicing and dicing it!

The demands on your life need to match your capacity and abilities and also fit into the time you have available. How do you get started figuring out what to cut out? In the next section, we'll get back to the moral inventory we talked about earlier. This will be the place for you to start.

Analyzing Personal Strengths and Weaknesses

Although we wouldn't presume to minimize the enormous task of recovering from alcoholism, in some respects it might be easier than recovering from ADD. As an ADD adult, your flaws are less apparent than those of the alcoholic's and may therefore be somewhat easier to deny and ignore. You have the power to take control of your life by looking squarely at your limits.

Acknowledging your limits offers an opportunity for you to grow far beyond them. By limiting the activities that stress your fragile skills, you will free up energy and time for those you do well. It's time for you get busy on your inventory to help you better understand your strengths and weaknesses. Use the following questions as an outline for this important job.

What Can I Do Well?

This first question may be the hardest to answer! Members of our local adult support group were initially stumped when they tried to describe some of their strong points. Several expressed that they couldn't think of anything positive because they were so accustomed to focusing on their mistakes. Over time, it became apparent that there was indeed a wealth of talent among us. After several months, group members gradually became less tentative about their strengths.

If you have a similar problem, we suggest that you work first on enlarging your thinking about what constitutes an asset. For instance, as some of our group shared particular talents in their jobs, one participant (we'll call her Sarah) was initially apologetic about not working outside the home.

As the sharing continued in subsequent meetings, it became apparent that Sarah was a virtual genius at living a balanced life. She had conducted her own elaborate "one-rat study" to determine her work capacity. She added up all the mental and physical tasks performed in a typical week to arrive at a total number of working hours. Her calculations were very precise. Sarah de-

termined that travel time to her son's school conference constituted work, and time spent at the support group was leisure. She
informed the group that she didn't count the time it took her to
get dressed in the morning, but if she had to change into her
grass-cutting clothes during the day, she counted it as work!

Sarah spent several weeks tracking her signs of stress as she manipulated the numbers of hours she worked in a given week. At
the end of her study, she concluded that she could work no
more than fifty hours a week without exceeding acceptable levels of stress. Since she already had two children, motherhood
wasn't an optional role, but she knew she could make decisions
about her other roles.

She realized that she could manage only a part-time job outside
the home, but didn't waste energy fretting about the lowered
family income. Instead, she turned her creative talents to devis-
ing strategies for living well on less money. She grows much of
the family's food in a backyard garden, swims in a small pool
dug with family labor and barters with friends for other goods
and services. She carefully considers the impact of labor and
money decisions on the family system, not only as financial expenses but also as the cost and value of energy and time.

The result is a family that is truly in balance. Sarah, whose particular gifts aren't easy to measure or define by societal standards, is
extremely successful. She could be a valuable consultant to many
harried, stressed families.

When you make your list of things you do well, go beyond the
obvious. Many of us with ADD measure personal worth by the
yardstick of people with more orderly or ordinary lives and
minds. We consider ourselves successful if we play tennis or golf
well, have careers with a steady upward climb and perform
tasks efficiently. Remember, our abilities are often more offbeat.

KK: "My younger brother has ADD and has always had an intense curiosity about how things work. When he was a kid, he

got in mega-trouble because he always took things apart and neglected to put them back together. He did, however, have a talent that was very useful. He could figure out how to open any kind of lock. We always called on him when family members had locked their keys in the car.

"He was a lifesaver when my dad, who worked for Colt firearms, accidentally locked my cousin Florence in a pair of police handcuffs one Friday night. Unfortunately, the key was in Dad's office, which was closed until Monday morning. Cousin Florence would have spent a very uncomfortable weekend had my brother not come to her rescue.

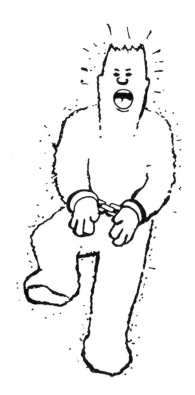

"My brother would have made a great burglar, but he might also have turned his unusual talent into something both income-producing and legal! I don't know. Maybe he could have designed security systems. Actually, he became a chef who happens to have many other untapped talents.

"When I was twenty-three years old and doing my own self-assessment, I was initially hard-pressed to figure out what I did well. A string of failures had left me wondering if I had any abilities at all. I sidestepped the question of my abilities by taking a look at what I liked to do. Identifying my talents followed logically from this starting point.

"The first item on my list was that I liked to spend time talking with my friends. I realized that not only did I like it, I was also good at it. People often called on me for help when they were in trouble or feeling unhappy. Bingo! I realized that I was an effective, albeit untrained, therapist.

"I added my love of reading to my list. I realized that besides books, I loved reading *people* and trying to understand them. My list grew to include attributes such as my tolerance and acceptance of others' faults and my problem-solving skills."

When you begin working on your own list, try starting with the things you like to do. Since we often prefer activities that come easiest to us, you may find yourself focusing on your talents without even realizing it. Include as many things as you can. Don't limit yourself to standard or marketable skills such as being a computer whiz or a good dancer. If you can tie a knot in a cherry stem with your tongue, include it on your list. If your talent is playing the "Star-Spangled Banner" on your teeth, don't hesitate to write it down. These abilities might not have any apparent value. But some creative thinking can lead to some surprising uses for seemingly useless and strange talents!

What Can I Do Adequately?
Your downhill skiing talents may not exactly qualify you for an Olympic gold medal. If you can manage, however, to get down the hill in one piece, add this item to your inventory. What about the costumes you sewed for your daughter's school play?

Maybe some of the seams ripped apart and had to be pinned together for the performance, but you did manage to get the
twenty-five costumes sewed together.

The point is, you should include each thing you can do *reasonably* well. These activities may not be your favorite things to do
and they may not be a showcase of your talent, but at least you
can get by with them. If you are a mediocre tennis player, include it as long as you don't play so poorly that you face humiliation each time you step on the court. If your cooking is fairly
routine and unexciting but edible, it belongs in this category.

What Can't (or Shouldn't) I Do?

This final section of your inventory is extremely important because it will help you make decisions about the things you should
simply stop doing. Do you remember Debra, who tries to hide her
deficits by doing everything? Not only does she try to do everything, she tries to do everything brilliantly! She continually feels
stressed and inadequate owing to her unrealistic expectations.

Even if you aren't trying to do it all, you are probably trying to
do things you shouldn't do. You may be a whiz in mathematics,
but that doesn't necessarily mean that you should do your own
income tax returns. Do you really have time to fit this into your
schedule, or should you pay an accountant to do it? What
about those things that really aren't your forté? If you are experiencing failure when your efforts don't accomplish what you
want them to, perhaps your only failure is in trying to do some
of these things at all. No one can be wonderful at everything.

Many ADDers try so hard to be *normal* that they are unrealistic
about their capabilities. If playing softball always results in an
agonizingly embarrassing experience, don't do it—even if your
three closest friends pressure you into joining them for this
great pastime. Bland, rather tasteless meals are acceptable, but
if you repeatedly burn down major sections of your kitchen, it's
time to reevaluate your cooking.

These activities should be added to your Can't/Shouldn't Do list. As you examine your assets and liabilities, be honest about your weaknesses. We certainly don't encourage you to focus exclusively on your deficits. But through the process of examining and identifying them, you can move on to the abilities they mask.

Balancing Acts Aren't Just for Circus Performers: Climb on the High Wire but Make Sure There's a Safety Net Underneath!

Not all high-wire circus performers use safety nets, but many do. We think they are an absolute necessity for most of us with ADD. Each of us needs a custom-designed net to break the fall from a life that is out of balance.

You'll use your inventory as a blueprint for organizing and simplifying your life and building your safety net. The wise folk who brought us the Twelve Steps were acutely aware that balance is a critical component of recovery. In AA, a repeated phrase is "Keep it simple." Balance can be achieved only by uncluttering your life.

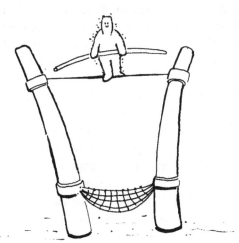

"An ADDer's High-Wire Act with a Safety Net Underneath"

If you support your rather unbalanced nervous system with a carefully planned lifestyle, the external structure will provide some degree of internal order. You need to figure out how you can do more of the things you do well and less of those that cause repeated failure. Be ruthless about eliminating the unnecessary from your life to avoid the overload that causes stress.

We bet you're thinking, "Come on, be realistic. I can't do what I want and get away with it." Of course you can't do exactly what you want all the time. But there are many things you can control and alter to suit your individuality. Let's look at a framework you can use for cleaning house.

Evaluating the "Should-Do's" and "Must-Do's" in Your Life

Refer back to the questions we posed about the balance issues in your life. Reconsider them as they fit with your assets/liabilities list and take another look at your schedule. Are the numbers of things you're trying to accomplish exceeding your capacity? To get them all finished, are you using the time you should be sleeping? Too little sleep can impair the quality of your concentration and performance. Is there little time left for doing things you enjoy, either by yourself or with your family?

Can you make some realistic adjustments to your list of activities and responsibilities? Consider the things you've listed as obligations. How obligatory are they? Can you work on being more assertive when other people make demands or requests? There are unlimited numbers of things we all *should* do in the sense that they are important and worthwhile. Somebody needs to work on the church committee, organize the Parent-Teacher Association or coach the soccer team. The question is, does it have to be *you*?

Many of us with ADD have worked so hard all our lives to stay afloat that we're unrealistic about our limitations. We're so

afraid of not measuring up to expectations that we drive ourselves to do anything and everything. Many times we're doing
more than our fair share but don't know what a fair share is.
Even if we aren't doing as much as our peers, we may be working to the limits of our capacities.

We can't answer any of these questions for you. Only you can
make a determination about the should-do's and must-do's in
your life. But we want to share some of our thoughts about a
couple of them. As you think about the ideas that follow, carefully consider the to-do's that are an accepted part of your
lifestyle. Reflect on them within the context of your inventory
and schedule—are you absolutely sure that they should be part
of your life, or do they throw the balance off?

Analyze Your Financial Equation

As you review your diary, take a hard look at your standard of
living. Is there a way to make changes in this area? Obviously, if
you're just meeting basic needs for food, shelter and health
care, there isn't anything to cut out. Many of us do, however,
have the flexibility to get by on less money. If you're stressed by
exceeding your work capacity, you probably need to look at
ways to reduce the demands. This may mean a reduction in income. Prioritize your commitments with these questions in
mind:

What is essential for survival?
What is important?
What can I do without?

As you try to figure this one out, think of it as an equation. On
one side of the equation are your needs and desires for a certain
standard of living. On the other side is the toll it takes to earn
that living. Only you can decide the best way to balance this
equation! You may decide to reduce your workload by shorten-
ing your hours or by taking a less demanding job. Use your creative ADD brain to come up with ideas for living well on less
money.

Analyze Your Simplicity/Complexity Equation

The key to simplifying our ADD lives is maintaining a proper equilibrium between too much or too little of each balancing act. Although we've been stressing the value of keeping it simple, it's possible to make it *too* simple. If you've been coping with your ADD by severely limiting yourself, you can tip the balance in the opposite direction. Without sufficient challenge, ADDers don't function well, either.

If you often feel bored, lethargic or depressed, you may be understimulated. You may need to push yourself a little more—just enough to function at an optimal level. Your task will be to figure out how to inject more challenge into your life without taking on too much. Ask yourself the questions again to determine if your problem is overstimulation or understimulation.

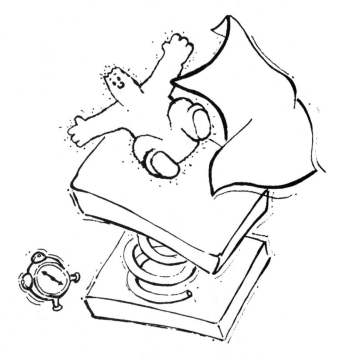

The Revolutionary Bed Ejector—A New Invention That Gets You Up and Moving in the Morning!

Are you getting too much rest or sleep? Experiment by cutting back on the number of hours you sleep each night. Do you feel better with less sleep than you have been routinely getting? If so, set your alarm clock every night, even on weekends, and make yourself get out of bed no matter what. Or buy a Revolutionary Bed Ejector!

Train yourself to hop out of bed at the first sound of the alarm even though your natural tendency is to shut it off and go back to sleep. Getting yourself going in the morning isn't easy, and if you think too much about it, you'll get cold feet! Once it becomes a habit, you may feel better and more productive during the day.

Making the process automatic helps. Just go through your morning ritual on autopilot. Do only things that require so little effort that you could do them when you're half-asleep—which might be how you're still feeling at midmorning! Ask your family not to talk to you or make any demands until you are fully awake. Also try to plan your workday so that the tasks that require problem solving are done later in the morning.

In looking at the other areas of your life, you need to examine ways you can inject spice and challenge. Would a job change or seeking a promotion be in order? Would a new hobby provide needed excitement? The choice is yours. Make changes gradually so you can find your optimal level of challenge. If you start experiencing anxiety or other stress symptoms, you've probably reached your limit and need to think about cutting back.

Analyzing Your Miscellaneous Should-Do's and Must-Do's

To continue paring down your overscheduled life, take a look at all the areas on your list. Can you cut down on the amount of time you spend on grooming? Do you have more social activities than you can handle? Are you carefully considering your need for breaks? Is there some way to ensure that you get them? Continue this process of asking questions and making appropriate modifications until you have a weekly schedule that's more manageable.

How-To's of Slicing and Dicing

We hope this discussion of balance issues can help you take a studied look at your lifestyle. The decisions you make about them will be the basis for constructing your safety net to reduce undue burdens. Only you can decide what a balanced life means for you and what methods will work in achieving it. But how can you make the changes you've decided will simplify your life?

Of course, we can't tell you exactly how you should proceed with your slicing and dicing. But some of the ideas that follow may give you some things to think about. We don't recommend that you impulsively start acting on them all! We do recommend that you try some of them and modify or toss out the ones that won't work.

Slicing and Dicing Techniques

Can You Make a Budget to Determine How You Spend Your Money?

This is a long process of reviewing your checkbook, bank receipts and bills for an entire year. If you can push yourself through it, you will gain invaluable information. Most people are surprised at the money they fritter away. It might actually save you money if you hire a financial coach to help you with the overwhelming details of making a budget.

Can You Cut Down on Impulsive Purchases?

Since one of the hallmarks of ADD is impulsivity, you may buy first and think later. Simply being aware of your tendencies may help. Train yourself to stop and think before you buy anything—"Do I really need this? Can I afford it?" Make a rule not to make any major purchase until you have discussed it with your spouse or family. If impulse buying is a problem, you may have to stay out of stores, cut up your credit cards or plan your shopping trips with an empty wallet!

Can You Resist the Pressure to Keep Up with the Joneses?
Many of us have lifelong habits of measuring ourselves against others. We worry so much about our inability to keep up with other people that it's easy to buy into the equation that "Competence equals Material Success." We rashly jump on the endless treadmill of consumerism, afraid we'll be left behind. Each of us can reduce stress by re-thinking our values.

**Can You Change Your Job Responsibilities
or Change Jobs for a Better Fit?**
What can you save in emotional wear and tear by working fewer hours or making a job change? Perhaps a different job would actually lower your commuting, child care or wardrobe expenses.

**Should You Get a Job Outside the Home
If Full-Time Parenting Isn't Your Forté?**
Not everyone is cut out for staying at home with her family. You may not want a full-time career, but maybe you need the stimulation of a part-time job. The rewards of a little extra money and connections to other people might make your life more interesting. You might find yourself in a bet-ter emotional state of mind to deal with family issues when you have some time away from them.

Can You Barter for Goods and Services?
Do you have a skill or talent that would benefit someone else? Exchange it for something you need. Bartering is a time-honored system for exchanging duties to save money and aggravation and to maximize your talents.

Can You Get Some Outside Help?
Babysitters, cleaning people, gardeners—anyone or any-thing you can afford or can barter for—can help make your

life more manageable. You don't have to do everything yourself.

Are You Asking for Help When You Need It?
Don't let pride stand in the way when you're overloaded. You can return the favor later. You probably have friends or family who would be willing to do some things for you. Why can't your sister pick up the milk you need when she's at the store? You don't have to attend every one of your daughter's soccer games. Ask another soccer parent to take her sometimes and cheer her on.

Are You Firm About Meeting Your Essential Needs?
If you need a half-hour of quiet at the end of your workday, take it without guilt or apology! If you are the ADD parent of an ADD child, you probably have your hands full managing the details of both your lives. Do you have to donate the little time left over to volunteering on the local library committee? Practice saying "No" to requests for commitments of your time. State politely, firmly and without apology that you are already doing as much as you can handle. If the request is made more insistently, repeat your refusal without anger or defensiveness and promptly end the conversation. If you want to help in some way, discuss possibilities with a clear statement of how much you are willing to do.

Can You Lower Your Standards?
Is a super-clean house really necessary or can you subscribe to the Dim Lightbulb Theory of Housekeeping? You may not be crazy about your spouse's ironing capabilities, but if he's willing to assume the chore, can you learn to live with the wrinkles in your blouses?

Are You Keeping the Sabbath?
You may be a Catholic, a druid or a dyed-in-the-wool atheist. Whatever your spiritual beliefs or practices are, there is wisdom in having a sanctioned day of rest. Your day of rest might include a trip to church, temple or mosque, or it might

not. Having some kind of spiritual renewal is important, while the form is irrelevant. Pick one day a week and put your "to do" list out of sight. Make a pact with yourself to run on inspiration that day. You can do an activity that may fall into the "work" category only if you really really *want* to do it. This day is yours, for rest and play. Many of our clients are pleased to find that the Sabbath attitude often begins to spill over into the rest of the week. They still manage to cross off many of those to-do's, but with a lighter heart.

Balance Maintenance

As time goes by, you'll become more skilled at achieving balance in your life. You'll need to continually update your plan to reflect new challenges and life changes. Each time you add a new responsibility or make changes in your life plan, reevaluate the equation and check the balance. Is your capacity for work and stress still roughly equal to the demands placed on it? If your life is out of kilter, you need to return to your drawing board for further adjustments. If you neglect to do this, your life can start to unravel.

Finding the right balance is a complicated process. If you decide to fulfill a lifelong dream to learn Chinese, keep in mind that it will be a slow process! It takes a good supply of mental energy to learn something new. After you've mastered the new skill, you can think about using your energy to take on a new challenge. The trick is to continue cautiously and not pile on too many changes at the same time. If you up the ante in measured steps, you can maintain your optimal level of stimulation, accumulate an impressive number of new skills and still keep your life in balance. You may also discover opportunities and choices that were previously unattainable.

As ADD adults, we need to apply the metaphor of the high-wire performer to our lives. Every day we face extraordinary risks and challenges as we attempt to balance ourselves above the crowd. One slip and we fear we'll find ourselves plunging to the ground. We can't eliminate our missteps, but we can build safety nets to catch us when we fall.

This book is about building personalized safety nets. We've already examined several steps in the construction process: educating yourself, dismantling unhealthy defenses, grieving and balancing your life. Education is probably the easiest step. We hope that you're using your new knowledge to erase faulty assumptions and to make some decisions about your life. The other steps require greater effort.

If you're still struggling with excessive sadness or anger about your ADD, you might need to reread this book later, when you're emotionally ready to begin making some changes. Until you can work through the grief process and achieve a degree of self-acceptance, it will be difficult to make a realistic assessment of your capabilities. Grieving is important work that takes a lot of energy. Don't add impossible burdens by making too many major life changes at the same time.

If you're feeling a bit overwhelmed, slow down, take a deep breath and remember that recovery is a slow, ongoing process. If you're squarely facing your ADD and your coping mechanisms and are taking a studied look at the balance issues in your life, you're ready to move on to some other steps in your recovery. So let's turn to Chapter 6 to begin exploring the dynamics of ADD in interpersonal relationships.

CHAPTER 6

The Art of Relating: In Groups and Friendships

This chapter marks a change in direction from the first part of this book. In educational jargon, the information in the first five chapters was *Readiness*. We were providing information that will be the basis for everything that follows. Since we want to be effective teachers, we need to remind you to periodically review some of the old material as you continue your reading. We will use the balance inventory again, so if you haven't completed it, we hope that you have at least been thinking about it. We hope that at a minimum, you've added it to your "to do" list!

In preceding chapters we talked about the impact of ADD on other people within the context of specific symptoms, differences and defense mechanisms. Now we're going to examine the impact of ADD specifically within the context of relationships.

Although much of the focus of the next three chapters is communication, we'll also consider other issues. In Chapter 7, for instance, we'll examine various factors that have an impact on an ADDer's ability to "relate" to his job responsibilities. Now that you know where you're heading in your reading, let's get busy examining the art of relating.

We all interact daily with other people. When we talk on the phone, participate in a meeting or share dinner with a friend, we're relating with other people. The success of these interactions, whether brief, onetime encounters or long-lasting relationships, depends largely on adequate communication skills.

Virtually everything we do as members of the human race is a form of communication. Volumes have been written about the art of *effective communication.* Family and marriage therapists focus on its importance and attempt to help people keep the *lines of communication open.* College courses teach *positive communication* skills. Based on all the attention given to issues of communication, one can assume that it must be considerably more complex and difficult than simply talking!

Of course, you already knew that. Relationships would be a breeze if this were the case. In reality, even the briefest of interactions can fall apart through a misunderstanding. So let's take a brief look at the dynamics of communication as a starting place for our discussion of interactions and relationships.

We interact with each other by transmitting our thoughts, feelings and desires through the medium of language. In its simplest form, language involves speaking and listening: I talk and you listen, and you talk and I listen. Sounds simple, doesn't it? Read on.

The Art and Science of Communication

Although Mom and Dad often frantically try to figure out exactly what the crying signifies, their one-second-old infant is already communicating. Long before the growing baby acquires real language, he uses squeals, gestures and facial expressions to "talk."

Unless we have a speech problem or a specific language disability, most of us learn to talk fairly early in our lives. We learn the *science of communication* rather effortlessly. We learn to pronounce words correctly and to use them to communicate our needs.

The *art of communication* is often considerably more difficult to learn. Successful interactions with the taxi driver or a spouse rely on a mastery of this art form. Similar to a painting, communication can be designed and interpreted in a variety of ways. It sends a message that includes multiple elements of form, color intensity and shading, subtlety and detail. Unless you are an art aficionado, you may walk away from an abstract painting as confused as you are after some conversations.

An adult with ADD can have real problems with communication and relationships because the rules of the art form continually change. As he tunes in and out, his deficits interfere with his ability to truly understand the meaning of conversations. He may communicate messages he never intended and misinterpret the messages he receives.

The Rhythm of Language
Unlike a painting, communication isn't a static art form. It has rhythm and movement. We have to synchronize ourselves to its flow and to know where, when and how much to contribute to a conversation. Similar to a ballet, a conversation has many elements. It includes a proper time to make an entrance, an awareness of what others are doing, allocation of time for a solo and rules for executing a graceful finale and exit. Many of us could really use some dancing lessons!

Verbal and Nonverbal Communication
Communication is an interplay of words and body language. In general, people from one country use words incomprehensible to foreigners. People in the same country may speak different dialects depending on the ethnic group or area they come from. It has also been suggested that men and women speak different languages.

ADDers and non-ADDers alike differ in their ability to read the interplay of verbal and body language. For some of us, the additional clues of body language help rather than hinder our communication skills. We can use observable gestures and fa-

145

cial expressions to fill in the gaps of words we would otherwise misunderstand.

Others may grasp the precise meaning of spoken words but misunderstand the message of nonverbal language. Years ago, during a visit to Australia, President George Bush (the daddy) held up his fingers in a "V," recognized by Americans as the classic symbol of victory. Much to his chagrin, he learned that an Australian uses the "V" to communicate the same thing as an American holding up his middle finger! President Bush really should have taken a crash course in the Art of Nonverbal Communication before he made his historic blooper!

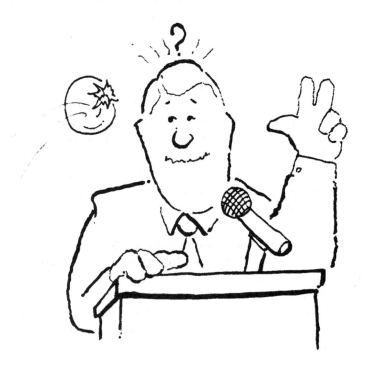

Communication is fraught with the potential for misunderstanding. You may know the meaning of the words "You should leave," but your response will vary according to your fluency in the art of communication. If you rely only on the words themselves, you might respond, "Yes, I probably should get going." But what about the accompanying body language?

You **should** leave: The speaker is relaxed and smiling. He looks at his watch and realizes that it's time for your next class, so **you SHOULD leave.** He is enjoying the conversation but is concerned that you'll be late.

You should leave: The speaker moves close to you and his face is expressionless. He looks at his watch and says angrily that **YOU should leave.** He isn't at all concerned about your punctuality. And at the moment, he doesn't care much about leaving for his class either. He wants *you* out. NOW!

You should **leave:** The speaker backs away from you and his eyes are little more than slits. His mouth is set and his lips barely move as he grabs at his watchband and hisses that **you should LEAVE.** The message is that you've done enough already—he doesn't want you to breathe, flinch or talk. He wants you to *leave* and never, ever think of coming back!

We think you get the message. Words, voice inflections, facial expressions, gestures, body posture and positioning all communicate subtle (or not so subtle!) messages. An ADDer can repeatedly face social slippery spots as he attempts to negotiate around the obstacles to successful communication. Let's examine just two particularly dangerous hazards before we move on to issues of various relationships in our lives.

Hazard—Social Slippery Spots!

Social Slippery Spot #1—Basic Manners: We would venture to say that most of us with ADD need to proceed very cautiously in this area. We're not saying that ADDers have cornered the market on bad manners. But societal conventions of politeness can be hazards because of our particular differences.

When people talk about good manners, they're usually talking about rule-governed speech and behavior. Grandparents brag about their well-mannered grandchild, and teachers admonish their students to show better manners. Good manners require adequate communication skills that include an ability to monitor behavior and pay close attention to detail. Since these skills can be shaky in an ADDer, he may behave in an unmannerly fashion, making errors of both omission and commission:

> Teacher: "I will thank you to keep those opinions to yourself!"
> You: "Oh, you're welcome!"
>
> Woman whose place in line you just took over: "Well, excuse me!"
> You: "Oh, am I in your way?"

An ADDer may fail to say "Excuse me" when he jostles someone (omission) and interrupt and monopolize conversations (commission). He probably knows the rules but haphazardly applies them. Since these skills may not come naturally to him, he needs to make a conscious effort to learn and practice the behavior expected of adults in our society.

KK: "When I first lived away from home, I remember being shocked that the rest of the world didn't function the way my family did. Since most of my family were affected to some degree by ADD, we developed a style of interaction based on behavior that came naturally to us. Mealtimes were a free-for-all, with everyone talking at once and no one listening. Interrupting was normal behavior. It was a revelation to discover that most people take turns talking and listening to each other!"

PR: "The ADD Council's hotline coordinator shared a humorous anecdote with me. He had a conversation with a repeat caller who usually spoke with one particular phone volunteer.

When he suggested that the caller speak with the volunteer she had previously spoken to, she replied, 'Oh, I don't have enough time to talk with "Melissa." She's been a great help but she'll talk so much and keep me on the phone so long that I'll forget the one question I needed to ask!'"

"I don't know who the phone volunteer was, but it could have been me! As ADDers sometimes do, if I'm not careful, I can get carried away with a one-sided conversation. I become so involved with sharing my advice and experiences that I forget the cardinal rule of effective communication: LISTENING!

"I have gotten much better at this but sometimes fall into old habits. I sometimes have to put my hand over the mouthpiece of my phone to cue myself to stop talking. Perhaps the Council's phone line coordinator should teach this trick to his talkative volunteer!"

Even if an ADDer avoids clearly rude actions and bad manners, his social life can be hampered by the general fogginess of ADD. He may be unable to clear the clouds sufficiently to really connect with other people. "Is anyone home?" . . . "Earth to Mark!" . . . "What a space cadet!" . . . He may be so vague and dreamy that he doesn't seem to exist in the real world.

He may be ridiculed for being out to lunch or rebuked for caring only about himself. He doesn't mean to be rude or uncaring, but his failure to respond can look like selfishness.

Social Slippery Spot #2—The Telephone: A great deal of daily communication is conducted by telephone. Telephones are a great invention, but they sometimes do a terrible disservice to ADDers. It's not that we fail to appreciate the convenience, but we're not too crazy about the uncanny ability of a telephone to change our personalities!

Have you ever met someone for the first time after talking to him only by phone and been amazed at the difference? Can this bright, fascinating person really be the same character who seemed so dull on the telephone? What about the sparkling telephone conversationalist who becomes almost mute in face-to-face encounters?

The telephone can also cause a remarkable change in our dispositions. Perhaps you can identify with this phenomenon of Telephone Transformation:

PR: "I suffer from TTTS: Testy Telephone Tyrant Syndrome! A ringing telephone can transform me into a mean, confrontational person. If you are the unfortunate individual who walks into the room when I'm on the phone, you will endure scathing looks. If you make the mistake of making noise or talking to me, you'll endure far worse. Simply stated, *I get nasty!* My children watch in continual amazement as their relatively even-tempered mother transforms into a screaming meanie!

"I have never understood the power this inanimate object wields. When the phone rings, I instantly go into a stance of defense or attack. I wait, hoping someone else will answer the incessant ringing. After the third or fourth ring, I reluctantly answer it, after announcing that 'Nobody better interrupt me during this call.' If my warning goes unheeded, my family is in for the assault of the telephone tyrant!"

KK: "Before either of us knew anything about ADD, my husband used to accuse me of having a disease he called Phone-a-Phobia. He claimed I inherited it from my mother, who has similar symptoms."

A phobia is a fear out of proportion to the actual threat in a situation, and people with phobias generally try to avoid the situations they fear. Some ADDers do avoid using the telephone. The avoidance, however, isn't a phobic reaction to inappropriate anxiety or fear—they have real problems with telephone communication.

The problem is sometimes an inability to process the meaning of words without the visual clues of body language. Telephone conversations may be peppered with silences, requests for the speaker to repeat himself and charming phrases such as "Uh" and "Um." An ADDer may forget to identify himself, leave out important information or abruptly end the conversation.

An inability to filter out background noise also contributes to the difficulty with telephone conversations. An ADDer can become a telephone tyrant as he fights to shut out noises and interruptions. Listening and making sense of communication is hard enough work without having to contend with outside interferences.

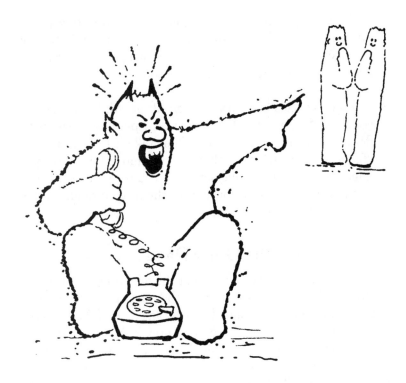

Survival Tips for the Telephone

The telephone may never be your preferred mode of communication, but there are some things you can do to make it more user-friendly. Here are a few telephone strategies that may reduce your Phone-a-Phobia and TTTS:

- Rehearse and write down what you're going to say before you make a call—your greeting, the major points you want to make and the way you'll politely end the conversation.

- Keep your notes in front of you during the call to jog your memory.

- Stick to your script to avoid the "wandering" conversation.

- Make your phone calls in a quiet, distraction-free place. Also, get yourself a cordless phone with a headset. This arrangement will cut down on the background noise and allow you to wander around while you talk.

- If someone calls and catches you off guard, briefly excuse yourself, saying you'll have to switch phones, answer the door or return the call later. Then take a few minutes to compose yourself and gather any written information you might need for the conversation. If you have taken the call in a noisy area of your house, take the time to request quiet or switch to another phone.

On the Other Hand . . .

You may be surprised to discover that the telephone can become your friend. We wrote this section on the trials and tribulations of the telephone many years ago, before doing a lot of ADD recovery work. Believe it or not, we both now happily spend many hours per day on the phone, coaching our clients. If you remove the surprise factor by answering the phone only when you are ready to take a call, the telephone can be neutralized as an instrument of torture. Phone headsets also make a big difference.

One of the big advantages of phone coaching is that the visual distractions are decreased. We also know from experience that it is a lot easier to talk about embarrassing things when you don't have to be face-to-face. Most ADD coaching is done by phone. Don't let your phone-a-phobia stop you from taking advantage of one of the most effective tools for ADD recovery.

With this general framework of communication and interactions in place, we'll turn our attention to the art of relating in group and one-to-one encounters. As you consider these issues, your guiding principle should be the theme of this book—maximizing your strengths and minimizing your weaknesses. Don't attempt to become like people with calm temperaments. You'll fail miserably and lose sight of the plus side of your inventory. Since we're advocates of the open-book test, we encourage you to keep your inventory notes handy as you continue reading! We'll test you at the end of the book. (Only kidding . . .)

Relationships: A Play with Multiple Acts and a Cast of Many Characters

If the world were filled with fellow ADDers, many of us would probably do just fine in our relationships. With our personal experience with ADD, we would understand the "quirks" of the ADDers around us. Of course, the world is made up of a variety of different kinds of people, many of whom can't figure us out at all! If we're going to fit in, we have to figure out how to communicate with and relate to others.

You may need to completely reprogram your mental computer to improve its interfacing capabilities. You may have unique strengths in this area and need only minor adjustments to your program. You may already be using your identified strengths to bypass any weaknesses in this area of functioning. You may have a keen sense of humor and vivid imagination that attract people and repair the damage of a social faux pas. You may be judiciously using your disinhibition—saying or doing things other people censor—to develop a frank and open communication style that disarms others and puts them at ease.

Act I: The Art of Relating in Groups

We live, work and play in groups—families, social clubs, meetings and committees. We can't avoid these interactions even if we wanted to. If you are like many bright, enterprising ADD adults, you may face group situations with about as much enthusiasm as you do a trip to the dentist! What can you do to prevent the social suicide you fear? To help you with this issue, let's observe some social situations in action.

Michael

Michael is standing in a cluster of four people who have been talking about a variety of topics. He hasn't added much to the conversation because he doesn't know anything about the latest software or the movement to protect endangered caterpillars. His brain is racing to think of *something* to say before somebody asks him something he won't know how to answer.

He is preoccupied with planning his verbal entrance to the conversation and vaguely hears a comment about recent activity in the Oval Office. Since he's a builder with a specialty in custom renovation, he eagerly jumps in with his account of an interesting circular room he once built.

It suddenly occurs to him, halfway through his story, that something isn't quite right. He looks up to see four faces etched with question marks! He gradually realizes the enormity of his blunder and slinks away with a halfhearted chuckle: "Oval Office . . . White House . . . I knew that. I just wanted to see if you were paying attention."

Amanda

Between bursts of small talk with her two companions, Amanda twists around to watch her friend Michael humiliate himself. She asks of no one in particular, "Can you believe he just said that?" She quickly switches gears as she observes that her companion's tie looks just like the one her uncle Joe used to wear. To her companion's comment about the benefits of using glass instead of paper products, Amanda asks, "Do funeral directors recycle the dearly departed loved one's clothing? The reason I'm asking is that your tie looks exactly like the one Uncle Joe wore at his funeral."

She laughingly assures both men that she's only kidding and wonders if they've noticed how many people have already left the party and if they have any suggestions about what she should say to Michael about acting so stupid.

Elizabeth

Elizabeth is standing with a large group near the buffet table. An animated conversation about the plight of the homeless is so engrossing that everyone ignores the delicious food. Elizabeth is the only person in the group who isn't saying anything. Her eyes look glazed and her face is expressionless. To the woman who asks her opinion about this serious topic, she replies with a yawn, "Oh, I don't really know." Someone else offers to drive her home in case she's been drinking too much and needs to sleep it off.

Notes: Act I

Mental Gymnastics: Do you remember the discussion about dividing attention and shifting gears? They are a kind of mental athletics. Successful group interfacing depends on an ability to shift gears rapidly. The exchange of conversation is a challenging task for an ADDer who can't make quick mental adjustments. He has to follow the flow of talk as it bounces from person to person. He has to concentrate enough to understand what the speaker is saying. He also has to be sure he doesn't get locked in. Otherwise, he comes to a grinding halt while the general conversation goes on without him.

Some of us take mental time-outs to process the conversation. Remember our slow reaction time? A break can give us time to deal with our less than trustworthy memories. We may be so intent on frantically rehearsing and remembering what we're going to say that we block out everything else. We do mental handsprings as fast as we can. Unfortunately, we often end up interjecting seemingly irrelevant comments. We're talking about spring soccer when the conversation moved on five minutes earlier to the winter Olympics.

Creative thinking also plays into the mental athletics. Rather than getting locked in and taking a time-out, an ADDer's mind may move at breakneck speed, taking a detour at the end of the track! A comment during the conversation stimulates an idea that sends him on a wild, imaginative journey. Several laps later he ends his little detour and shares some tidbit. His comment is greeted with either raised eyebrows or replies of "What the hell are you talking about?"

The comment that makes perfect sense to him is incomprehensible to the rest of the group. They didn't go on the mental journey with the ADDer and don't know where he's been. If he's among friends, they'll probably just shrug it off. If he's with strangers, they might wonder what planet he comes from!

Running Out of Gas: There are other reasons for an ADDer's difficulties with group interactions. The atmosphere of a group can be intensely stimulating. Impaired attention and a defective sensory filter can be pushed beyond their capabilities. Attention can jump from a companion's perfume to the crackling fire across the room. Where should he focus—on the speaker's words or on the body language of the person standing next to him? Bombarded with sights and sounds from many different directions, his senses rapidly reach an uncomfortable level of overload. Similar to a car climbing a long mountain road, he quickly uses up his reserves of fuel. He may run out of mental gas.

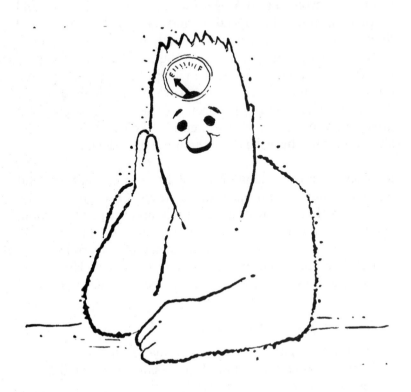

Have you ever been in a stimulating group situation feeling as if you've just taken a sleeping pill or gone into a coma? We have. It's as if the body stays in the same spot while the brain goes off to a quiet corner somewhere to rest and regroup. That's just great for your brain, but what about you? You end up standing there with a blank look and a yawn. You may not exactly endear yourself to the speaker who is sharing fascinating information.

It's not that the conversation is boring, although it might be! It's that the overstimulation of a group situation causes mental fatigue. Simply put, an ADDer might either tune out or fall asleep. That's precisely what happened to Elizabeth, who attributes her poor social skills to a lack of sleep.

Cruise Controls Set on Mega-Speed: Conversely, the mental cruise control may be flipped on and set way above the speed limit. The Porsche is revved and ready to go! Foot-in-mouth disease escalates out of control as the ADDer barrels around the track, heedless of anyone who might be in his way. With a poor sense of boundaries, he may careen, literally and figuratively, into other people. He fidgets too much, talks too fast and drives everyone crazy with his intensity. The people around him alternately view his behavior as amusing or annoying.

Impulsivity and disinhibition are sometimes attempts to fend off mental fatigue and maintain alertness. Of course, no one else knows that! Many of us often talk and act first and think later. As Amanda does, we may fill up physical and emotional space with our presence and chatter. Inappropriate, rude or silly remarks are out of our mouths before we know it! How many times have you said to yourself, "I can't believe I just said that."

Synopsis: Act I

It might seem that you process information too slowly when you're in a group conversation. Is it possible, however, that you process the information *in greater depth* than others do? Do you make connections that elude everyone else and have real value? It might seem that your mental detours are inappropriate, but that doesn't mean they're worthless. Perhaps your tangents and wild leaps of imagination can lead the group to creative problem solving.

And here's something interesting to think about. Are your problems in groups caused by your deficits or by *the rules for interaction that are ill suited to your style of thinking?*

KK: "With professional experience as a group leader, I mentally geared up for a difficult challenge when I agreed to start an ADD adult support group. I pictured a group of people talking nonstop, interrupting each other and jumping from topic to topic. I figured my main function as the facilitator would be to referee.

"What happened is vastly different from what I imagined. The flow of ideas does jump around a lot, but this doesn't seem to be an obstacle to the group process. Generally, the group as a whole is able to follow the logic of the conversation and sometimes moves it off into wonderful, productive tangents. The tempo is much faster than I have encountered in other groups. But group members, often left behind in 'normal' groups, are able to keep up with the speedy conversation."

The logic of an ADD thinker is a different brand from that of linear folks. His logic, formulated by the generalizations and connections of his distractions, may in some ways be superior to the logic taught in school. It makes sense that if he could play by his own set of logical rules, his communication would flow more freely.

The dance of conversation in an ADD group seems to move to music entirely different from that of other groups. It seems to have its own unique rhythm, tempo and patterns. Perhaps we ADDers don't need dancing lessons after all. We may just need to dance to our own ADD beat!

If you have an ADD friend, get together and enjoy the dance you share. Of course, you can't always dance to your own beat, just as you can't always do what your impulses drive you to do. Since you can't avoid being in groups of non-ADDers, you'll have to learn some of the conventional steps. Here are some survival tips that might help you on the dance floor.

Survival Tips: Act I

Be Prepared: Before you arrive at the social gathering, make sure you're prepared. Start taking notes as a newspaper reporter would. Find out who will be there and write down their names, occupations, interests, etcetera. If you're lucky, somebody else who loves radio-controlled race cars as much as you do will be in attendance. Ask about the dress "code" so you won't arrive in jeans while everyone else is wearing suits and ties. Make sure you write down the date and time of the gathering! Arriving for a dinner party an hour late will definitely not win rave reviews from your host.

Do Your Homework: If your mind and mouth inexplicably shut down in group settings, rehearse ahead of time. Part of this rehearsal can be keeping up, at least superficially, with current events. This doesn't mean you have to sit down on a daily basis with the lengthy *New York Times*. It does mean that you might want to know that "the changing nuclear family" isn't a topic about folks glowing in the dark with radiation poisoning!

The value in having an awareness, however vague, of names, places and events in the news is that it provides a file of information on which you can draw. If the subject turns to the primaries, you won't interject a comment about your son's experiences in the primary grades of your local school. Instead you might offer, "Campaign activity is really heating up, isn't it? I haven't seen the paper the past few days. Is there anything new going on?"

Practice: Rehearsing means just that. Write a script. Rehearse. Practice. When you arrive, what will you say to the host? How will you join a conversation? What words will you use? How will you introduce yourself? How will you respond to the inquiry "What do you do for a living, Don?" Develop a standard script for these questions that come up in groups. Then practice it with a spouse or friend or in front of a mirror.

When you work on your script, consider ways you can respond to information shared by others. After you've answered the inquiry about what you do for a living, how do you respond when somebody tells you about his job?

> *Someone asks: "What do you do for a living, Don?"*
> *You start your script: "I restore antique furniture. What's your job, Fred?"*
> *Fred replies: "I'm a media center specialist."*
> *You comment: "Oh, really . . ."*

The conversation stops dead in its tracks. What happens now? Rather than feeling uncomfortable and trying to fill the dead space with rambling, you can refer to your memorized script of canned responses. Questions are excellent because they keep the conversation going and draw attention away from you. Generic comments can bail you out if you have no idea what a media center specialist is. A rehearsed list of questions and comments can also help with any problems you have with monopolizing conversations. Try some of these scripts and add some of your own:

> "How did you get interested in that area?"
> "I don't know very much about that field. What exactly does your work entail?"
> "Have you always done this work or did you start off in a different field?"
> "That sounds like an interesting job. Can you tell me more about it?"

The focus of the conversation will probably come back to you after this question-and-answer period. By then you should have found some familiar territory and will be able to talk comfortably about a subject you know. You may get in a bind and exhaust the items in your script. If this happens, you can excuse yourself to make a phone call or to ask the host something. Include these *emergency exit* techniques during your rehearsal. Also include your spouse or friend in your practice sessions so you'll have someone to bail you out when you need help.

If you're a member of a support group, you can learn about your behavior by watching yourself. Arrange for a video or audio recording of your group's interactions. Although the camera might be somewhat distracting, you can learn a lot when you review the tape.

This is a valuable process for reviewing what you did well, not just the areas marked "needs improvement." If you're a member of an ongoing support group, you might be able to tape a series of sessions. You can use the tapes to monitor your progress as

161

you practice new ways of behaving. Of course, this idea presupposes that you feel comfortable in the group and that none of the members objects to being taped.

Watch and Listen: When you're with an unfamiliar group of people, initially keep a low profile. Look and listen a lot and talk very little. Watch the others to see how they behave. Find out how much personal information people share with each other and try to figure out any unspoken rules. Most groups have informal codes of conduct that govern the behavior of members. The hidden code may tell you which subjects are taboo, where to sit or even how to dress.

We don't advocate blind conformity to rules or buying into the idea that you must fit in. It will be up to you to decide whether to continue your association with a particular group. You can, however, make a reasonable attempt to be cordial and respectful of the group's rules at least for one evening. If nothing else, use the evening to practice your conversational skills.

Watch Your Watch: Focus on the speaker. Force yourself to make eye contact. Pay close attention to the dance of conversation and don't give a solo performance. Before you start talking, make sure you aren't interrupting. Make it a practice to ask the speaker if he has finished before you jump in and cut off his next thought.

Wear a watch with a second hand and unobtrusively note how long each person speaks. When it's your turn, time yourself. Set a mental alarm clock to *turn yourself off* if you exceed your allotted time. Watching your watch can also help you maintain focus as it gives you something to do. In case somebody notices you watching your watch, you can always claim that the battery seems to be wearing out. It's better to wear out your battery than your audience!

Watch Your Wandering: Pay close attention to the number of tangential journeys you take so you won't start jumping all over, monopolizing the conversation. In a safe group of friends, ask someone to signal you when you're getting off track. If all else fails and you're off and running before you know it, acknowledge your rambling. Say something like, "Boy, my mind is really on a mental marathon, isn't it? Sorry about that . . ."

Work on Your Reading Skills: Remember that people communicate through verbal and nonverbal channels. You'll need to practice reading both kinds of language. The verbal channel uses the voice as the instrument to produce words, while body language and facial expressions provide valuable clues about the impact of your behavior.

If you notice a look of horror, it's a good bet that your words sent an unintended message—unless, of course, you wanted that particular reaction! Immediately apologize if you know your words were impulsive. If you hate to apologize, grit your teeth and do it anyway! Think of it as balancing your checkbook or doing push-ups. It's not fun but it makes life easier in the long run.

If you don't know what caused the negative reaction, ask! You could say, "I noticed you frowned when I said such-and-such. Is there a problem?" An alternative is to make a joke about your impulsivity. You could say something like, "I have a bad case of foot-in-mouth disease today. Please let me know if I've said or done anything out of line." A lighthearted approach can make it easier for the other person to provide feedback about your behavior.

Welcome the Feedback: When you receive the feedback, *listen to it!* The advice is three simple words. Responding appropriately to comments about your behavior, however, is anything but simple! Your tendency might be to put up your shield and go into *automatic defense-and-attack mode.* Leave your shield at home or in the trunk of your car. Remember, you can't do this all by yourself. You need help.

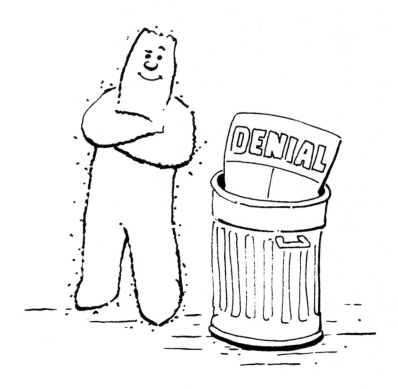

Think of this learning process as therapy. In physical therapy, for instance, the slogan used to inspire patients is "No pain, no gain." And of course, comments don't have to be negative. Don't be afraid to ask for positive feedback as well, and don't forget to thank the person for taking the time to help you.

Careful listening is hard, accepting criticism is harder and changing your behavior is the hardest of all. But these are essential parts of your recovery. Using feedback to change your behavior can have a powerful, positive impact on your social success.

Carefully Choose Your Social Activities: If you feel washed up and worn out after every social event, it might be time to reread the section on balance: Be honest with yourself: Do you attend these functions because you want to or because you feel compelled to? When an acquaintance shares his very full social calendar, do you feel somehow that you just don't measure up socially?

There may be some social events that you must attend. Prepare carefully for these and do the best you can, but *Just say "no"* to the others. Be selective, and base your decision on a realistic assessment of your abilities and disabilities. Small-group gatherings may work better for you.

This doesn't mean we are suggesting that you give up on learning and practicing your relating skills. You will need them everywhere from PTA meetings to office planning sessions. Just remember that there isn't a rule requiring you to be a social butterfly.

Act II: The Art of Relating in One-to-One Encounters

Some of us prefer large-group interactions that enable us to remain somewhat anonymous. We may feel far less comfortable in one-to-one relationships because it's impossible to hide. Our carefully constructed shields don't work well in close relationships that illuminate our shortcomings.

Even if your experiences in relationships have been unsuccessful, don't resign yourself to solitary confinement. If you've been working hard at your recovery, you have knowledge and skills you may have lacked before. Your newfound understanding about your balance sheet can support you as you risk the self-disclosure inherent in developing close relationships. You can be successful if you're aware of the potential pitfalls and design strategies to avoid them.

In Act II, we'll study some other relationships in action. These are the one-to-one encounters with friends and acquaintances. Let's see what we can learn from them.

Ken

Ken looks up to see Paul walking down the aisle. He runs over to him, expressing surprise and delight to see him again so soon after their first meeting. He asks if Paul received the three messages he left for him on his answering machine yesterday. He invites Paul to dinner that evening and without waiting for an answer, begins asking what his new friend would like to eat. Ken begins telling his new friend all about the cooking classes he's taking and what he's learned about designing healthy menus.

Carolyn

Carolyn invites Jason, her new neighbor, to join her for a cup of coffee. She talks briefly about the neighborhood and comments that she's sure he'll like it much better than where he used to live. Jason tells her that he'll miss the cookouts he used to have with his three neighbors. Carolyn responds by telling him not to worry about it. She tells him that in this neighborhood, fifteen families share a block party every summer! Carolyn refills her coffee but doesn't notice that Jason's is empty. She responds to his story about the tree house his son built in their old yard, by gazing out her back door. She advises, "Well, I bet with my son's help, your boy will be able to build a really great tree house in his new backyard."

Notes: Act II

Many of the rules for interactions are the same for both group and individual encounters. We must take turns listening and speaking, watch for nonverbal behavior and monitor verbal and nonverbal communication. Beyond these similarities, though, individual interactions require somewhat different skills.

Is your friendship mode similar to Carolyn's or Ken's? Don't worry if you identify with either of them, because they have a lot going for them. With some refinements, they could develop good interaction skills.

Ken shows genuine affection for Paul and is willing to work hard at developing this new friendship. What he needs to do is work equally hard at not working so hard! He needs to learn to redirect his focus from his needs to his friend's needs.

Then there's Carolyn. Desperately wanting her new neighbor to like her and his new neighborhood, she overwhelms him with her intensity. She needs to think about her words and review the messages she sends. She needs to watch Jason's body language and note his attempts to add comments to her one-way conversation. By singing the praises of her neighborhood, she's trying to help him adjust to his new home. Jason's body language would give her a good clue that she's sending an unintended message of boasting and "one-upping."

Synopsis: Act II

There's both good news and bad news for an ADDer in one-to-one social interactions. The good news is that these encounters put fewer demands on the ability to switch gears—there are fewer details to track and fewer people to read. The bad news is that tuning out is more obvious—the focus is on him with no one to run interference! He can't afford to take mind detours because there's no one to pick up and carry the conversational ball.

If you haven't come to terms with your disorder, one-to-one communication can be particularly scary. You might talk yourself into failure.

"What if she doesn't like me?"
"I don't have anything interesting to say."
"He's a professor and I barely finished high school!"
"What if I forget her name?"
"What if I run out of things to say?"

Engaging in negative self-talk is destructive because you look at only one side of your equation. Never forget the other side of your balance sheet! Henry Ford said, "Whether you think you can or whether you think you can't, you're right." If you run from potential friendships, you're acting and believing *you can't*. On the other hand, if you affirm yourself as a capable person who happens to have some disabilities, you are acting and believing *you can*.

Many of us have excellent people skills. We can learn to be great listeners, locking in our focus to give a flattering level of attention to the other person. The rhythm of the exchange is slower and easier to follow in one-to-one encounters. We can focus intently, noticing things that others miss and offering sensitive and empathic support.

You may be fortunate to have a close friend. You may have several close friends. But if your friendships are rocky or shorter-lived than you'd like them to be, you may need to get to work. As you think about your own skills in one-to-one relationships, consider these tips. They may be useful and give you added confidence in these situations.

Survival Tips: Act II

Relax and Listen: Don't feel you have to fill every second with conversation. ADDers tend to go to extremes, talking a mile a minute or completely tuning out. Some silence is okay. If you check out altogether, your companion will think you're not interested in what he has to say.

The key to maintaining a correct balance between the two extremes is active listening. Active listening enables you to interact without filling up the conversation with your words. Send a message that you are listening and interested in what your companion has to say by nodding your head, leaning forward and maintaining eye contact.

Watch his body language and pay attention to the message it sends. Interject comments that let your companion know you are listening.

"Go on" . . . "Tell me more" . . .
"Could you explain that a little more?"

If you find yourself talking excessively or feeling uncomfortable at a lull in the conversation, share your confusion:

"Am I talking too much?" . . . "I've run out of things to talk about" . . . "Do you have any ideas?"

Clarify the Message: Remember that communication is an art form. The clarity of the message has an impact on the listener's understanding. Moreover, each of us interprets language from an individual frame of reference. The intent of the message can be misinterpreted regardless of how clearly it is stated.

Statement: "Things are a mess in this house."

Possible Interpretations: "He's accusing me of being a slob."
"He's telling me to clean up the house."
"He's just noticing and commenting on the state of the house."

Although history may support the first statement, don't jump to conclusions. To avoid communication misunderstandings, clarify the way you interpreted the message—restate it in your own words.

Restated Interpretations: "Are you trying to say that I should do something about the mess in the house?"
"When you said that, I thought you were criticizing me. Is that true?"

Effective Clarification: "I thought you said . . ." or "Were you saying . . ."

Avoid "Fightin' Words": We talked about the importance of active listening. To ensure that your companion will interpret your message accurately, take great care with the words you use. One surefire method for shutting down the channels of communication is using the words "you always" or "you never." Strike them from your vocabulary unless you want a full-scale battle to erupt! These words feel threatening and accusatory. They assign blame and create feelings of defensiveness. Even if your spouse rarely remembers your anniversary, he has been around for fifteen years and remembering dates may be difficult for him.

A better technique is to rephrase your words as *I-messages* to communicate your feelings about how something affects you. When you use *You-messages*, you direct the focus to your listener and force him to argue his position. Here are some examples of the differences between these two kinds of messages:

I-message:	"When you didn't call yesterday, I wondered if you were mad at me."
You-message:	"You never call when you say you will."
I-message:	"When you start talking before I'm finished, I feel that what I have to say is unimportant."
You-message:	"Why do you interrupt me all the time?"

Watch your listener's body language. If he looks puzzled, stop talking. Ask him to clarify his understanding of what you said. He may be hearing something very different from what you're trying to say.

There are many other useful communication techniques, but we hope you get the idea from these examples. It might be helpful to increase your learning experiences by taking part in a class or group that practices these skills. The communications department of a local university would be a good place to look for this kind of training.

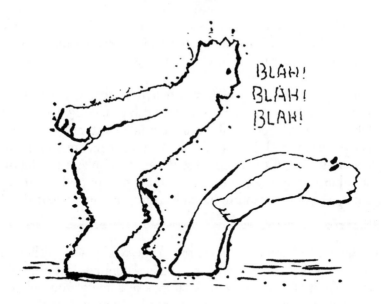

Watch Your Intensity Level: ADD adults can be intense, passionate and single-minded about personal interests. If you're not careful, you can scare a calmer person to death!

Be cautious when you find yourself discussing one of your favorite subjects or pet peeves. If you find the other person mentally or physically backing off, lighten up! Tell a joke, ask a question or change the subject.

An ADDer can get carried away with a topic because of his intensity. It can also cause a more general problem that pervades the whole relationship. He often overwhelms other people with the ferocity of his friendship. He might shower a friend with sincere but excessive flattery that leaves her feeling embarrassed or wondering if he's really teasing. As Ken does, he might get physically too close, oblivious of the other person's need for space.

Slow Down: Even if an ADD adult is adept at verbal and nonverbal communication, he can have difficulty maintaining a friendship over the long haul. He doesn't want to wait for the natural progression of phases in developing relationships. He may not be attuned to the pacing and gradual easing into involvement, trying to get too close, too fast.

If this is a problem for you, it may help to keep a diary or calendar that tracks your behavior in friendship-making. Don't just pick up the phone to call your new acquaintance until you check your journal. Pencil in when you make a contact and jot down notes about the encounter, paying particular attention to the other person's response. Indicate in your journal a date for your next contact, and don't call or drop in before that date!

In the next chapter we move on to the workplace. Although our focus will be on issues of relating and communication, we'll also do a brief task analysis. We'll look at some of your *jobs on the job* and offer some suggestions for improving your skills in some of them. We'll also look at your *relationship to your job,* to help you analyze any failures you may be experiencing. This analysis will include the important question: Are you failing on your job or is your job failing you?

CHAPTER 7

The Art of Relating: Getting Along on the Job

Careers can be made or destroyed based on how well we get along with other people on the job. There are elements of both one-to-one relationships and group interactions. The one-to-one relationships of employees aren't close friendships but require similar maintenance over time. Likewise, the group interactions of employees are different from social gatherings in that they are ongoing.

In the one-to-one relationships of friendships you can choose the people with whom you'll share your time and personal involvement. The same is true of the social gatherings you attend—you can choose to skip a party if you aren't crazy about the people who will be there. But you can't choose the employees with whom you'll interact and you can't choose the meetings you'll attend. You have to interact with your coworkers in a variety of settings.

The workplace is a social arena and arguably a political one as well. Success on the job requires good interpersonal relationships and an ability to understand the "politics" within the work setting. These dynamics create some unique problems for an ADDer with shaky communication skills. With her friends, she can count on a degree of understanding about her ADD. With her colleagues, she has to manage her deficits with great finesse.

As an adult with ADD, your success in the work world is also largely dependent on how well you get along with your job. Because of your particular deficits and differences, you have to carefully build a safety net for your job as you do for the other parts of your life. Are there some strategies you can use to improve the quality of your work? How can you make your job work for you? Is your job the best match for your particular abilities and disabilities? In this chapter, we'll expand our discussion to include these specific aspects of job management.

Act III: Getting Along on the Job

Diane

Diane found her niche in sales and quickly became a top saleswoman. Single-handedly she increased the sales volume of her department after being on the job only a few months. Her hard work and talents were rewarded with large commissions, bonuses and a promotion to the position of Sales Manager.

Three months later, Diane started taking aspirin on a daily basis and considered getting back into therapy. She recently found a crumpled piece of paper on the floor and is trying to figure out what to do about it. The paper is a caricature of her drawn by one of her salesmen. In the picture she is towering over her sales force, clutching a huge megaphone in both hands. Words are shooting out of the megaphone and raining down like fireworks on her "subjects" below.

Notes: Act III

Diane is a hardworking, energetic and creative ADD woman. She's an excellent employee whose performance has been noted and rewarded by her superiors. So what is going wrong for her?

There are probably a number of explanations for the problems Diane is experiencing in her job. The most obvious is that her managerial skills aren't as good as her selling skills. Selling a product isn't the same as selling people on one's ideas for managing a sales force. Diane's social deficits may have caught up with her. Although she rose rapidly to an administrative position, she is learning that staying up there is tricky.

Diane's impulsivity may play a role in her problems. She is a can-do woman who is used to getting the job done—now! When her salespeople don't solve problems as fast as she does, she grabs her megaphone and starts issuing directives. She greets a question about her policies as a hindrance to her sales figures. She can't understand why some of her employees refuse to work the same fifty or sixty hours she does every week. She rants and raves that she has to do the work or it would never get done.

Synopsis: Act III

The work environment is a minisociety governed by rules formulated to protect the rights and establish the responsibilities of the people who work there. The relationships in a work environment are affected by the positions people hold, individual personalities and job responsibilities and multiple interpersonal relationships. Although ADD adults may have some unique problems in this work setting, they are only one part of the equation.

Large, complex organizations have a great potential for breakdown. Many people are part of work relationships and some of them also have ADD or other disabilities. This makes for some very interesting situations! Consider, for example:

> *The boss who never seems to listen and who asks the impossible of you.*
>
> *The coworker who doggedly sticks to her job description even when deadlines loom and colleagues are desperate for help.*
>
> *The boss who continually makes his emergency yours.*
>
> *The coworker who adamantly refuses to take responsibility for a screwup.*

There isn't much you can do about the hidden agendas of fellow employees. If you remember that you're only one piece of the puzzle, you can view a situation from its proper perspective. When a work relationship unravels, don't assume that it's exclusively your fault—or your unreasonable colleague's. Perhaps she's struggling with deficits similar to yours. As an adult with ADD, you should be sensitive to the needs of colleagues who might also have hidden disabilities.

What does all this mean for you? It means you really have your work cut out for you! To be successful in the world of work, you'll need to review many of the things we've talked about in previous sections of this book. Review your inventory and pay close attention to your balance sheet. It will be an invaluable framework as you begin to develop your management strategies. If Diane paid attention to hers, she might decide to give up the higher pay and executive title to do what she does best—sell products. Let's take a look at some ideas for dealing with problems in the world of work.

Survival Tips: Act III

Rules, Procedures and Policies
Many ADDers hate to swallow these bitter pills; unfortunately, there's no way to sweeten them! Unless you own your own company, you will be playing by someone else's rules.

Much as you may hate your policy handbook, study it anyway. It outlines your company's system of government and chain of command—such as who reports to whom and areas of individual responsibilities. It's not a good idea to leave this homework undone! Get very clear about where you fit within the overall structure, to avoid overstepping your bounds or failing to carry out your responsibilities.

Make Sense of the Rules: Try to understand their rationale. When you're away from work, talk with your spouse or a close friend about them. Make a list of all the policies you disagree with and analyze each of them. Do some have validity for the organization as a whole even though you personally disagree with them? If so, you may need to bite the bullet and learn to live with them, sigh!

Perhaps you can set up a reward system as a motivating tool. You may decide that not being allowed to listen to rock music in the office is totally unfair. You can't change the rule, but you can reward yourself for following it by treating yourself to a favorite tape during your break.

Question the Rules Carefully: You've probably heard the adage "Rules are made to be broken." We suggest you modify the words slightly: "Rules are made to be changed." If a rule doesn't seem to make sense for you individually or for the company as a whole, question it. Make sure your communication skills, particularly your listening skills, are solidly in place. Think through the rule you're disputing and approach the appropriate person with your question. And then *listen.*

If you receive the response "because I'm your boss," you can forget about doing anything beyond swallowing your objections and toeing the line. On the other hand, if your superior offers information you had overlooked, thank her for entertaining your ideas. At least you'll have a reading on her as someone who is willing to negotiate. The door will be open for future exchanges.

Sell Your Ideas: Although it's unwise to challenge authority at every turn, questioning policies and procedures can be a positive quality. Just don't move too fast. Keep your impulsivity in check and proceed s-l-o-w-l-y and tactfully. Don't start shaking things up after you've been on your new job exactly forty-five minutes!

No one in the company will buy your ideas if you are an unknown quantity. First, demonstrate your loyalty and dependability. Work on building positive relationships. Spend time keeping a low profile and doing what you're expected to do. Arrive at work on time, take one hour for lunch and not a minute more, and don't take advantage of your sick days. After you've earned the respect of your superiors and coworkers, you can start making suggestions for change.

If you have a great proposal, try it out on a trusted person in the informal office network to see if it's workable. She can help you evaluate its merits and confirm that you've included all the necessary facts before you formally present it.

Letting the boss think she came up with your idea is a time-honored method to facilitate change. A carefully conceived proposal that focuses on the benefits for her as an individual and the company as a whole, can also work. Make sure you do your homework first. If you come up with a new system for order processing without bothering to find out that the old one is your boss's "baby," you probably won't be in her good graces!

Unwritten Rules, Procedures and Policies

You won't find everything you need to know in the company's policy handbook. Much of the vital information is unwritten and is part of an informal network of office politics. This network is the office grapevine that reflects the complex dynamics of the people who work together. It holds the inside information about the real power structure in an organization. For instance, a secretary who isn't officially high on the chain of command may wield enormous power. With detailed knowledge about the company and ready access to the boss, she may have great influence within the company. The real chain of command may operate through her, bypassing the vice president who is simply a figurehead.

Get Inside the Inner Circle: If you have trouble figuring out the informal network, develop a relationship with someone who seems to know what's going on. Gradually draw her out to learn how the company operates. Take it easy, though. Usually the employees "in the know" are old-timers who have earned their status and play their roles to the hilt. If you try to make an instant friendship or start grilling someone over lunch, you may find her unwilling to divulge her knowledge. You'll need to earn her respect to enter the inner circle.

Follow the Unwritten Rules: If written policy dictates that memos should be sent to Mr. S and Ms. T, don't fail to send one to Mr. R if the unwritten rules call for it. Make a list of these informal procedures. Use your checklist to be sure you're following proper formal and informal procedures. Better still, you may want to carry a small calendar or notebook where you keep these confidential materials, especially if employees at your work site don't lock their desks.

Technology and Communication

Since we've already talked about the dynamics of communication in various relationships, we won't repeat ourselves. Review the information about communication skills and continually practice and rehearse. Our discussion and suggestions here will cover the dimensions of communication that are somewhat unique to work settings.

Communication is the transmission of messages from one person or group to another. We've focused on communication as spoken words and body language, but in the workplace it is frequently in the form of written expression. Businesses have always relied on written documentation and record keeping. Now there's a high-tech twist—the price sheet is faxed, the ad is scanned, the memo is e-mailed and the report is networked! This is another good news/bad news situation for ADDers.

For the Good News: High-tech equipment, particularly the computer, may be the best thing that's ever happened to an ADDer. It won't put gas in your car before your business trip but it can remind you to do it! It will check the spelling and grammar of your letters and send the contents, already formatted, to the printer. You don't even have to wait impatiently at the door for the mail carrier. In a flash, your computer or fax machine can send inquiries and receive responses.

For the Bad News: *Have you heard the joke about the employee who got his tie caught in the fax machine and ended up in New York?* Three things may have happened when you read this little tidbit:

1.**Nothing:**   You have no idea why this is funny because you have no idea what a fax machine is.

2.**You laughed:** If fax machines had this capability, you can think of at least one person in your office who would routinely end up in another state.

3.**You cried:**   If fax machines had this capability, you know that the person routinely ending up in New York would be you.

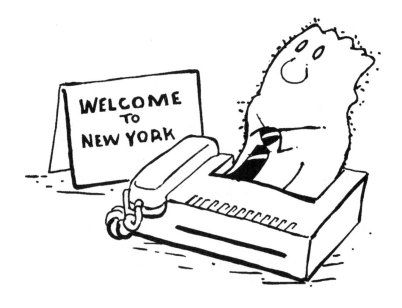

Each of these responses illustrates the disadvantages of modern technology. E-mail, networking, scanning and faxing may still evoke a fear response, never mind that these technologies have been around for a while. This isn't a reflection of your IQ! It's mind-boggling how rapidly new methods for transmitting information have developed.

While this book isn't a training manual for high-tech equipment, it wouldn't be complete without a discussion about technology's impact on communication. Even if you approach a TV remote control with fear and trepidation, you might have to use a fax machine and telephone that have more buttons than the front of your shirt!

Office Equipment and Cheat Sheets: Many people have trouble using mechanical or technical equipment. This isn't exclusively a problem for folks with ADD. But some of the ADD differences do compound the problem.

You've seen how increasing complexity has an impact on your performance. This is true whether you're doing math problems, interacting with large groups of people or figuring out how to use a complicated telephone system.

Related to this is an impaired memory. How many times have you approached the duplicating machine to hand-feed a two-sided document and couldn't remember how to do it? Ten tries later, with the wastebasket overflowing with pages reversed and printed upside down, you finally get it right! Not only have you wasted an entire package of paper, you've also wasted valuable time.

It's a good idea to make a cheat sheet for yourself. Make a list or chart of the procedures and tape it to the top of the duplicating machine. If you share the machine with others, you may need to keep your set of directions in your desk drawer. Do the same thing for the fax machine, computer, telephone, etcetera. You might find that this memory bypass system ultimately helps you to memorize the procedure because you use multisensory learning as an anchor. You *see* the directions as you *perform* them.

Written Expression—Memos, Letters and Reports: A computer can perform incredible feats if you are *computer comfortable.* You may find it very helpful in your job. It can relieve you of the tedium of details and become your personal secretary. Even if you use spell checkers and word processing programs, however, you might continue to have problems with written expression.

If the writing requirements of your job are primarily internal memos and business letters, consider buying an easy-to-use software package of templates. Templates are prepared generic letters for everything from order confirmations to congratulations for a colleague's job promotion. With the software, you choose a template that matches your need, change the names and dates and presto—you have a polished business document.

If your responsibilities include writing reports and other more complex documents, you can still use various templates as your framework, but you will need to do the actual writing yourself. Remedial writing classes may help you work on shaky writing skills. Consider working with a tutor, or check out continuing education classes at your local university.

Remember to use some of the bypass strategies we talked about in previous chapters. If you have a secretary, dictate your letters. Otherwise try using a tape recorder to "write" your first drafts. Your ideas may flow more easily if you talk first and write later. Show your work to a sympathetic colleague for a critique before you send it out.

Don't forget to use bartering as a tool to bypass your weak writing skills. For example, you can collaborate with a coworker who writes clearly but has problems generating original ideas. Together you may be able to write reports that outshine anything either of you could produce alone.

Work-Related Stress and ADD

An ADDer's boss may compliment her on the quality of her work but express concern about the quality of her relationships with coworkers. Superiors and subordinates alike might complain that working with her is difficult. They are probably commenting on her general irritability and moodiness, which are, of course, symptomatic of her disorder.

These symptoms typically get worse as demands from the environment increase. Their severity can be minimized by managing stress levels in the work environment. The general strategies taught in stress-management programs are useful, but there are others more specific for the unique problems of ADDers.

Noise, Doors and Telephones: First, try to figure out the source of your stress. If the source is everything about your job, you might be in the wrong vocation! Our guess is that noise probably contributes a great deal to your stress. Intrusions of noise can be very distracting and irritating.

If you have an office with a door you can shut for periods of time, take advantage of it! There are important reasons for keeping your door open. An opened door sends the message that you are available as an active participant in the work environment. But you have to balance the need to maintain work relationships with your need for quiet to handle the details of your job.

Explain to your coworkers that you can't concentrate on detailed work when there is excessive noise. Then close your door. You don't have to tell them about your ADD. Many people are bothered by noise and will understand your need to work without interruption. Just make it clear that this is *your* problem. You haven't closed your door because you don't like your coworkers!

You will win brownie points if you're available only during certain hours but are calm and welcoming when your door is open.

Even if this means taking some of your work home, it may be worth it if you can minimize your stress during work hours.

The same principle applies to the telephone. Your work quality and telephone manners might improve if you schedule a designated time for handling telephone calls. You'll accomplish much more without the constant interruptions. Before your scheduled telephone time, you'll have time to gather everything you'll need to handle the calls in a friendly and efficient manner.

You may be thinking "These ideas sound great, but I don't have any control over my schedule," or "I don't even have my own office." If you work in an open area where you can't close the door, is it possible for you to wear headphones when you need to concentrate? You could listen to music as you work or a tape of white noise if music is distracting.

Your boss might be more amenable to suggestions if you offer them as ways to improve your efficiency. Document your increased productivity to convince her that these strategies really work. Again, you don't have to share your diagnosis unless you're confident she'll act on your disclosure in a positive way.

If you feel that you have no control over your schedule, are you absolutely sure that's the case? A number of corporations have experimented with designated hours for employee phone calls. They have found that the decrease in interruptions throughout the day improves productivity. Approach your boss about this. Ask if your office or group could experiment with designated phone hours or even designated quiet time for work that requires heavy concentration.

Talk with coworkers to find out if noise and interruptions bother them. Chances are they probably also have trouble with excessive distractions. Enlist their support. You may be able to make changes in your workplace that will make the environment more user-friendly for everyone. It may be surprising to you, but these strategies are taught in time-management courses. You may elicit support for these changes under the guise of wanting to manage your time more effectively.

If you try everything and still can't control the noise and interruptions, think seriously about looking for a new job or even a different line of work. The stress level from a highly distracting environment can be a threat to your mental health. Are you failing, or is your work failing you?

Miscellaneous Strategies

For ease of reading we've tried to group the management strategies into categories. The ones that follow don't really fit anywhere else, so we've included them together in this section.

Take Your Medicine: This probably goes without saying, but if you need to take medicine to manage your symptoms, make sure you take it during your work hours. Your ability to handle details and interruptions will improve. Moreover, the condition of your fingernails and the anxiety of your office mate will probably also improve! As an ADD adult, you may not be in perpetual motion anymore but may have mastered the art of foot tapping, finger drumming and knuckle cracking. This constant fidgeting can be extremely annoying to other people. These behaviors are definitely not conducive to improving interpersonal work relationships.

Manage Your Symptoms: Actively work on your problematic ADD behaviors to decrease them or make them less noticeable. Try substituting a behavior that is less distracting to other people. Can you move your hands or swing your leg under the desk so that no one sees you doing it? Tapping your fingers against each other is quieter than kicking your desk or drumming your fingers on the desktop. Can you gnaw on the top of your pencil so you look as if you are deeply engrossed in your work?

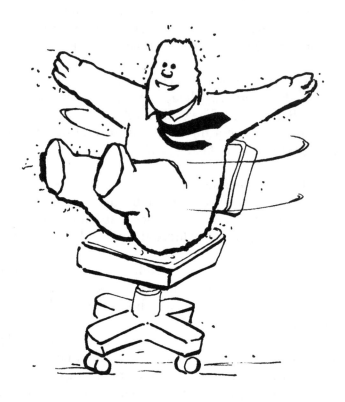

How about using your "closed door time" to spin happily on your desk chair? What about carefully spaced trips to the water fountain, file cabinet or duplicating machine? Volunteer to run needed errands. Find acceptable excuses to get up from your desk periodically.

Watch Your Foot-in-Mouth Disease: Have you ever filed a medical insurance claim for Foot-in-Mouth Disease? It may not be on the list of covered medical conditions, but if you have ADD, you probably have it! This condition causes an ADDer to spend most of her life with at least one foot in her mouth because she doesn't monitor what she says before she says it! It's no wonder she stumbles along in work relationships. Hopping on one foot while extricating the other from the mouth makes it difficult to manage the details of a job!

Of course we're talking about that troubling impulsivity of our ADD that keeps getting us in hot water. It got us poor grades in conduct on our school report cards and gets Diane an unsatisfactory grade as a manager. A thoughtless remark or a poorly worded memo can make enemies and even contribute to the loss of a job.

Our advice to you on this one is to be an **S.T.A.R.** Before you speak, act or approach someone, remind yourself to stop and think, look and listen. When you take action, reflect on the results of your actions. If necessary, glue a large **S.T.A.R.** on your desktop as a memory teaser for **S**topping, **T**hinking, **A**cting and **R**eflecting. It will take some effort to pull this off. You may need to reward yourself by finding a like-minded individual you can trust. Together, you can let off steam at lunch or during breaks.

Review Chapter 6 Again: All the issues we discussed in group and one-to-one relating apply to the work setting. Refer to the strategies in the previous chapter for continued work on interpersonal relationships and communication.

The remainder of this chapter is a departure from the format we've been following. We'll use this discussion to explore the question we posed earlier: Are you failing in your job, or is your job failing you?

What Do You Want to Do When You Grow Up?

Have you ever pored over the want ads in the newspaper looking for a job that matches your qualifications? How many times have you closed the newspaper without responding to even one inquiry because you couldn't find a match? Let your ADD imagination roam for a moment and pretend you've just seen the following ad:

WANTED
Fast-growing company looking for one special employee!
The perfect candidate will be someone who has:

difficulty with rules and authority,
ineffective communication skills,
trouble switching between tasks,
an intolerance to noise,
an inability to handle interruptions,
an irritable, moody, unpredictable and impatient personality,
an intrusive, impulsive and hyperactive behavior style.

Now, there's a job designed for ADDers! But let's get back to reality. The chances are slim to none that you'll ever come across an ad like that. Don't just toss it aside, though, until you take a closer look. To do this, you'll need to refer to your inventory again in Chapter 5. Use your creative thinking and growing awareness of your ADD advantages to hypothesize about ways to use both sides of the equation.

Negative OR	Positive Qualities?
difficulty with rules and authority	develops possibilities and solves problems
impaired communication skills	only with excessive complexity
trouble with switching gears	super focus + ability to get one job done well
intolerance to noise	super focus + ability to get one job done well—if it's quiet
inability to handle interruptions	super focus + ability to get one job done well—in small setting

188

irritability, impatience	shaking up complacency; getting things done
intrusive and impulsive	not so bad in a small setting; energizing
hyperactive	getting things done: stimulating

Whether you're twenty, forty or sixty years old, it's not too late to reassess some of your life choices. Your asset and liability sheet may help you evaluate the question about job failure. Perhaps the job you're in is dead wrong for you.

Vocational Planning: For our young ADD adult readers who are considering their future professions, pay careful attention to our want ad and list of positive and negative qualities. You may decide, based on your interest and math aptitude, that accounting is an obvious choice for you. Before you spend substantial time and money on a college education, give plenty of thought to your balance sheet. You may love math, but do you love details and paperwork? If not, the painstaking detail of accounting work may bore you to tears. If your real love is the creative, problem-solving aspect of mathematics, you might be happier in certain kinds of engineering or computer work.

If you can get by without the earnings of a summer job, consider using your free time to do volunteer work in your field of interest. You'll learn a great deal more about a profession by experiencing it firsthand than reading about it in a book.

Talk to people in the profession you're considering. Ask them detailed questions about what they do every day. Find out what they like and dislike about their work and think about how this fits with your new self-knowledge. Are you cut out for spending much of your working day writing lectures, grading papers and going to endless committee meetings? If not, you may need to rethink your decision about using your love of literature to become a college professor. Perhaps becoming a freelance writer would be a more rewarding choice.

If you want to attend college but have only a vague idea of your future career interests, try to attend a university that offers a variety of degree programs. Talk with a college counselor about the course work in various programs. Credits often apply across degree programs. You can use credits you've already earned in a new program if you decide to switch your major. If you plan carefully, you can save wasted time, effort and money.

You're Grown Up and Still Asking: "What Do I Want to Do When I Grow Up?"

Even if you've invested tons of money and time in your career and current job, you don't necessarily have to throw it all away. Before you decide to jump ship, thoroughly examine your current situation. In many careers there is latitude for change within the profession. Psychiatric and community health nursing, for example, require creative problem solving and a gestalt approach. Unlike hospital nursing, they don't include extensive detail work. In teaching, possibilities exist for a change of grade level or subject matter. There are also options for supervisory or counseling positions.

Find Your Niche: Perhaps the job you need is the one you already have, with a twist. You might be able to find or negotiate a job description that fits your abilities and offers unique benefits to your company. You may be thinking about beginning a degree program in counseling because you feel that you're wasting your people skills. Before you act on your decision, consider possibilities within your current organization.

Many businesses offer training and consultation services to their employees. Can you become the in-house trainer or consultant? With your individual talents and some seminar training, you can offer your services at a fraction of the cost your company typically incurs in hiring outside consultants. Your company may even be willing to pay for the additional training you'll need.

Match Yourself with Your Job—Start Your Own Business:
Maybe you're not a perfect candidate for someone's want ad
and will need to design a job to fit your qualifications. Is the
oversupply of rules and regulations, coupled with the snail's
pace of change in a large organization, unbearable? Perhaps you
could explore ways of working by and for yourself. The difficulties you experience in someone else's business may disappear
when the business is your own.

You may be able to use the niche you developed within your organization as a jumping-off place for other business opportunities. As
you continue to collect a paycheck and gain invaluable experience,
you can begin networking outside your company. You may at some
point decide to go off on your own and contract with your previous
employer and other related businesses to offer your services.

As a consultant, you have the advantage of being your own
boss. It can be easier to ignore arbitrary rules and rigid people if
you aren't a permanent employee. You don't have to get caught
up in the office politics and can move on when policies and
people start getting on your nerves. And it's usually easier to be
on your best behavior when you're in a new situation for only a
short time. You may also be able to retain some of the benefits
of working for someone else—use of office equipment, secretar-
ial support and the established network of business contacts.

If you choose to join the ranks of many ADD adults who start
their own businesses, do it carefully. Take a hard look at your
balance sheet and your list of perceived financial needs. Can
you afford financially and emotionally to live with less while
you work at developing your own business?

If you decide to take the calculated risk of working for yourself,
use your list of assets or positive qualities to explore possibilities
that offer the best match. Keep in mind that working on your
own offers flexibility but requires long hours in the initial stages
of establishing your business. It also requires the ability to design and follow a plan to stay on track.

With no boss or time clock, it is important to establish your own schedule and set of rules to keep from sliding into the ADD Standard Time Zone, where all bets are off in terms of the actual date that *any* project will reach completion. An ADD coach who also has expertise in small businesses can help you maximize your chances of success.

Temporary Work: Rather than establishing your own business, you might try temporary work as a satisfactory compromise between self-employment and working for someone else. In temporary work, you "rent" your skills by the hour, day or longer, but usually work for an agency that employs a number of temporary workers.

Temporary work offers several advantages. The ADDer can satisfy a restless nature by changing job settings frequently. Another advantage is the ability to control the hours of work. Many of us find a standard forty-hour, five-day workweek incompatible with our unique capacities. Some of us find full-time work too taxing. Others prefer working for long stretches and then taking large blocks of time off. Many ADDers are also night people, unable to function well until the afternoon. In temporary work, unusual working patterns can often be accommodated.

If you're fairly adaptable and can get along with people for short periods of time, temping may work well for you. Of course it doesn't offer carte blanche to do anything you please. If you don't follow through with completing tasks or develop a reputation for being difficult, you'll stop getting assignments.

If you have had a history of employment failure, use your new self-knowledge to reassess the reasons for it. Your awareness of your strengths and challenges can help you realistically analyze your situation, sorting out the problems that result from your behavior and those that are related to the behaviors of others. You may be in a better position to figure out whether you have failed on your jobs or your jobs have failed you. Your new insights may even help you become more accepting of the quirks of your colleagues.

Your main goals should be to improve your work relationships and limit the time you spend in interactions that are difficult for you. You may decide that you can and should make some behavioral changes. You may decide that you should change your job or career. You may decide that you've already made the correct choices and are happy with them.

If you decide that some changes are in order, move slowly and thoughtfully. Although you need to base your decisions on your individual strengths and weaknesses, don't forget to include your family in the decision-making process.

Maintaining friendships, surviving in group encounters and interacting on the job aren't easy tasks. But developing intimate relationships can be even more challenging. In the next chapter, we'll turn to the Art of Relating, Acts IV and V. We'll watch some scenes taking place in dating and family relationships. These higher-risk relationships share some elements with the ones we've already examined. But they are unique in their depth and complexity and require special care and nurturing. We'll offer some specific ideas you can use to make them work successfully.

CHAPTER 8

The Art of Relating: In the Dating Game and the Family

The "rules" of dating and family relationships are similar to those of group and one-to-one relationships. The level of complexity and emotional investment is very different, however. And the stakes are much higher if the relationships fail.

Act IV: The Dating Game

Sharon and Brad

Sharon returns from work to the four messages Brad left on her answering machine. She told him last week that she doesn't want to see him anymore, but he is unwilling to accept her decision. He's sure that she doesn't really mean it.

He drives to her apartment complex late each night and leaves notes under her windshield wipers. He calls her at work several times a day and shows up at her door with flowers and gifts. Brad is heartbroken because he knows that Sharon is the only woman with whom he wants to spend the rest of his life. Sharon doesn't know it, but she is Brad's third "only woman I'll ever love" in the past year. Brad falls deeply in love—again and again.

Angela and Simon

Angela and Simon spend every waking hour together. They are truly in love, and Simon is planning the perfect time and place to propose to her. He met Angela just a few weeks ago but wines and dines her almost every day.

As weeks turn into months, Angela begins to orchestrate some conflicts that prevent her from seeing Simon. When they are together they have a wonderful time, but Angela is beginning to feel a bit closed in. One afternoon she asks Simon to stop by her house. When he arrives, another man answers the door. He tells Simon that Angela is busy and can't see him now.

Notes: Act IV

With the exception of Sharon, all the actors in the preceding scenes have ADD. We can only speculate about why Brad, Angela and Simon feel compelled to behave as they do.

Brad may approach his new relationship as he approaches projects at work—with intensity and impulsivity. He may be accustomed to making quick decisions and getting things done in a hurry. Unfortunately he doesn't understand that he can't control the women in his life the way he does the facts and figures on his sales plans.

Brad's problems with his relationships may also result from his battered sense of self. He may be one of the walking wounded, believing that he can be emotionally whole only when he has a "better half." Men and women alike can have unrealistic expectations about being saved by a relationship.

Angela's behavior reflects her insatiability. Although she genuinely enjoyed Simon's company during the first months of the relationship, she became bored. She has an ADDer's tendency to become absorbed quickly in relationships and to become bored by them just as quickly. As the initial, intense stimulation of her romance has dwindled, so has her interest in it. Although Angela probably doesn't chart her conquests, she may leave a trail of discarded partners, including Simon, as souvenirs of her frequent, intense affairs.

Simon's impulsivity may also play into the demise of his relationship with Angela. He drives the relationship with his need for closeness. Angela's insatiability aside, she may be terrified that Simon will "swallow" her individuality. Given time, it's possible that her love for Simon would win out over her fears of closeness. But she never gets the chance because Simon's intense need for closeness tips the precarious balance of their relationship much too quickly. Angela would rather lose her love than her identity.

Synopsis: Act IV

It sounds pretty gloomy, doesn't it? Is it time to head out to a hermit's hut? Well, if you've been paying attention—sorry, we couldn't help it—you know how we feel about doom and gloom. It's fine for disaster movies on the big screen but it's counterproductive to your recovery.

Dating relationships are vulnerable to an ADDer's intensity and impaired communication skills. His enthusiasm or sparkle can be a strong magnet that initially attracts his love interest. But over time, his level of intensity can suffocate his lover. She's left gasping for breath and backing away to get some space. The ADDer, comfortable with the intense pace, may not recognize his lover's need for a gradual progression to closeness.

In a romantic or sexual relationship, an individual risks revealing himself big-time! The risk can be greater for the ADDer who has failed so many times and in so many different ways. His generalized feelings of inadequacy, born of differences he's never understood, can explode when he bares his soul and body to a partner. When he dares to reveal himself to a lover who subsequently rejects him, he can suffer a serious blow to his fragile self-worth.

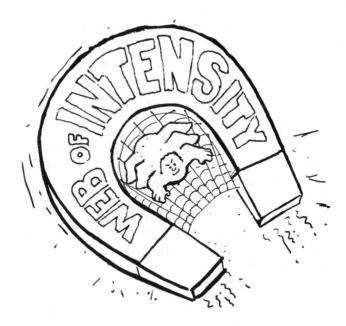

Some adults experience ongoing difficulties in intimate relationships because they regard them as safe ports from their feelings of inadequacy. Even with our changing society, many families still condition their daughters to believe that the roles of wife and mother will protect them. An ADD woman's life of negative experiences can reinforce this myth. She may believe that the only escape route from her demanding life is through a wedding ring and then a diaper bag. She comes to view a partner as a lifeline or safety net and may scare suitors away with the weight of her clinging dependency.

We didn't use these stories to illustrate what *will* go wrong in your relationships but what *might* go wrong. An ADD adult's differences can contribute to problems in maintaining intimate relationships. By understanding the dynamics of your disorder you will have taken a step in the right direction. If you're aware of potential hazards, you can be prepared the next time you meet someone special, to stop and think before you act.

Having clarified our message—an important part of positive communication—we'll look at some ways to avoid the pitfalls and improve the quality of your relationships. Here are a few pointers on successfully playing the dating game.

Survival Tips: Act IV

Play Hard to Get: It is not a good idea to utter the words "I love you" after just a few dates! Watch your partner's signals for clues about the progress of the relationship. Use the dynamics of approach and withdrawal behaviors to your advantage. Even if you immediately set your sights on your new love interest, play hard to get for a while. This keeps the desire and fear of closeness in proper balance until the other person has time to catch up with your willingness to make a commitment!

This approach may sound somewhat manipulative but it doesn't have an evil intent. Let's face it, an ADD adult has to carefully plan many aspects of his life to make them work. Why should relationships be any different? After all, the hard-to-get approach is just a variation of learning to stop, think, act and reflect, right?

Monitor the Relationship: Spontaneity is a lovely thing but ADDers can get in trouble when freedom reigns. To a certain extent, you'll need to approach intimate relationships as you do everything else—with careful planning and ongoing monitoring. Keep your finger on the pulse of the relationship. If your partner seems skittish, back off and lighten up! When the intensity level is too high, be less available for a while.

Don't swing too far in the other direction either. You can chase a love interest away with your apparent indifference. Relationships require continual work and maintenance. The challenge for an ADDer is to sustain attention to the relationship over the long haul.

Work at your communication skills. Remind yourself to listen to your partner, ask questions to draw her out and pay attention to moods and nonverbal clues.

Don't Lose the "Me" in "We": Be sure to maintain your usual interests when you begin dating someone new. This will help you keep a reasonable distance from the relationship, to prevent your total immersion in it. This will also help you maintain your own identity.

Watch Your Impulsivity: Impulsive behavior can create an assortment of problems in an ADD adult's life. In a sexual relationship, it can cause life-threatening trouble! In this day of serious sexually transmitted diseases, more than emotional well-being is at stake. It's wise to wait a while before beginning any sexual relationship.

You may need to make some rules for yourself to prevent impulsive decisions. Talk to a trusted friend who seems to be in control of his life. Ask for his advice. How long does he think a person should wait before having sex, saying "I love you" or living with a new romantic interest? Ask how long he thinks a person should know a lover before marriage.

Use this information to make a vow to wait X amount of time before taking any of these steps. Enlist your friend's help with your vow. In many support groups, a sponsor helps the individual stick to his *program*. Your friend could become the sponsor you call on when you're having trouble sticking with your program—that is, your rules for dating behavior.

Stop and Think: If you're feeling restless just thinking about such an unbearably slow pace of a relationship, use your imagination and consider this: Visualize a *whole lifetime of restlessness* with a spouse who bores you to death! Visualize a giant vise systematically tightening down and squeezing out all your hard work at recovery and rebuilding your sense of self. You are worth too much to throw away your progress by impulsively hooking up with someone who is wrong for you. The consequences of an impulsive marriage can be heavy, particularly if children are involved.

Act V, Scene 1:
The Art of Relating in the Family

Now we'll examine the most complex kind of relationship. We'll introduce you to the Baker family to help us explore the unique issues of family interactions. The family includes Jan, Tom and their three biological children, Amy, Zachary and Jennifer. Each of the five members of the family has ADD, although each has slightly different problems associated with it.

Tom

A successful real estate broker, Tom is extremely restless, hyperactive and irritable. He earns a good living but the family experiences ongoing financial crises. Everyone in the family spends the money as quickly as he can earn it. Tom has a Jekyll and Hyde personality that changes at the drop of a hat. He flips back and forth from an enthusiastic, fun-loving man to an irritable, withdrawn grouch. Jan and the children are always a bit afraid of him.

Jan

Jan isn't particularly moody or hyperactive. She is more of a gentle space cadet. She has trouble organizing the household and disciplining the children. She is so overwhelmed by the demands of life that she just lets them wash over her. Having few reserves of energy to gain control of her life, she manages to do little more than survive each day.

Amy

The oldest daughter, Amy, is an extremely bright, chronic underachiever. She has always been a maverick. She has problems following rules and fitting in with other children. She's continually in trouble at home and at school. Amy shares her dad's symptoms of moodiness, impulsivity and hyperactivity. At thirteen, she's becoming increasingly rebellious, refusing to take her Ritalin and hanging out with a group of kids who take drugs.

Amy and her dad have an explosive relationship since they both regularly fly off the handle. She and her mom don't argue a lot but they have a tenuous relationship. Amy treats Jan with contempt, not even attempting to hide her low opinion of her mother. She can't understand why Mom is so wishy-washy about everything.

Zachary

Ten-year-old Zachary is quiet and rather passive. He doesn't make waves. He struggles in school and receives only mediocre grades despite putting in long hours doing homework. He's anxious most of the time and has a number of health problems including asthma, severe allergies and frequent stomachaches. He's shy and has trouble making friends.

Zachary was evaluated and diagnosed with multiple learning disabilities and ADD. His psychologist recommended intensive tutoring but the family never has enough extra money to hire anyone. Jan has taken on the job but can't do it with any regularity because she's so overwhelmed by the details of her life. So Zachary struggles along without the educational help he needs.

Jennifer

Jennifer is the baby of the family and her parents treat her that way. They place few demands on her. At eight years old, she's a delightful child with a sunny personality and an engaging sense of humor. She's fairly hyperactive but doesn't display the irritability and moodiness of her father or sister. She channels some of her excess energy into gymnastics, cartwheeling or dancing around the house much of the time.

At school she has become the class clown, entertaining her peers and keeping her teachers so busy laughing that they ignore her difficulties with schoolwork. Her grades are even worse than her brother's, but no one gets on her case about it. Her teachers assume that she just isn't very bright. Her parents are busy arguing with each other and with Amy. They work so hard at just surviving that they don't have time to worry about their youngest child. They figure that at least they have one normal child even if she isn't any smarter than the rest of their kids.

Notes: Act V, Scene 1

Marriage and child rearing present all the challenges we've already discussed and then some! The intricacy of the dance of family relationships is dramatically more complex than that of groups, friendships or romantic interactions. In this regard, we would like you to consider these new math facts. Are you ready?

$$1 + 1 > 2$$
$$2 + 1 = 4$$
$$2 + 2 = 11 \ plus$$

We're not going to tell you quite yet what these equations mean, but the answers are correct . . . sort of. It depends on the questions you're asking. We'll get back to this in a few paragraphs.

As soon as two individuals become a *legal we*, the rules change and the complexity and intensity of the relationship increase whether or not either has ADD. There are often unrealistic expectations that the spouse will fulfill the roles of Savior, Mother, Father, Best Friend, Expert Lover, Tower of Strength, Therapist, etcetera.

Further complicating the relationship of a couple, particularly as time goes on, is the history they have shared. Communications are colored with memories, both good and bad. An innocent remark can spark an argument about a past hurt or unresolved conflict that had an impact on the relationship. If we add a spouse with ADD to the picture, the relationship can change unpredictably.

Jan and Tom were delighted to find each other and had an exciting courtship. Jan loved the spontaneity of impulsive trips to the beach and phone calls at 3:00 a.m. Tom loved having Jan help him remember to put gas in the car and agree with his opinions.

When Amy was born in the first year of their marriage, they seemed to become totally different people. The transformation they experienced is certainly not unique to ADDers. Virtually all parents, even those who carefully plan their families, say it's impossible to imagine the magnitude of the changes that occur with the birth of a child.

This brings us back to the answers in our equations. They are correct if we ask the following questions:

What does one spouse plus one spouse equal?
What does one couple plus one child equal?
What does one couple plus two children equal?

Jan and Tom assumed that their problems resulted from baby Amy's constant crying. A difficult infant can definitely add stress to a relationship. Even if Amy had been a calm, placid baby, our couple would have experienced a transformation in their relationship.

With the addition of each child, the relationships between and among family members become increasingly complicated. The complications grow not arithmetically but geometrically. This may be why parents often say a second child adds more than just double the work of an only child. The extra work doesn't have nearly as much to do with extra laundry or meal preparation as it does with an exploding number of relationships. Let's look at what happens to the number of relationships when you add children to a family:

The Couple = husband and wife
(plus their individual
and collective "baggage")

The Couple + One Child = husband and wife
husband and child
wife and child
husband, wife and child

The Couple + Two Children = husband and wife
husband and first child
husband and second child
wife and first child
wife and second child
first and second child
husband, wife and first child
husband, wife and second child
husband, first and second child
wife, first and second child
husband, wife, first and
second child

Synopsis: Act V, Scene 1

Although it is now easier for different kinds of computers to talk to each other, making the PC and the Apple worlds more compatible was quite a challenge. We wonder what those programmers would think about the task of interfacing a family unit. They would have to program individual personalities to interface with the multiple relationships among family members. The dyad of husband and wife alters the one-to-one relationship of premarriage days even before children add to the complexity of interpersonal relationships.

Since ADD tends to run in families, it dramatically alters the dimensions of the family unit and exponentially ups the ante as children are born. Raising ADD children is a challenging job that taxes the resources of non-ADD parents. Many adoptive parents can attest to this. In a family like the Bakers, where everybody has the disorder, the potential for discord and communication breakdown is enormous.

Does this mean that the equation of ADD adult(s) + children = disaster? Absolutely not! You may be a wonderful parent! ADDers are lively people. Many can respond to the challenges of child rearing with incredible enthusiasm and avoid the pitfalls by leaping energetically over them!

The Job of Parenting: ADD adults have strengths and weaknesses when it comes to parenting. A typical balance sheet for an ADD parent may look something like this:

Strengths	Weaknesses
active	impatient
creative	moody
open-minded	intolerant of noise and chaos
compassionate	careless with details
sense of wonder	shaky communication skills
curious	limited capacity for work and stress
enthusiastic	easily bored
passionate	impulsive
good sense of humor	disorganized

How does this balance sheet play out when you become a parent? It's hard to say with certainty. Your child's personality and the interrelated profiles of you, your spouse and your offspring all have impacts. You might become a parent who yells a lot or is grouchy much of the time. The added noise and stress of having children may push buttons that weren't pushed before. You might look at your reflection in a mirror and wonder where the mean, angry person came from.

On the other hand, you might take advantage of the wonderful "immaturity" everyone used to criticize. With your children in tow, you can giggle, climb on the monkey bars and sing aloud in the grocery store without questioning looks from other people. You might effectively use your compassion and open-mindedness to roll with the inevitable punches of parenting.

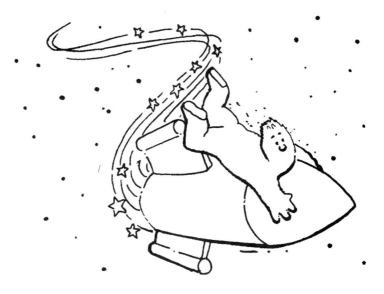

Your effectiveness as a parent will be tested by the genetic probability that one or more of your children are likely to have ADD. Their high-strung temperaments will require special handling. In some respects your own ADD uniquely qualifies you as a provider of special handling. You have insight unavailable to your non-ADD peers. If you haven't yet achieved a workable balance in your life, however, you will need to consider your own needs for nurturing. You will be more available to your children if you are also taking care of yourself.

Parenting has been compared to a scary, exciting, unpredictable roller-coaster ride. We submit that when ADD is an issue, parenting becomes an even wilder journey. It's like guiding an out-of-control rocket ship at the speed of light toward an unknown destination! Is this necessarily so bad? Just think of all the teacher conferences and emergency room visits our parents would have missed if it hadn't been for us! What would they have done with all that extra time? Just think how boring the world would be without us.

Can we learn any lessons from this survey of the family dimension? We think the most important one is the need for planning. Your parents and teachers probably complained so often about your poor planning that the very word makes you uncomfortable. As much as you may dislike planning, it's probably the single most important thing you can do for yourself. Use the following considerations as a framework for your "Planned Parenting." The job of parenting is too important to leave to chance.

Survival Tips: Act V, Scene 1

Spacing of Children: Carefully consider the spacing of your children. This has nothing to do with the psychology of spacing as it affects a child's adjustment. Rather, careful spacing allows you to absorb the impact of each child on your capacity to handle the additional demands. If you have several children in the space of a few years, you may be pushed beyond your limits before you know it. Spacing buys you the time you need to make a wise decision.

Personal and Financial Resources: If you and your spouse want to continue full-time employment, can you both emotionally handle the second shift of parenting? If not, can you survive financially if one parent has only a part-time job or stays at home? Of course, if you're a single parent, you won't have an option in this regard.

Realistic Assessment of Effort and Money: Do your homework. Ask other parents, especially parents of ADD children, about the work and money it takes to raise children. Everyone knows that children are expensive. But when ADD is part of the financial picture, you'll need to think about the added expenses you may incur. Your child may need extra help. He may need, among other services, tutoring, speech therapy, medicine or psychological counseling.

General Strategies: What resources are available to lighten the load? Are there relatives living nearby who are willing to help? Can you reduce your financial obligations? Can you organize the workload so each parent can have periodic breaks? When you add children to your life, you need to be even more ruthless about simplifying it to maintain balance.

Act V, Scene 2: The Art of Relating in the Family

In the following scenes we'll offer a glimpse of the Baker family's interactions. They are illustrative of the complexity of family relationships when ADD is added to the mix.

Jan, Tom and Zachary

Jan is tutoring Zachary at the dining room table. Tom walks in and starts to tell her some exciting news about work. When she doesn't respond, he becomes increasingly exasperated by her seeming uninterest. When his raised voice finally elicits Jan's request to "wait a minute," he leaves the room in a huff.

Tom, Jan and Jennifer

Tom sits bleary-eyed at the breakfast table, drinking his first cup of coffee and trying to read the newspaper. Jan, who is a morning person, chats to him nonstop and reminds him that it's garbage day. Tom finally looks up from his paper and announces that the garbage needs to be taken out. Jan testily replies that if he'd been listening he would know that she's aware of that fact. Jennifer suddenly appears out of nowhere to give her startled parents bear hugs. She is scolded for being so rough and slinks out of the room wondering why her parents don't seem to want her love.

Jennifer, Amy and Zachary

Jennifer rushes into her sister's room and pounces on the bed to give Amy a morning kiss. Amy, who is just beginning to wake up, shoves her off the bed and feels only mildly remorseful when Jennifer scrapes her knee on the way down. Now fully awake, Amy heads down the hall for a shower and lets loose a string of epithets when Zachary walks in to brush his teeth.

Notes: Act V, Scene 2

The Baker family includes five people whose individual differences collectively combine to create Chaos on the Cul-de-Sac. All families share some of their problems—balancing the rights of individual members with the needs of the larger family unit. The Baker family has an extra layer of shared ADD challenges that makes this balancing act particularly difficult.

Families who live under the same roof share both physical and emotional space. If the family is to live peacefully together, each member needs an adequate amount of both. Each of the Bakers has a poor sense of physical and emotional boundaries and impulsively invades each other's territory. Acting on autopilot most of the time, they bump, jostle and literally step on each other's toes as they repeatedly miss both obvious and subtle requests for space.

A closed door or a sign that says Keep Out is a fairly clear statement of a desire for privacy. Most of us understand its obvious significance, but what about the subtle, nonverbal requests for privacy? Many of us with ADD misread these "signs."

These nonverbal signs are the invisible circles that people draw around their bodies for privacy and protection. The circles define the perimeter of personal space and convey the message "Don't come any closer than the circle I have drawn around me."

These circles aren't fixed in time and space. The diameter of your own circle constantly changes according to your mood, circumstances and relationship to the other person. The circle narrows to encourage a lover or a beloved child to get close, and widens to keep the stranger or someone you dislike at a safe distance. If you're angry or depressed, the circle may become huge even for loved ones as you send out the message Stay Away. For an ADDer, the circle sometimes inexplicably widens when he can't stand to be touched or to allow anyone in his immediate vicinity.

Synopsis: Act V, Scene 2

Awareness of and respect for these invisible circles requires good nonverbal communication skills. Lacking these skills, the Bakers impulsively trounce on each other's feelings and invade personal physical spaces. Since the whole family has ADD, each person has a unique need for space. Each person also has an inability to prevent his needs from colliding with the needs of everybody else. Privacy is as hard to come by in this family as peace and quiet are. The experience of living in this kind of family is one of feeling intruded upon and overwhelmed.

Most ADD families experience some degree of difficulty in their interactions. What can an ADD family such as the Bakers do to make their home more of a haven for the people who live there? The first order of business is to see a family therapist.

This family has been in trouble for a long time. They need an objective outsider to analyze and balance the needs of the family as a unit with the individual needs of family members. The therapist's job is to help the family system become healthier so it can better meet the needs of each member. Right now, the family is too stressed and chaotic to provide the necessary structure and nurturing.

We can't emphasize enough that treating a troubled family is not a do-it-yourself enterprise! A Band-Aid approach may temporarily slow down the bleeding, but it won't stop the hemorrhage! *If your family is really in trouble, get professional help ASAP!*

If your family is basically okay and needs only minor adjustments, that's wonderful. There are several techniques you can use to support and build your family system. The following discussion includes specific suggestions for improving communication and managing boundary issues.

Survival Tips: Act V, Scene 2

Creating Living Space Large Enough for the People Who Share It

When we talk about living space, we're not suggesting that you increase the square footage of your house or apartment! We're talking about carefully designing sufficient *emotional* living space so that family members can coexist with relative harmony.

Teach Respect for Boundary Needs: Suggest that your family visualize a boundary as a Hula Hoop. We know we're showing our ages—many people under thirty-five have never even played with one! Anyway, if you have a Hula Hoop lying around, put it around you to demonstrate your personal circle. Ask each family member to picture himself surrounded by his own personal hoop.

The room suddenly starts to shrink in size as people and Hula Hoops begin to take up space. As everyone starts to move around in the space, the inevitable happens. There's a fair amount of confusion as Hula Hoops start bumping into each other.

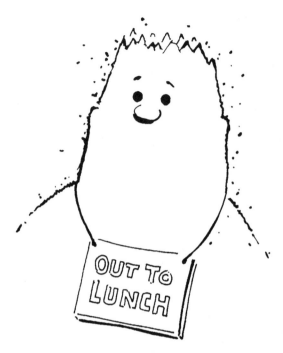

Each family member should put this image in his memory bank for future reference. The next time he starts to intrude on someone else, he may be able to call up the Hula Hoop image in his mind. "Seeing" Dad in a Hula Hoop might just be enough to make Junior Stop, Look, Listen . . . and Laugh!

Design Rest and Relaxation Zones: In many families, there are unwritten rules regarding private space. The den may "belong" to the parents—the children understand that this space is Mom and Dad's retreat. Similarly, the children often use their bedrooms as escapes from the demands of the family.

ADD families need to establish written rules regarding the boundaries of privacy. Each member of the family should have his own designated zone. In a small apartment, this space could be the balcony, the hall or half of a shared bedroom. Each family member has a right to privacy and needs a private retreat— a place that is off-limits to everyone else. "Out to Lunch" or

"Temporary Shutdown" signs can indicate current occupation of a personal zone.

This provision for *down time* is essential to forestall the negative behaviors of frustration. Each person has a right to state his need for space. When a family member makes a request for quiet time, for example, the others are to refrain from talking to him.

Designated Quiet Zones: Designate specific quiet zones in your home as places for reading, studying or resting. Place the television and stereo in an area with a door that can be closed. This area should also be as far away as possible from the quiet zones. A soundproof room for noisy equipment would be ideal, but most homes don't have this luxury. One option is to establish a rule that TV or stereo users must use earphones.

Rules for Communication and Respect for Boundaries: You can't take anything for granted in an ADD family! You need to design structured rules to protect the emotional and physical circles of family members. Some of these suggestions may be helpful:

- **Set Aside Specific Periods for Quiet** when the TV should be turned off and the answering machine turned on. Develop a family schedule with designated times for studying or other quiet pursuits as well as times to be together as a group.

- **Observe a Period of Silence** when the noise level is too high or emotions are getting out of control.

- **Require Each Family Member, Including Parents, to Ask Permission** before borrowing anything from someone else.

- **Impose a Stop—Look/Listen—Speak** procedure for all communication between family members. When a conversation is in progress, the person entering the room is expected to wait until he's invited to join in. If someone is doing something that requires concentration, such as reading or paying bills, he shouldn't be interrupted except for an emergency.

- **Determine What Constitutes an Emergency.** An untied shoelace can be an emergency for an ADD child. You may need to discuss and make a list of real and perceived emergency situations. Insist that everyone refer to the list before interrupting a conversation in progress. If an interruption is necessary, establish the following rule: Get the person's attention by gently tapping him on the shoulder, wait for a response and then excuse yourself before you begin to talk.

- **Prohibit All Long-Distance Conversations** except for announcements that the house is burning down! Yelling up the stairs or shouting from another room to find someone is a no-no. There are two reasons for this. First, if family members have to strain to hear, they will frequently misinterpret the message. An ADDer can have enough trouble sending and receiving messages without the added burden of trying to talk to someone in another room. Second, it's not the most respectful means of communication. Yelling upstairs to get someone to come down is a lot like calling the dog—and it feels like it too!

- **Use Intercoms.** You might want to invest in some intercoms to communicate with people in other parts of the house. Be careful not to overdo it. A buzzing intercom every five minutes can be as annoying as a bellowing voice!

- **Prohibit All "On the Run" Conversations.** Talking to someone while you rush to finish a task isn't conducive to effective communication. The intended recipient of this one-way conversation has to listen to a program that fades in and out or follow the speaker around on his travels. On-the-run conversations contribute to miscommunication.

- **Enforce a Rule to Prohibit Unwanted Teasing or Joking** about individual family members. ADDers often read the literal meaning of messages and miss the intended meaning. Since impulsive ADD family members often fail to notice the discomfort of others, their teasing can quickly escalate into perceived full-scale attacks. All requests to stop teasing are to be respected. If a joke hurts someone, it's not funny.

- **Set Up a Message Center** in a prominent place. The kitchen may be a good place for this as it's often the center of family activities. The best location is near a phone with an answering machine. Preferably, the space will have a counter or desk for a writing surface. The center should include a bulletin board, a method for filing mail and important papers, a large calendar and an ample supply of paper and pens.

The bulletin board needs to be sufficiently large to provide a specific section for each family member and one for the whole family. Keep extra colored paper tacked in each section or use color Post-it pads. Each family member can have a personalized color that makes it easy to post and retrieve messages. A white board may be a good backdrop for the colored notes. Be sure that everyone, including small children, can reach the bulletin board.

The *General Messages* area is for anything the whole family needs to read. The rest of the board can be divided into sections for individual family members. Each message is to include the signature of the person who posted it, the date and the time. Whenever possible, telephone calls should be handled at or switched to the message center phone.

Encourage family members to make a habit of checking the message center several times a day and every time they come home. As soon as someone reads a message, he removes it from the board. This will reduce visual clutter and improve the odds that the family won't overlook posted messages. If someone adds a general message to the board, he should initial it at the bottom. As each person in turn reads the message, he adds his initials. The last reader will know that everyone else has seen the note and that he should remove it from the board.

Besides looking for posted messages, each person needs to check his mail slot and listen to the answering machine or voice mail. Phone calls can be added to the board and the tape rewound. Before making any plans, everyone should check the message center's master calendar for important family dates.

We're not suggesting that families do all their communicating by way of the message center! Putting things in writing can be a big help, however. Otherwise, an ADD child might forget to mention that Dad is stranded with a flat tire and sister is in the emergency room with a broken arm! A disorganized ADD family can truly benefit from a structured system that tracks family messages and appointments.

- **Monitor Your Family's Emotional Temperature:** Monitoring your personal stress level is important, but in your excitable, roller-coaster ADD family, the effect of workload or stress snowballs. It's similar to what happens to the number of relationships when you add new family members: 2 + 1 is greater than 3.

This is how it happens. One of the children comes home after a bad day at school and is bouncing off the walls. Mom arrives an hour later in a bad mood after a difficult day at work. In a matter of minutes, Mom and the hyperactive child are at each other's throats as the child's noise and activity irritate a mother who has no reserves of patience. The fight that erupts puts everyone in the family on edge, and before long the house feels like a war zone.

Because the stress level of each person has such a profound effect on the family, it's important to monitor the demands on the family as a whole. If an individual family member is pushing himself too hard and feels irritable as a consequence, it isn't just an individual matter. If the family as a whole is trying to do too much, the stress makes relaxation and downtime impossible.

Before we close this chapter, we want to at least mention the wider family circle—the extended family. Grandparents, in-laws, aunts, uncles, etcetera, will all have an impact on the dynamics of your family. Their support or lack of support can be a powerful influence on your efforts to be a successful ADD family. We can't examine this issue in depth because the subject is too complicated to address in a few sentences. These chapters just scratch the surface. We'd like to write another book that focuses exclusively on ADD family relationships.

But there are some other important family issues we're going to address in the next chapter. With family relationships as the backdrop, we'll revisit the Baker family to examine some management issues unique to the functioning of the family.

CHAPTER 9

From Mealtime Mania to Outing Ordeals: How-To's of Decreasing Discord

The family is a microcosm of society. It includes individual and group rights, responsibilities and rules. It's a system of multiple interpersonal relationships that need to be carefully managed.

Hundreds of sociological studies have explored the entity of the family and how it functions. Since we are neither sociologists nor family therapists, we don't presume to be experts in these fields. We do, however, consider ourselves experts in two specific areas: the ADD families of Kelly/Pentz and Ramundo. Our experiences could fill volumes, as we're sure yours could too.

When we use the word "expert," we use it humbly as a reflection of our lifetime experiences, not as a measure of our expertise. We can't give you all the answers about ADD families because we don't have them! We can share some of our observations and the collective experiences of other ADDers and their families. We'll rejoin the Baker family to help us do this.

Our previous visit with them provided a glimpse of a family living in the sitcom *Chaos on the Cul-de-Sac*. If you recognize your family in the description of the Bakers, do you have to resign yourself to being part of the neighborhood? Is there anything you can realistically do to make your family life more manageable? We're going to take on the role of the Baker family's therapist to find some answers.

To begin unraveling the family's complex problems, we'll encourage each family member to communicate her own version of the Baker family story. This sharing will happen over time and within an atmosphere of mutual support.

Tom: "I feel helpless, angry and worthless most of the time. I know I lose my temper too much and it hurts people, but I just can't seem to help it. The angry words are out of my mouth before I know it. I feel lonely too. Jan doesn't seem to know I exist unless she's cringing because I got mad. She's always busy with something. She doesn't look me in the eye and never pays attention to me when I try to talk to her. I'm scared all the time. I worry that I can't keep pretending I'm in control. Work just takes it out of me. When I get home, I don't have any energy left for my family. I'm supposed to be strong—the man of the family— but sometimes I feel as though I'm just barely hanging on."

Jan: "I feel as if I'm underwater all the time, fighting to swim to the surface but never getting there. No matter what I do, I never seem to get anything accomplished. I work hard to take care of the house and family but I never have anything to show for it. The place is always a mess and we never seem to have a moment of peace. Everyone is always fighting. I'm a failure. Tom and Amy are always yelling and putting me down. I probably deserve it. I'm pretty useless."

Amy: "Everybody thinks I'm just a rotten kid but they have no idea how I really feel. I'm scared that I'll never be able to make it as a grown-up. I know I'm a 'smart-ass' but that's just a cover-up. I'm mean, have terrible moods and can't seem to get it together to do anything worthwhile. What am I going to do when I finish high school? With my grades, I probably won't make it to college and I'm not fast enough to do something like waitressing. Sometimes I wish I were more like Zachary. I make fun of him for being a wimp but he's a nicer person than I am. Sometimes I wish I were dead."

Zachary: "I hate the fighting at my house. Even when my family is laughing or joking, I'm always waiting for something terrible to happen—for Dad or Amy to start a big screaming match. I can't stand it when people yell because the noise hurts me. I don't know how to protect myself. I get so mad sometimes I just want to yell at them to shut up but I can't get the words out. It's hard enough to talk when I'm feeling calm. When I get upset, I get so confused I can't think straight. I feel like a dope. I work harder in school than anybody I know but I still get mostly Cs. My dad gets impatient with me because I'm not good at sports and I won't stick up for myself. Mom seems to like me better but never has enough time to help me with schoolwork. I hate to even ask her because she seems so busy and tired most of the time. I know I cause a lot of trouble because I hear Mom and Dad fighting all the time about my doctor bills. I wish it was more peaceful at my house."

Jennifer: "It's crazy at my house! I especially hate dinnertime because it takes too long. Everybody's always telling me, Sit down, Jennifer . . . Be quiet, Jennifer . . . Stop falling off your chair, Jennifer. I can't stand to sit there all that time. I'd rather be outside playing. I like it when my family tells jokes but a lot of times people yell and get in fights. I hate the yelling. Most of the time I don't think my family even notices I'm there. My mom and dad don't even seem to care when I bring home Ds on my papers. They do say that it's too bad I don't get grades for my talking because I sound so smart. I wish they would watch me dance and do gymnastics but they're too busy talking, doing other stuff or fighting. I don't like going to school either. My teachers make me be quiet and sit in my seat until I want to jump right out of my skin!"

It's obvious that nobody in this family is happy with the way things are going! There's one common thread that weaves through everyone's story in the Baker family: the noise and emotional levels are too intense. Tom and Amy don't directly complain about the noise, but we can observe their sensitivities to it. Their hot tempers escalate in direct response to sensory intrusions. They also have some awareness of the impact of their yelling on other family members and don't feel very good about it.

Families who deal with the dynamics of ADD face numerous challenges every day. We can't discuss them all but we can examine two that are illustrative of several fairly common problems in an ADD family—Mealtime Mania and Outing Ordeals.

Mealtime Mania

It's Mealtime Mania at the Baker house. There are several poorly trained dogs who bark, jump up and beg for food throughout the meal. Amy and Tom, who are both sensitive to noise and touch, constantly yell at the dogs and push them away but do little else to train them. Jennifer adds to the general discord and busyness of the family meal by jumping up and down to dance or turn cartwheels.

Three separate, one-way conversations go on as Amy, Tom and Jennifer talk nonstop to no one in particular. Zachary and Jan try to follow the conversation but quickly tune out as they become overwhelmed by the chaos.

Jan rarely sits down at the table. She spends dinnertime wandering absentmindedly. She fetches the forgotten items of silverware, napkins or food that took longer to cook than the rest of the meal. Zachary quietly fades into the woodwork, trying to eat his dinner without getting a stomachache and hoping that a big fight doesn't break out. He knows that his mother won't be much help in averting the battle that will inevitably ensue between his father and sister Amy.

The anticipated knock-down, drag-out fight between Tom and Amy is a common occurrence at some point in the meal. Both have hair-trigger tempers coupled with foot-in-mouth disease.

This lethal combination means that each of them frequently makes careless remarks that touch off an explosion in the other. Both Tom and Amy tend to hear only half of what is said and to misinterpret the other half.

Sometimes the chaos is fun with lots of joking and fooling around. When Tom's in a good mood, he likes to become a kid again, telling silly jokes and instigating animal noise contests and food fights. Jan and Zachary don't participate very much but they laugh and enjoy the antics of the others during these happy times. They're always a little nervous though, knowing that when things get out of hand, the party atmosphere will rapidly and disastrously change. They know that Tom and Amy, the instigators of much of the rowdiness, are unpredictable and irritable. The mood of the gathering can change abruptly if either of them becomes annoyed with the noisiness or by someone stepping on their toes.

Easily enraged, they quickly generalize their anger to everyone else in the family. They frequently yell at Jan for burning part of the dinner, at Jennifer for leaping around like a frog and at Zachary for sitting like a bump on a log. Invariably, Amy stomps off before the meal is over since she has been grounded to her room "for the rest of her life." Zachary feels sick to his stomach and can't eat, and Jennifer dances around at a manic pace. Sometimes the atmosphere at dinner isn't so much chaotic as it is deadly silent and chilling, with everyone brooding and poisoning the environment with silent misery.

Notes: Mealtime Mania

With their difficult temperaments, Amy and Tom seem to dominate the picture in the Baker family. But they're not solely responsible for the impaired family interactions. Each of the family members has shaky communication skills and a limited capacity for stress and stimulation. Individually and collectively, these behaviors contribute to the family chaos and stress level.

If you plug the individual behaviors into a chart of family inter-actions, you can understand how things get so out of hand for the Bakers. As family tension escalates, Jan becomes increasingly more disorganized and disengages herself from the family. Tom gets more stressed out as the burden of discipline falls on him. With his short-fused temper, he's ill-equipped to handle it. He feels increasingly angry at Jan's failure to take charge of the house and children. Tom is not a sexist pig—he and Jan had agreed on the division of labor when she quit her job to stay home.

Tom gets burned out easily. After a day at work, he can do little but collapse. Amy desperately needs firm, calm, structured discipline but doesn't get it. Zachary doesn't actively bother anybody but, through no fault of his own, puts great demands on family financial and emotional resources. Jennifer contributes to the noise and chaos level with her clowning and hyperactivity.

The Baker family is a group of related individuals who have compelling needs for structure, support and understanding, but there doesn't seem to be enough to go around. Having fewer children probably would have helped, but it's too late for that option. It isn't too late, however, for the family to make some important changes to reduce the chaos and turn the volume down. If Mealtime Mania seems to be a way of life for your family, think about these ideas and consider trying them.

Survival Tips for Decreasing Discord

Reduce or Eliminate Unnecessary Distractions: Take the phone off the hook during meals. Turn the TV and radio off and put the newspaper in another room. The family dogs can be trained to stay away from the dinner table or kept in another room until the meal is over. To further minimize the extra distractions, the family might consider finding a new home for one of its dogs.

Establish a Family Signal: The signal cues everyone that the noise level is getting too high. Make a family rule that a moment of silence will be observed if anyone, including the youngest child, signals for less noise.

Make a "No Arguments at the Dinner Table" Rule: Conflict isn't all bad, but mealtime battles aren't very good for the digestive system! Arguments can be shelved and resumed at a designated time and place for discussion.

Plan a Weekly "Work Detail" Ahead of Time: This should include a list of individual responsibilities for meal preparation and setting and clearing the table. Family members can rotate these jobs from week to week. Preplanning eliminates much last-minute confusion. There is nothing more chaotic than an ADD family trying to work together without the direction of a plan! When other family members pitch in to help, the cook is free to join the family instead of aimlessly wandering around fetching things. The family can follow a rule that no one sits down to eat until the meal is on the table.

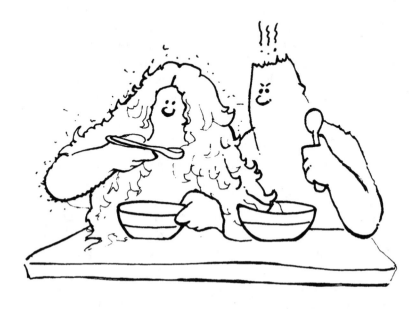

Maintain Order by Establishing Structure: Structure, order—what is this, boot camp? What happened to the idea of home as the place you can let your hair down and be yourself? *Letting your hair down is fine as long as you don't drop it in someone else's food!* In families with ADDers, there is a good possibility that letting one's hair down will disintegrate into a family free-for-all.

Structure and order can take the form of a family ritual or tradition. The ritual signals the beginning of special, shared family time. It can help family members put aside the stresses of the day, concentrate on being with each other and become aware of the comfortable haven of home. When the family has gathered, say grace, recite a poem or sing a song. Try a show-and-tell time for sharing anecdotes or telling jokes. Begin your meal with word games, trivia or threaded stories that each person builds on in turn. The ritual can be *anything.* The idea is to impose structure so family members take turns and learn to listen to one another.

Change the Rules: If someone is having a difficult day or is particularly hyperactive, she should have permission to leave the table. Just be sure to have an established procedure for requests to miss family meals.

If All Else Fails, Eliminate Family Meals: They are a lovely convention and can help families connect. In an ADD family, however, the disadvantages of a family meal can outweigh the advantages. When temperamental characteristics come together in a small space, the mixture can be combustible!

PR: "During our initial visit to a therapist, we decided that family meals, our nightly ritual, frequently destroyed an otherwise reasonable day and had to be eliminated.

"Our family meals resembled a hotly contested sporting event with angry opponents. My hyperactive son is particularly sensitive to smells and as a child was an extraordinarily picky eater. Jeremy spent most of our torturous dinner hour falling off his chair and using his gifted verbal skills to compare the smell of the meal to various decaying animals. Dad performed as head coach of the opposing team. He spent most of the mealtime describing the lack of food in his parents' mountain village in southern Italy. He used every means at his disposal to force Jeremy to eat. I donned my referee's cap, quoting scientific research to support my assertion that our son would not die of malnutrition—and I attempted to maintain order.

"The compromise that Dr. Melowsky helped us reach reduced the stress and brought peace to our kitchen. We decided that we would invite Jeremy to dinner but he wouldn't have to join us. The dinner rule was that he could decline to eat with us but had to refrain from character assassination of his mother's cooking. When he finally got hungry, he would be responsible for fixing his own sandwich and cleaning up after himself.

"I suppose one could argue that we gave in to our son by letting him skip the family meals. But the key is that we didn't eliminate our rules. We simply changed them to meet our family's needs. The family harmony was well worth the skeptical and disapproving looks of outsiders who didn't understand the dynamics of ADD."

We're going to leave the family dinner and join the Baker family in an Outing Ordeal. We invite you to join the scene already in progress.

Family Fun: An Evening at the Movies

The Baker family is getting ready to go out for a movie and Jan feels more anxious with each passing moment. As usual, she feels perplexed that she's always late for everything. Before the children were born, she had always managed to get to appointments on time. She doesn't stop long to ponder this because Jennifer interrupts, asking where her purse is, and Amy engages her in combat over the outfit she won't be caught dead wearing.

As she begins to put on her makeup, Tom demands a consultation on his slacks and the color of his sweater. Amy's discovery that her blouse is wrinkled sends Jan running to the laundry room to iron it. Now immersed in distractions, she momentarily forgets the time deadline and decides to pick up the dirty laundry on her way downstairs. When she gets to the basement, she starts working on a stained pair of jeans and throws Amy's blouse in the washer instead of ironing it.

The timer she set as a warning for the family to finish their preparations goes off. Jan realizes with a start that she has gotten off track again! She arrives back in her bedroom to Jennifer's bloodcurdling screams for protection against Amy, who has threatened her with death if Jennifer doesn't stop hiding her shoes. As the time ticks away and the stress mounts, the yelling gets louder as everyone blames somebody else for the problems with getting ready on time.

Finally all the members of the Baker family are ready to leave—everyone except Jan. Zachary, the only person who took care of himself, attempts to come to his mother's aid as the rest of the family accuses her of making the family late again!

Notes: Outing Ordeals

Many of us with ADD aren't well known for our punctuality. With our time sense, or lack thereof, we regularly set new records for travel time from point A to point B. Somehow we manage to climb into our cars precisely at the moment we're supposed to be arriving at our meeting on the other side of town! We have trouble organizing, we get distracted and we routinely forget things.

Getting oneself organized to be somewhere at a certain time is difficult, but getting an entire family organized is infinitely more complicated! If your family is anything like either of ours, getting dressed and out the door for an outing is a major production. Jan can't figure out why she's always late, but it really isn't hard to understand. If you multiply the difficulty by the number of people in a family, the extra time required grows exponentially as family relationships do when each new member arrives.

This scene is avoidable if the family designs an action plan. Without a specific plan, an ADD family's Outing Ordeals will continue. The following suggestions might be useful for your family's action plan.

Survival Tips for Outing Ordeals

Identify Individual Dynamics: The first step is for each family member to identify her unique contributions to the family's disorganization. It's easy to point the finger at someone else—each family member does contribute to the general disorganization and chaos. A more productive approach would be to help each family member decide what he or she needs to do to be ready on time. Then the whole family can come together and figure out an action plan.

For instance, Jan may require an uninterrupted half-hour to get herself together, and Tom may need help choosing his clothing since he's color-blind. If Tom and Jan discuss their needs in advance, they can strike a bargain. Tom can agree to give Jan the time she needs by running interference with the kids and saving his own requests until she's ready. Jan can agree to give Tom her undivided attention to help him choose an outfit after she's ready.

Establish Family Responsibilities: The family needs to think through the chores that must be done before anyone can leave. Who will feed the dog and put her in the basement? Who will have the responsibility for turning on the porch lights? The division of labor should be explained and assigned in advance to each of the family members.

The planning may even need to include things such as a bathroom schedule to avoid the problem of everyone trying to get into one or two bathrooms at the same time. It would also help if everyone gets dressed and ready in separate areas so they don't distract one another. Clothing can be assembled and laid out well in advance, so there's time to do needed laundry or repairs.

Prepare a Work Detail for the Family: To reduce the number of "I forgot's" or "What am I supposed to do's," give everyone their own checklist of responsibilities.

Reduce Distractions: It never fails that the phone rings in the middle of preparations. Take it off the hook. This isn't the time for reading the newspaper or watching TV either. The "No Distractions" rule for mealtimes applies as well. The television should be off-limits, the newspaper or other reading material set aside and the stereo turned off. Anyone who operates more efficiently with background music can wear headphones to reduce the distractions for other family members.

Set a Timer: Jan's use of a timer is a good idea, but it's best to set it to sound a warning and then a final signal when it's time to leave. To allow for a margin of error, set the departure time earlier than is really necessary. It's nice to have extra time to clean up the dirt from the flower pot Jennifer knocks over when she cartwheels into it!

If it's important to get to an event on time, set a prewarning signal. This gives everyone plenty of time to get dressed and ready before the second warning rings. Family members can read, watch TV or play short games during the extra time.

If all this careful planning seems like too much work, weigh it against the stress and conflict your family experiences when they operate in the usual fashion. Try it both ways before you decide.

In the next chapter, we will go deeper into the realm of relating with a discussion of sexuality, the most intimate kind of relating. In addition, we will explore the topic of ADD and gender issues, including the impact of hormones on ADD symptoms.

CHAPTER 10

Gender Issues and Sexuality

ADD comes in a rainbow assortment of flavors. We have the "bouncing off the wall" hyperactive types, the "never seem to wake up and get activated" folks and many varieties of activity level in between. Some of us, using almost superhuman effort, keep our noses bolted to the grindstone most of the time. Others are distractible butterflies who can't stay with a single focus to save their lives. When you add in different learning styles, personality factors and other human differences, the variety is infinite.

One of the most striking differences in how ADD presents itself has to do with gender. In the history of ADD awareness, the focus has been almost exclusively on males. That was because women and girls tend to have a more hidden, subtler form of the disorder. Only recently have researchers begun looking at how ADD manifests in girls and women. It used to be thought that there were as many as nine times more males than females with ADD. We now have research indicating that the ratio may be closer to two to one. There is not enough space in this book to go into great depth on the subject of gender and ADD, so we refer you to the excellent books by Sari Solden and by Patricia O. Quinn and Kathleen G. Nadeau (see Suggested Reading) for more details on this topic. Here are some of the highlights.

Sexy Brains and Hormones

Got your attention? Actually, this is not about the brain and sexual activity, but the fact that male and female brains are different. Of course, you knew that. No doubt you have read or listened to news stories on the latest brain research. We now know that even sexual preference can be linked to variation in size of parts of the brain. We know that there are brain-based differences in ADD. In 1990, Alan Zametkin demonstrated that ADD brains functioned differently from the brains of people without ADD. The frontal lobes are not as active (measured by glucose metabolism on a PET scan) when a person with ADD does a task that requires concentration. Since then, a number of studies have been done that examine various parts of the ADD brain. Two other examples of brain differences in individuals with ADD are (1) the relative size of brain hemispheres (are the right and left hemispheres the same size or different?) and (2) the size of the basal ganglia.

Both of these brain features are *also* different in males and females. Although the research on gender issues and ADD has barely begun, it is clear that there are biological factors that contribute to the ways ADD shows up differently in men and women.

Hormones: Okay, first we had the anatomy lesson, now it's time for a minilecture on physiology. Hormones have a profound effect on both form and function in the human body. Testosterone, a male hormone, has an impact on both brain development and behavior. During brain development, testosterone acts on brain hemispheres to create differences between them. In males, gray matter on the right side of the brain is thicker than on the left. We are all aware of the most dramatic effect of testosterone on behavior—aggression. On the female hormonal side, the most valuable player is estrogen. In contrast to the effect of testosterone, estrogen decreases aggressive behavior, impulsivity and hostility.

231

Well, you guessed it, if you didn't already know this: ADD males are generally more aggressive than ADD females. They also tend to be more impulsive and inattentive. Does this mean that women with ADD have an easier time of it than ADD men? If their symptoms are less severe, ADD is not such a big problem for women, right?

Of course, it's not that simple. Women have certain characteristics and challenges that can magnify the impact of their symptoms. In the next few sections we will take a look at how the more subtle women's form of ADD can create as many problems as the out-there/in-your-face male variety. It is important to add that there are many men and women who do not fit the general pattern for their gender. There are gentle, spacey, inattentive men, and women who really know how to put the "H" in hyperactivity. Each person with ADD is unique.

The Squeaky Wheel Gets the Grease

The most obvious challenge for ADD women is that it is harder to recognize the syndrome when it is more subtle. That sweet little girl in the back of the classroom doesn't bother anyone. No one notices that she isn't really tracking what the teacher is saying. She is lost in daydreams or her mind has flown out the window to play with the birds. The boy across the aisle from her is a different story. He is loud, easily angered and always in hot water for getting out of his seat to stir up some excitement. Yes, he gets in a lot of trouble, but he also gets some help in the form of a diagnosis and treatment.

The little girl gets passed on in school with mediocre grades. She grows up thinking she is just not very smart. Or maybe she is another type of girl with ADD, very bright and very motivated to please others. She manages to get good grades, but at great cost to herself. She borrows heavily from sleep and play time to carve out the long hours she needs to keep up with classmates who do the work in half the time. This little girl feels like a failure too . . . she must be stupid if it takes her so long to get things done.

Little ADD girls who are unrecognized and untreated grow up to become women who never feel "good enough" no matter what they do. The legacy of struggle without an explanation takes a huge toll on their confidence and self-esteem.

Self-Esteem

Research tells us that ADD women have more problems with self-esteem than ADD men. Why would this be so? The following is a list of possible (or likely) suspects:

1. One piece of the puzzle, as we just mentioned, is that women with ADD are less likely to be diagnosed and treated.

2. Men are encouraged to focus on areas of strength at an early age, while women are expected to be generalists. We know that when you have ADD it is important to focus on areas of strength and spend less time in areas of weakness.

3. There is more tolerance for males with ADD behavior— the "boys will be boys" attitude.

4. Relationships are the coin of the realm for females—they are "expected" to be social experts. The impact of ADD on relating skills is huge . . . and women take it to heart much more than men do.

5. Do men lie on those questionnaires? Well, "lying" is a pretty strong word. Men are not as likely to *admit* to problems . . . even to themselves. We know that women are much more likely to seek therapy than men.

6. Mothers are more critical of their ADD daughters than their ADD sons. To our knowledge, no one has yet published research on the "why" of this finding, but we have a hunch that it has to do with the mirroring effect. Your ADD son or daughter is a mirror held up to you, demonstrating your own ADD behaviors that you are less than proud of. When the

child is your own gender, it is much closer to home and thus harder to deal with.

7. Girls with ADD experience more peer rejection than do boys with ADD. This may be the result of higher expectations for females in the social realm.

8. Impulsive risk-taking behavior is less acceptable in girls. We will elaborate on this in the next section.

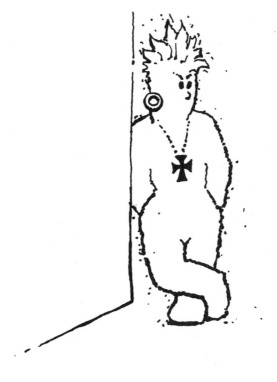

The Impact of Sexual Risk Taking

In 1994, at the second ADD adult conference, we cooked up a happening that was entitled "The Bad Girls' Break-Out Session." There was a lot of speculation and rumor buzzing around the event, especially among men, who were not invited. Years later, we are finally ready to reveal what went on behind those closed doors. To the accompaniment of a jazz pianist playing "The Stripper" and other related tunes, women told their stories of the "wickedest" thing they had ever done or thought about doing. Well, they didn't tell them personally. The women wrote them on a piece of paper and put them into a hat. The bolder, more "stagey" personalities in the group volunteered to read the stories to the group anonymously in a dramatic fashion. As I am sure you have already guessed, most of the tales were about sexual activities. We laughed, hooted and even shed a few tears. After the conference we received a number of letters from people who thanked us for providing the most healing experience of their lives to date. We all left a ton of shame behind in that conference room.

ADD women often struggle with baggage about their sexuality. We all know that one of the cardinal symptoms of ADD is impulsivity. Sexuality, of course, is a common arena for impulsive behavior. Research tells us that adolescent girls with ADD are sexually active at an earlier age, have more risk of pregnancy and more partners than girls without ADD. They are also at greater risk for STDs. Studies also reveal that, once the impulse-ridden teen years are past, women are more likely than men to feel shame or humiliation when they look back on their behavior.

In spite of the great advances made by women in the past few decades, the double standard lives on in the minds of midlife and older folks, who absorbed it in their formative years. The impulsive girl who has many partners is stamped with the proverbial scarlet "A." At best she is considered misguided, at worst she is a worthless slut. Many of the formerly "loose" ADD women we have coached now live responsible mainstream lives. They have husbands, jobs, children and mortgages. You would be hard-pressed to guess their history of a "misspent" youth. Some of them remember those days rather fondly, wistfully longing for a sense of freedom and adventure that is now missing in their lives. Others struggle with a profound sense of shame. If you are one of those who are troubled by their sexual past, don't let it hide in the dark corners of your mind. A good therapist can help you become more comfortable with yourself and your sexuality.

Housekeeping Is the Job Description from Hell for ADDers

This phrase was coined by Sari Solden, in her groundbreaking book *Women with Attention Deficit Disorder*. Of course, she was right on target. Think about it. What do ADDers hate but need desperately? Structure. What is completely lacking in the job of household manager? You guessed it, structure—unless you make it up yourself and then follow the blasted plan. As we all know, follow-through is not high on the list of ADD strengths.

There are a few men out there who have taken on the house-husband role, but most household managers are still women. Women with ADD may initially welcome the opportunity to leave the stresses of the workplace behind to be a stay-at-home mother. Often, however, they find they have simply exchanged the frying pan for the fire. The following is a Help Wanted ad for a household manager. Does this sound like a good job fit for your ADD self?

Wanted: Full-Time Household Manager for Busy Executive

This position requires endless handling of boring details. You will be constantly interrupted by phone calls, delivery people and the whiny demands of small children. Lunch hours and coffee breaks not guaranteed— in fact, it is doubtful there will be time for such frivolous activity. You will be expected to cook meals, clean a four-bedroom house and manage the lives of one adult and three children. Two of the children have special needs and thus will require extra help with homework, structuring daily activities and driving to various appointments with specialists. There will be daily crises, involving trips to the emergency room with the accident-prone children and calls from the school demanding that you pick up the suspended child *this instant!* This is a 24/7 job, but excellent performance will not earn you any time off. In fact, no one will notice your performance unless you screw up. In that case, you are unlikely to be fired outright, but you will be subjected to endless recrimination. You are expected to take care of your own needs in your (ahem) spare time, and to do so without complaint. In addition to your basic responsibilities, you will be expected to organize events for extended family members and the executive's work colleagues. Your job description can expand at any time without prior notice. Compensation for this sought-after position is hardly necessary—after all, it is not a real job and you will be receiving room and board in a lovely home, not to mention basic expenses. Only the seriously masochistic need apply.

Oops, got a tad sarcastic there. Makes it hard to find any reason to get out of bed, or do anything but sit in front of the soaps eating bonbons. Still, it is a pretty accurate description of the household managing experience of many women. Most of the traditional women's jobs have a lot in common with the household manager role. Consider the working conditions for nurses, teachers and administrators. You have a lot of responsibility and very little control, which translates to "anything that happens is your fault" even if there is nothing you could have done to avert the disaster. You are expected to process an incredible number of details, and you are on call for your entire workday. Hiding in an office to take a breather or some quiet time is not permitted. You don't even have an office . . . the best you can get is a little cube, in the case of administrators. Noise levels are high and the pay is not that great. We could go on and on. If you are the proud possessor of one of these ADD-unfriendly positions, we are not advocating that you hand in your notice immediately. We all have to eat. At the very least, stop beating yourself up because you struggle in your job. It is a lousy fit, with working conditions that are unfriendly to human beings, let alone ADDers. In addition, give some consideration to developing a plan to transition into a work life that serves you.

Women with ADD Are Likely to Have Children with ADD *and* Be the Primary Parent

We touched on this one in the last section. The job description from hell includes a mention of those special needs children. If you have children, we bet at least one of them has an ADD diagnosis, not to mention some of the other differences that often travel along with ADD. Your child may also be dyslexic, have Aspergers Syndrome, a language disability or a number of other challenges. Special needs are expensive, in terms of time and energy as well as dollars. As an ADDer you have limitations on the amount of energy in your mental fuel tank. The demands of your special needs children can quickly burn through the reserves in your personal fuel supply.

The biggest trap in this situation is guilt. You have an ocean of compassion for your struggling children, especially since they are faced with many of the same stresses you experienced as a child. Watching your kid being teased and rejected by peers feels like someone just slammed a sledgehammer into your heart. As a mom, your greatest desire is to eliminate all pain and suffering from your children's lives. It doesn't matter that you're a wise woman who knows she needs to master challenges in order to grow and evolve—it still hurts to watch the process. So you go overboard in your attempts to nurture and protect your fragile offspring. You burn yourself out—after all, you can't possibly do enough for them. Taking time for self-renewal is just not an option.

We are here to tell you that it is likely your quirky children will survive . . . and even thrive. Between us, we have three children, all of whom are now adults. Each of them has ADD and a number of other disabilities. We are still stunned by the miracle of transformation we have witnessed in these children. Someone somewhere waved a magic wand and turned our hopeless kids into mature, loving people who actually take responsibility for themselves. Kate's daughter Tyrell has even shared with her mother (on more than one occasion, so it wasn't just a fluke) that Kate was the perfect parent for her. She said something to the effect that "you hugged me when I needed it, and you kicked my behind when I needed that too." Both of us felt guilty when we were not able to be there 100 percent of the time for our children—when we were so burned out that we had no choice about taking personal time. Later we learned to take breathers before reaching the point of no return. The times we had to check out due to overload turned out to be growth opportunities for our kids. They learned to be more self-reliant. The very best thing you can do for your children is to make sure you take care of yourself.

Women Want to Know

Why Do Women with ADD Have a Greater Tendency to Believe That Events Happening to Them Are Their Fault?

A research study tells us that women with ADD *do* tend to blame themselves more than women without the disorder. This research did not compare ADD women and men, but we do know from other studies that men with ADD have more externalizing symptoms, while women with ADD have more internalizing symptoms. In plain English, this means that men are more likely to blast out their distress so that the rest of the world can see it. Women have depression and anxiety, but they take it out on themselves. Men often struggle with rage, for example, while women take their anger and frustration and turn it inward.

Why, though, would a woman with ADD think everything is her fault? Well, perhaps not *everything,* but we have heard a lot of clients express exactly that on "bad brain days." In the study comparing women with and without ADD, a couple of the examples given were car accidents and the boss yelling at you. The women without ADD would express that the car accident was due to weather, with poor visibility the major culprit. The boss yelled because he was having a bad day. The women with ADD, however, blamed only themselves for the car wreck and thought that the boss was yelling because they did something wrong. These women did not seem to consider the possibility that something outside themselves might at least be partly responsible for the outcome.

Women with ADD, then, get a double whammy. They think that the negative events in their life are their own fault, and then take their frustration out on themselves. It is not hard to imagine how women with ADD come to believe that they are always the guilty party. They already have a more negative self-image than men with ADD. Owners of an unpredictable brain that is prone to "oopses," they learn to mistrust their actions and perceptions. The self-talk starts with "I have made mistakes," expands to "I make a lot of mistakes" and then, finally, "I always make mistakes."

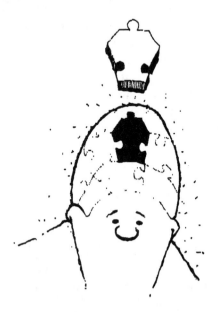

Estrogen — the Missing Piece

Hormones Again . . . ?

Hormones have a powerful effect on both mood and cognitive functioning. In an earlier section we mentioned the impact of the male hormone testosterone on aggression. We humans all have the same hormones in our bodies, but the mix is quite different in males and females. More estrogen and progesterone for women, for example, and more testosterone for men. Women, however, have a hormonal challenge that men simply do not. Creatures of the moon, we follow roughly lunar cycles as our hormonal balance ebbs and flows each month. This cyclic pattern starts at puberty and continues until menopause is complete.

We all have some familiarity with the impact of hormonal fluctuations on women's mental/emotional state and behavior. It is no accident that PMS jokes are stock in trade at the comedy clubs. Better that we laugh than tear our hair out . . . or we tear our hair out and then laugh when we feel somewhat better. In addition to the monthly roller-coaster ride, women also have to contend with the hormonal storms of puberty, the childbearing cycle and perimenopause/menopause. The temporary imbalances of hormones that happen during these times of fluctuation cause the unpleasant "symptoms." Some of these symptoms are a lot like the ones we contend with as ADDers, such as fluctuating moods, irritability, short fuses, forgetfulness and difficulty concentrating.

Years ago, when we were promoting the original version of this book, we showed up for a radio interview and were greeted by the same woman who had had us on her show the previous year (let's call her Susan). Susan was effusive in her welcome—acted like we were long-lost best friends, as a matter of fact. She revealed that she really didn't "get it" about ADD the first time around. In the past year she had entered perimenopause and had her first experiences ever with lack of control over her functioning. Susan, who had always been organized, articulate and calm, was now having difficulty locating her keys, finding the right words to say and keeping her cool on a day-to-day basis.

Well, if hormones wreak that kind of havoc on women without ADD, just imagine what they are doing to us. Dr. Pat Quinn, who has done groundbreaking work on the issues of ADD women, has found in the course of her clinical work that hormones have a significant impact on the symptoms of women with ADD. Falling estrogen levels turn out to be the biggest problem for ADDult women. Unfortunately, it is not a simple matter of taking a blood test to determine if you have the correct level of estrogen in your body. It is possible to have an estrogen level that falls in the normal range but is low for you as an individual. Low estrogen states occur in the phase before menstruation and during postpartum and perimenopause/menopause.

What Does This Mean for ADD Women?

First, it is important to recognize that a fixed dose of stimulant medication may not do the trick for you. The hormonal factor needs to be taken into consideration. Essentially, if there is not enough estrogen in your system, stimulant medication will not be as effective. For some women, low-dose birth control pills have been used to keep estrogen levels steady for a longer time during the menstrual cycle. In other cases, estrogen replacement therapy has been used *before* perimenopause to increase the effectiveness of stimulant medication. Dr. Pat Quinn has studied eighty-five women with ADD, several of whom are postmenopausal. These women reported a worsening of ADD symptoms in menopause and an improvement when treated with estrogen replacement therapy.

What Can You Do to Be Proactive in Your Own Treatment, Given This Information on Hormones and ADD?

First, keep a record of your cyclic changes and share it with your doctor. Dr. Pat Quinn has her patients keep a two-month record, rating their symptoms of attention, concentration, focus and organization on a scale of 0 (good) to 4 (poor) during the first four weeks of their menstrual cycle. After two months, if it is determined that ADD symptoms worsen during the third and fourth weeks, the dose of stimulant medication is increased.

Second, share information about ADD and the hormone connection with your prescribing physician. You can refer him or her to the chapter on hormonal fluctuations in *Gender Issues and AD/HD*, by Drs. Pat Quinn and Kathleen Nadeau.

What About Pregnancy—What Can You Expect as an Expecting ADD Woman?

Well, the bad news is that taking your stimulant medicine is not recommended during pregnancy. It is possible to continue with antidepressants, however, as the safety of tricyclics and SSRIs in pregnancy has been established. The good news is that pregnant women with ADD report that their functioning improves, sometimes dramatically. This makes sense, given that pregnancy is a high-estrogen state, as is the breastfeeding period. Be aware, however, that you may experience a crash when the hormones shift, either postpartum or during the weaning process. Make an appointment with the person prescribing your stimulant medication before delivery if you plan to bottle-feed so that you can be ready to take your medicine immediately after childbirth. If you are breastfeeding, have your supply of medication on hand before you begin the weaning process. Since stimulant medication is not approved for breastfeeding mothers, you are advised to wait until the baby is weaned before starting medication. But at least you will be prepared. Being a new mother is disorganizing enough, even when ADD is not a factor. We are sure that you have had some experience with how long it can take to get an appointment. A little advance planning on this one is well worth it.

Do Men with ADD Have More Issues with Anger Management?

The answer to this question is a qualified "yes." Men in general are more likely to express anger than women, and ADDers in general have more difficulty managing anger in an appropriate way.

One big piece of this may involve the differences in how our society responds to men and women in identical situations. While men in many Western societies have been discouraged from showing emotion, one great exception is anger. In some instances, it is even seen as a sign of strong leadership for a man to demonstrate his anger. Women, however, operate under a different set of expectations. Some of the first female executives to reach the higher rungs of the corporate ladder were called "bitchy" or "manipulative." They were surprised to find that the same behavior displayed by a male colleague was called "persuasive" or "being a real go-getter." In the same way, you may have heard someone defending an angry outburst by a male authority figure in terms of his being "passionate about that subject." He could be praised for "rallying the troops" behind a cause, while his female counterpart may find herself described as "scary," or even "unstable." While this type of attitude is definitely changing, it is often useful to recognize that years of cultural conditioning are difficult to undo in a short time.

Of course, there are exceptions to the standard male-female differences around anger. We know a woman (one of our clients, actually) who just signed up for her *third* round of anger management. She loves it. In contrast to the other folks in the class, her attendance was not mandated by the court. They spend their time being pissed off about being forced to take the class, while she does the work. Despite this example, in most cases it is true that ADD men (and men in general) have more difficulty controlling anger. One of the things we know about folks with ADD is that we often find it difficult to inhibit our words and actions. Also, as we mention in the chapter on meditation, the limbic system, which is the seat of the emotions, is often overly reactive in ADDers. When you add the hormone testosterone into the mix, the results can add up to a hard-to-manage cocktail for men with ADD.

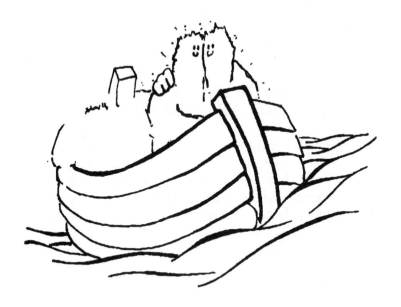

Sex and the ADDult

A number of years ago there was a psychopharmacology update floating around the Internet about a woman who experienced a, well, unusual reaction to taking an antidepressant. Actually, she was taking two antidepressants. One of them was Wellbutrin and the other was an SSRI, which stands for "selective seratonin reuptake inhibitor." Whew! What a mouthful. We have changed the meaning of those initials around to reflect our experience (and those of our clients) taking the darn things. We now think SSRI stands for "suppressed sexuality reduces intercourse." Some of the SSRIs are better than others, but basically they have a dampening effect on sexual functioning for most people.

Wellbutrin (bupropion), on the other hand, can counteract the sexual dysfunction caused by an SSRI. The woman in the Internet story reported that she had a spontaneous orgasm while shopping. This had never happened to her before. The report did not mention what kind of shopping she was engaged in at the time, so that is one of those pesky unknown variables. Obviously, this is not a controlled scientific study, but it does make you wonder . . .

Spontaneous Orgasm Brought on by Combination of Buproprion and Sertraline

. . . Female patient (35 years old) with recurrent depression was placed on sertraline (Zoloft) 100mg/d. After two weeks she complained of impaired sexual function, which prompted the addition of buproprion (75 mg/d) as adjunctive therapy for this condition. Her sexual condition improved considerably after one week and greatly after four weeks. At six weeks on this regimen, she experienced a spontaneous orgasm while shopping. She found the experience pleasurable, but socially unacceptable, and so she stopped taking the buproprion . . .

A friend sent this little tidbit from cyberspace, and also added a few comments of her own:

This has been haunting me ever since I read it. What store do you think it happened in? Did she moan and pant over the sausage counter in her local grocery store? Was she mooning over the men's jockey shorts when the experience "came" upon her? Just exactly what did she do? Perhaps she was in the women's underwear department and enjoyed a moment of rubbing a silky negligee across her cheek? How about the tool section in Sears? Would the sight of a power tool set her off? I just might order the *Psychopharmacology Update* just so I can get more exciting articles like this one!

This is not a chapter on medication . . . that comes later. The point of including this little anecdote is to underscore the relationship between brain functioning and sexuality. In Chapter 2, How Are We Different, we talk about how brain chemicals (neurotransmitters) are culprits in producing the symptoms of ADD. If you have had the delightful experience of having your libido turned off (like a water faucet) via the wonders of modern pharmacology, we don't have to tell you that tinkering around with those neurotransmitters affects your personal plumbing too.

To our knowledge, there is no research that specifically looks at ADD and sexuality, but here are a few tidbits from studies of the neurology of sexuality:

- Having sex increases dopamine activity in the brain. Of course, the studies that reveal this fact talk about copulating rats, guinea pigs and the like. However, almost everything we know about the human brain is the result of neuroscientists scrutinizing the behaviors of various rodents.

- On the flip side, dopamine is a major player in the creation of sexual desire. So we have a variation on the chicken or the egg issue. More sex equals more dopamine, and more dopamine equals the desire for more sex.

- Norepinephrine facilitates orgasm, while serotonin inhibits ejaculation and orgasm. In plain English, norepinephrine opens the door to the big "O," while serotonin closes it.

- It is not a matter of taking a lab test to determine the correct level of each brain chemical—it isn't even possible. Healthy sexual functioning is a matter of the *balance* between the different neurotransmitters.

What does this information mean to us ADDults who are far more interested in our own sex lives than we are in the bedroom behaviors of laboratory rodents? Well, we know that dopamine, norepinephrine and serotonin are big factors in producing the symptoms of ADD. The jury is out on exactly how these brain chemicals interact to produce the symptoms, but the balance between them is critical to optimal human functioning.

Since we know that these neurotransmitters are out of balance in ADD, and we know that they are important to sexual functioning, it stands to reason that ADDults would experience "differences" in the sexual realm. That is exactly what we have discovered in the course of our work with ADD adults. The following information is anecdotal:

- Many ADDults have revealed that taking stimulant medication for ADD boosted their libidos dramatically. This makes perfect sense, since stims are known to increase dopamine activity, and dopamine increases sexual desire.

- For some, the increase in desire led to more frequent and varied sex, while for others it fostered a more intense and pleasurable fantasy life.

- Quite a number of ADDults reported differences in sexual desire on different doses of medication. In other words, the changes are dose related.

- Of course, as we have stated previously, most people (up to 80 percent) experience a decrease in sexual functioning when taking SSRIs. In some cases there is a lack of desire, while in others the problem is with reaching orgasm.

Clearly, the optimal scenario for treatment of ADD that preserves sexual functioning is using stimulant drugs without the sexually troublesome SSRIs. What do you do, however, when the stims are not enough? There are a host of Web sites devoted to the topic of SSRIs and sexual side effects. Many of the people posting to those sites said that while they were not happy with sexual changes, it was better than living with the symptoms of depression.

Is the only option a disheartening choice between two evils, or are there ways of working around the problems?

Fortunately, the answer is yes. The following is a list of ways to vanquish the "suppressed sexuality reduces intercourse" demon:

1. Ask your doctor about trying Wellbutrin (buproprion) instead of an SSRI. Wellbutrin is an atypical antidepressant that increases dopamine as well as serotonin. Don't be overly concerned about the risk of having a full-blown climax while shopping for oysters. The woman described in *Psychopharmacology Update* was a very unusual case. On the other hand, some of you might consider it more of a benefit than a risk.

2. If your depression (or anxiety or impulsivity . . . whatever the specific symptom for which you are seeking help) is not relieved sufficiently by Wellbutrin, adding Wellbutrin to an SSRI may do the trick without creating troublesome sexual side effects.

3. Some people find that they adjust to the SSRI in four to six months and the sexual side effects improve or go away. Of course, this may be a long time to wait while your love life is on hold.

4. A few people have told us that they are able to reclaim their sexual functioning on SSRIs by increasing the frequency of masturbation for a time.

5. The "little blue pill" is another possibility. Viagra is not just for men. There is evidence that it helps some women with SSRI-induced delay in or inability to have an orgasm. The downside of this choice is that it is expensive.

6. Talk to your doctor about gradually reducing the dosage of your SSRI antidepressant, since the sexual side effects are dose related.

7. Case reports and a few studies have shown that the herbal supplement ginkgo biloba is somewhat effective in reducing SSRI-induced side effects.

8. A vigorous exercise program can help symptoms of anxiety and depression. This may enable you to decrease your SSRI dose.

Of course, it is important to keep your partner(s) in the loop about antidepressant-related sexual changes. Without this information they may assume that your lack of interest has something to do with them, or the relationship.

ADD and Sexual Differences

It may seem to be backwards—to talk about the sexual effects of medication treatment first, and then the general effects of having ADD on sexuality. Well, we don't pretend to be linear thinkers, so please bear with us. In this section we will just highlight and touch upon some issues ADDults experience in the bedroom (or the car, or the chandelier . . .).

Fluctuations in Desire: Of course, human beings are not raring to go at all times and in all situations. We all have normal variations in our level of interest in sexual activity. When you have ADD, however, those fluctuations may be more extreme and hard to explain. As we mentioned before, you may find that your libido is enhanced on stimulant medication. This, of course, is fabulous news. However, some ADDults find that having an increased sex drive creates new challenges. Their partners are used to the old level of frequency and are not interested in changing it. You may want to consider using masturbation as a means of discharging excess sexual energy in this case. If low desire is the issue, first take a look at your medication to see if that might be a problem.

Touchy Touchability: In the chapter about differences, we discussed tactile sensitivity, which is experienced as an aversion to being touched, or being touched in certain ways. As with most brain-based differences in ADD, the symptoms are variable; sometimes they are there and sometimes not. It can drive your partner crazy, not to mention yourself, when the moves that had you burning with desire on one occasion are like fingernails on the blackboard the very next day.

The first step in dealing with this pesky problem is to clue your partner(s) in. Frame it as a challenge rather than something horribly wrong with either of you. Experiment with various kinds of touch to find the sweet spot or spots for a particular lovemaking session. Of course, since the touchiness varies, the solutions will also change. Try out different levels of touch, from light feathery strokes to deep pressure. Engage with your partner verbally so that he or she has feedback on what is working or not working for you. There will be times when the best approach is to put the lovemaking aside for another day or time, without making anybody wrong for it. You can also decide to concentrate on stimulating your partner, if you are the one who is "touchy" on a particular occasion.

ADD and Kinks: A number of ADDults we have worked with have made a connection between "kinky" sexual practices and their ADD symptoms. Most of these folks were into what we call "S&M lite." Playful flogging with soft leather implements, for example, or tying each other to the bed. That sort of thing. We are not talking about pain here. A number of these folks said they found that the extra stimulation from these practices not only enhanced their love life, but also seemed to enhance their brain functioning. They were more focused after certain kinds of love play. This sort of activity may or may not work for you, but the need to try something different is worth considering.

The Need for Novelty: S&M may not be of interest to you, but do consider the need for variation in your bedroom activities. It is well known that the ADD brain craves novelty. The reason for this is that our brains are motivation dependent. This means that we need more incentive to get interested or stay interested in anything. Something new, of course, is always more fascinating than the familiar. Use your ADD imagination to keep your sex life snazzy. The chandelier might be a bit daunting if you're not in prime athletic shape, but what about the kitchen table, or the car? Changing the location is one possibility, as is a change in position. Browse through one of the gazillion sex manuals available if you are stumped for ideas. Spend some time with your partner sharing your fondest sexual fantasies and create some exciting sexual games. Do you fancy being the parlor maid who is seduced by the lord of the manor? How about playing the duchess and the chauffeur? Let your imagination take flight.

Managing the Stimulus Level for Both of You: Of course, the need for variety is one aspect of the larger issue of finding an optimal level of stimulation. That sweet spot, just enough and not too much input, will vary from person to person and from time to time. We already talked about the impact of ADD on our sense of touch, but what about the other senses? Visual stimuli, for example, are an important factor in sexual arousal, particularly for men. Making love with the lights on is one way to enhance excitement, as is watching videos. You may have a partner, however, who is not turned on by the films, or who prefers to make love in the dark. Your partner, ADD or not, may also be trying to find the right personal stimulus volume. ADD is not some bizarre set of behaviors dropped from an alien planet, but an exaggeration of certain human tendencies. Your "lights out" partner might be dealing with a sense of shame about sexuality, or he just might need to shut off the visual channel in order to focus on tactile sensations. It is not necessary to get into a struggle over this difference. One way to handle it is to use a blindfold. We recommend that you practice using the blindfold while maintaining a dialogue with your partner. The person who is blindfolded needs to feel secure, as this is a vulnerable position. Let him or her know what you intend to do, and ask permission first. What about the partner who is not interested in viewing sexual DVDs? Can you make a deal that you will view them by yourself before bedtime? You may want to share reading this section with your partner. He or she may be thinking that your need for more visual stimulation has something to do with their attractiveness or worth as a person. Viewing this issue through the lens of stimulus management can take the personal punch out of it.

Sex and the Laundry List: One of our dearest friends does a screamingly funny rendition of her inner dialogue during sex. Of course, like most of our friends, she has ADD. This woman (we'll call her Jenna) fights valiantly with her independently willful mind, trying to keep it from veering off into irrelevant topics, such as laundry or shopping lists. She knows that she is supposed to be directing her attention in the vicinity of her partner, but she just can't seem to make it happen. Jenna is convinced that her partner would be horrified if he realized that she was running down a list that included words like "Tide" or "Cheer" rather than, say, focusing on the incredible size of his equipment.

We can't always manage our distractibility. Sometimes we just have to let 'er rip. If you suffer from the sexual laundry list problem, suffer no more! If we took a poll, we bet the vast majority of people (ADD or not) don't have their attention strictly glued to their partner at all times during sex. Many people find their minds wandering to different images and even different sexual partners during the act. If you feel comfortable sharing this with your lover, a conversation or two about it may enhance your connection. If not, there is nothing wrong with keeping it to yourself. Stop beating yourself up for something that is out of your control and harmful to no one. If you absolutely must beat yourself up, consider asking your partner to use one of those soft floggers instead. Who knows? It might be more fun.

Losing Focus—for Men: Men have the additional challenge of greater performance pressure. It may not be an optimal situation, but at least women can engage in intercourse without full arousal. It is just not as obvious when women lose their focus during sex. Well, we know something about the balancing act involved here from our general struggles with ADD and attention. As ADDults we have learned to use a kind of mental force to shore up a, shall we say, flaccid attention. People observing us from the outside see all this stress and strain, and they wonder about the "why?" of our single-minded gluing of

253

attention to the focus du jour. They don't understand that we feel vulnerable to getting off track, and don't think we can afford to take a break or shift attention to something else. When it comes to sexual functioning, this dynamic can play out as a perceived lack of caring for or awareness of your partner. We are going to go out on a limb here and suggest that a partner who insists on performance above all else is going down the wrong road. They are not the one for you. Of course, you need to share your struggle with him or her before you come to the conclusion that they are judging your prowess in bed. It is possible that you are making it all up in the privacy of your mind. Do you really think that an ever-ready erect penis is the true measure of a man?

Jumping Your Partner's Bones: Have you ever had the experience of having your bones jumped? This is a sexual advance that seems to come out of left field. We are not talking about sexual assault in this instance, because the person coming at you is someone with whom you already have a sexual connection. There is also no intent to force or overpower or otherwise impose unwelcome maneuvers. Have you ever considered that the person who comes at you in a seemingly insensitive fashion might be under the influence of an "ADD oops"? Have you been the one who did the jumping, but you didn't realize that's what you were doing? Were you mystified at your partner's reaction?

Here is how something like this can happen in ADD-land. Actually, it can happen to anyone, but it is more likely when the mental connections are a bit fuzzy. Let's assume that the person making the advances is ADD. Let's make it a "he" and call him Jack. Jack has been living in his head all day, and his mind is populated with the usual junkyard assortment of thought-bites, images and so forth. One of the ways Jack has learned to jump-start his wandering brain is through sexual fantasy. We know from the previous lesson on the neurology of sex that this is a very effective strategy. So Jack goes there (at least in his mind) quite a lot. He spends a good part of the day generating steamy mental film clips.

When Jack gets home he is raring to go. He has had more than enough mental foreplay and is panting to get on with the main event. We know that the folks out there without ADD may have a hard time wrapping their minds around this, but Jack has a fuzzy sense of time and doesn't always completely grasp that the other people in his world have not lived the events that unfolded in the privacy of his mind. His wife, Susan, did not have a great day. She is lusting for a sympathetic ear or, barring that, a bit of peace and quiet. Jack is hurt and disappointed when his insistent ardor is met with stone cold disbelief. He is baffled: "How could she have forgotten the hot time we had in the old town last night? Where did that wonderful, wanton woman go?"

The Untouchable Syndrome: By the time we get to adulthood, our sense of self-worth is at least a little raggedy, having taken a beating as we grew up with a hidden difference. Most of us learn to paste on a mask of competence, and at least the outward appearance of confidence. However, that scared little kid who was tormented on the playground is still there, lurking just behind the mask. If you weren't exactly singled out for schoolyard torture, you may have done the deed yourself, in the privacy of your own mind, when you failed to measure up to your own expectations.

Our sexuality, of course, is at the core of our being and thus a part of us that is most vulnerable to assault. Anyone who has ever had the experience of a sexual betrayal knows that this is a huge and painful "hit" to the psyche. Feeling defective—lazy, stupid or crazy—is a state of mind that colors all aspects of our lives. When we are having a bad day, in terms of self-concept, we often don't want others to come too close to us. We feel infested with virtual "cooties" and are convinced, at some level, that anyone who gets too close will end up recoiling in horror. On those days, we don't want anyone within three feet of us, let alone the intense intimacy of sex. The untouchable syndrome is not the same as touchy touchability—that experience is neurologically based and one of feeling annoyed or irritated by touch, while this one is about feeling unworthy. If you have an intimate partner, it is a good idea to fess up when you are feeling like this rather than leaving the erroneous impression that there is something wrong with them.

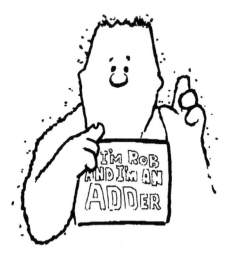

What He's Not Telling You: He's Also a Sex Addict

Sexual ADDiction: When we wrote the first edition of this book, we made an educated guess that ADDults might make up a large percentage of people in the "anonymous" groups. In the years since then, research has indicated that ADDults do have a greater tendency to struggle with addictions in many forms. Sex and Love Addicts Anonymous, as the name implies, is a twelve-step group that offers help to those who have an addictive relationship with sex.

At its core, addiction to anything is about feeling not good enough and trying desperately to grasp at something outside yourself for a "feel good" fix. Of course, from that initial impulse arises a cascade that eventually takes the individual's actions out of the realm of their personal control. Biology, for example, is a major player. Those "feel good" neurotransmitters are in short supply in people vulnerable to addictions.

As we discussed in the lesson on the neurology of sex, sexual activity is very effective at creating a feeling of well-being, in the brain as well as on a physical level. The big problem with using sex in this way is that when an addictive pattern is set up, the other person involved becomes an object, a means of satisfying desire, rather than a whole living, breathing soul with thoughts, feelings and desires of their own. The relatively short-lived "highs" experienced by a sexual addict are outweighed by the fallout from intense shame and guilt. As ADDers, we already have an unwelcome overabundance of those emotions. If you suspect that your relationship to sex has slid over the line into addiction, do yourself a big favor and check out the fellowship of those who have been there, Sex and Love Addicts Anonymous.

Speed Demons in the Bedroom: Hyperactivity, of course, is not simply a matter of squirming in your seat in the classroom or the boardroom (feels like bored-room to us). It can happen in any situation. It is also not a matter of absolute speed. If, for example, both you and your partner are satisfied with the tempo of your lovemaking, there is no problem, even if someone else might judge the pace to be too wildly frantic, or unbearably slow.

We are not talking about the pace of intercourse, in this case, but the progression from wooing to foreplay to the main event. Whoops! Did we really slip up and use the words "main event"? That kind of thinking helps to create the problem in the first place. If we are hyperfocused on going for the big "O," the connective steps leading up to it are given short shrift. Our partners are not happy when they end up feeling more like a target than a person, and that kind of approach doesn't serve us either. A frantic gotta-get-there energy is our enemy in all situations, and it is often most apparent in the bedroom.

What happens to sexual functioning when we are tense or anxious? Make no mistake about it, hyperfocus comes with a high level of tension. Now, we know that some of you are saying, "Huh? They don't know what they are talking about, hyper-

257

focus is my friend." Well, being totally focused on the present moment is a good thing, as long as you are relaxed. That way of being would more accurately be called the flow state. Hyper-focus is when you glue yourself to an object of attention with great effort. The excess tension generated has its consequences.

Both men and women shut down sexually when there is too much gotta-get-there energy. At the extremes, men may have symptoms such as premature ejaculation and impotence. Women can lose the ability to become aroused and/or reach orgasm. Both men and women may experience a decrease in sensation as well. These less than positive alterations in sexual functioning are the result of tension and speed. A certain level of relaxation is required to experience sensual pleasure. If you are hurrying too much you don't even allow yourself the time to feel the pleasure—it has come and gone before you know it. Even if you are functioning okay (able to become aroused and have an orgasm), you shortchange yourself when the focus is entirely on that orgasm. A much more satisfying full-body orgasm can be ours if we learn to slow down and feel the sensations in our entire bodies.

This is not new information. The ancient practice of tantric yoga teaches practitioners to slow down their sexual practices in order to reach higher states of consciousness. Students of tantra have spiritual goals, but the side benefit of having a great sex life certainly helps with the motivation to keep practicing! Actually, tantra doesn't separate sex from spirituality, which makes it a "terrific religion" in our estimation. In the secular realm, Masters and Johnson were pioneers in the field of human sexual response. Their program has helped countless people recover from sexual dysfunctions. In a nutshell, their methods are designed to help people slow down and take their focus away from achieving orgasm. Couples are prohibited from having intercourse for a time, and they are given homework involving a series of sensual exercises. Without the pressure to perform, the resulting relaxation response allows normal sexual functioning to surface. You can try this with your partner. Make an agreement that you will refrain from intercourse for a period of time. Set regular (say, every other night) appointments to get together for couples massage and sensual touching. Start with nonsexual touching and progress slowly to stimulating breasts and genitalia. We know how hard it is for ADDers to wait for anything, but isn't a wonderful sex life worth waiting for?

If There Seems to Be a Lot of Sex Going On, Do You Feel Like You're Missing Out? If we take our cues from popular culture, it is easy to come to the conclusion that everybody is f—ing like rabbits all the time. Like the kid who was alone on the playground, we feel that we are the only ones who can't get any action. This is simply not true. Remember, the images you see in movies and on TV are the product of someone's imagination. As coaches we have been privy to the intimate lives of many people, and our experience is that an awful lot of people have a pretty scanty sex life. Our busy, stressful lives are certainly part of the problem, and when you have ADD the life stress factor can get very intense. There are other issues to consider, however.

Are you hyperfocused on "getting some"? (this kind of energy is a big turnoff to potential partners)

Do you need to work on personal worthiness issues?

Are you afraid to get close to someone else?

Do you fear that, if they get close, they would find you wanting?

Does sex seem like a great idea (I think we could all agree that a great sexual experience is high on the list of peak experiences), but you really don't have the time or the energy for it?

Do you have some issues to work on with your partner before you can connect in an intimate way?

We promise that you will not have to wait forever. If you settle down and put your focus on healing, your energy will change. You don't have to be perfect or even close. Give it a try. When you are more accepting of yourself you will naturally attract others to you.

We've spent several chapters discussing the dynamics of ADD and relating in a variety of settings. We could probably continue adding things as they pop into our brains but it's time to move on to some other issues.

Throughout the book we've made references to organization, memory and learning. Many adults with ADD manifest unique differences in these areas—differences that can compromise the quality of overall functioning. In the next two chapters we'll examine the interplay of attention, organization, memory and learning. Our goal will be to help you identify the strengths you can use to compensate for any weaknesses in these areas.

CHAPTER 11

Dynamics of ADD in Organizing: Mechanics and Methods

In this last section of the book, we'll talk about everything we haven't had a chance to say yet! We'll look at many *"how-tos"* for an ADDer—how to work around specific skill deficits, how to make medication decisions and take care of yourself and how to move forward. Now that we've properly prepared you for your reading, let's get busy talking about the bane of many an ADDer's life: disorganization.

Life Is Difficult for the Organizationally Impaired

We saw this on a greeting card and wondered if an ADDer had designed it! Disorganization seems a way of life for many of us. It makes us wonder if perhaps researchers have been missing an important diagnostic tool—a questionnaire that might go something like this:

1. When you go to a bookstore, do you head for the self-help aisle in search of books with titles such as *Five Steps to a More Organized Life* by Ima N. Disarray or *Systematizing Stuff* by R. U. Tidy?

2. How many of these kinds of books do you own?

3. Do you decorate your rooms with Post-it notes instead of wallpaper?

4. Do you try a new filing system several times per month?

5. How many reminders do you have written on your left hand? Your right hand?

6. How many times do you search for your missing car keys every day?

7. How many times do you arrive at the grocery store without your shopping list?

8. How many piles of unopened mail are there in your house?

9. How many items have you listed on your "to do" list? Do you have a "to do" list? Do you have a "to do" list for your "to do" list?

10. How many times were you late for an appointment in the past week?

11. Do you frequently say the words "I forgot"? How many times did you say them in the past twenty-four hours?

12. How many times does your child go to a soccer game with wet socks because you forgot to put them in the dryer?

13. How many days after a business trip do you leave your suitcase still packed in the corner?

14. How many times do you get to your hotel and remember that your suitcase is thousands of miles away on the floor of your bedroom?

15. How often do you have to call hotel room service for a toothbrush or shampoo because you forgot to pack yours?

16. Do you wear a waterproof watch in the shower to keep track of time? Do you set the timer on your watch as a reminder to get out before you drain the hot-water tank?

We haven't standardized the diagnostic criteria of our test, but we think we might be on to something here. We're guessing that readers who "failed" this test know who they are. So, just how many times a day do you lose your keys, your child, your mind? We hope you know that this means you are in good company with many other wonderful, distractible ADD adults.

Although we began this chapter with a reference to (dis)organization, it's impossible to separate it from the larger issues of learning, attention and memory. The jury is still out regarding the specific reasons for the ADDer's problems with time and space. Are they symptoms of the disorder? Are they specific learning disabilities that come packaged with the ADD? Or are they a result of a basic difficulty with selective focus?

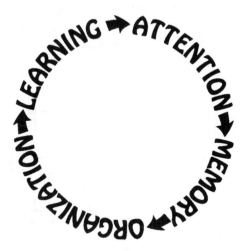

Creating Order—Where Do You Start?

Regardless of the specific causes of ADD adults' time and space problems, life is indeed difficult for the organizationally impaired! Feeling perpetually disorganized may be a daily reality. Many of us never seem to know how to manage the time and stuff of our world and often feel at the mercy of forces beyond our control.

Decide Whether the Disorder in Your Life Causes Stress: Your messy closets and desk aren't problems simply because your spouse thinks they're disorganized. If you can find what you need relatively easily and are comfortable with the seeming disarray, you don't have a problem.

If you decided that a messy house is a satisfactory trade-off for extra free time, you don't have a problem. Of course, it's important that this trade-off is acceptable to the rest of your family. Their needs should be a part of your balance sheet.

If disorganization isn't a problem for you, skip this discussion and focus on the other areas of your life that require your attention. If you scanned the table of contents and immediately flipped open to this chapter, you know you have a problem with organization. If you're constantly putting out fires and your life is cluttered with missed deadlines and paperwork pileup, you need to make a conscious decision to work at developing a sense of order.

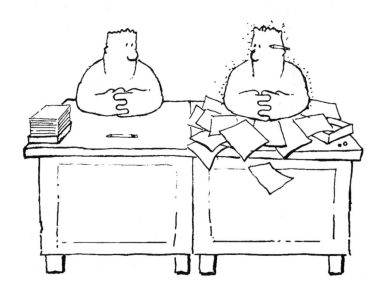

Remember That There Is No Such Things as a Perfect System: Although you may feel that organizing your life is an impossible task, it really isn't! With some creativity, work and planning, you can create order in your life. Don't worry, though, about coming up with the correct organizational system, because there is no right or wrong method.

Although you're an adult, you may still operate with parental admonitions ringing in your ears: "Put your soccer shoes in the closet as soon as you get home . . . Don't hang your jacket on the doorknob." Maybe hanging your jacket on the doorknob is a great system because it jogs your memory about the errand you still need to do. Perhaps leaving your shoes by the front door reminds you to polish them. The point is, you need to toss out the old "shoulds" and do what works for you.

Review your balance sheet. Think about your list and consider some of the following general time-and-space issues:

What are the spaces in your home and how do you use them?
Do you feel comfortable in the spaces you live and work in?

What objects fill your home and your life?
How often are these objects used—frequently, occasionally, never?

What things have remained unused for a long time?
How much time do you spend trying to figure out how to get started?

Do you have trouble controlling: Time? Stuff? Both?

To Get Organized, Approach Your Disorganization in an Organized Way: For starters, divide the global idea of order into smaller pieces. When you characterize yourself as a disorganized person, what do you really mean? Identify the problem areas, prioritize them according to severity and then design a plan for dealing with a reasonable number of them. By establishing a limited number of goals, you're already on your way to becoming more organized.

Approach the reading and digesting of this chapter in the same fashion. We realize this section is chock-full of suggestions, some of which may not apply to your individual situation. The volume of information may also be overwhelming. Break this chapter down into smaller chunks, tackling a piece at a time. If you find yourself becoming confused or overwhelmed, close the book for a while and come back to it later.

Organization Begins with a Pencil and Paper: To figure out your specific organizational problems, start with a pencil, a planning notebook and some quiet time. If you can find all three of these things, you may not be as disorganized as you thought you were!

Think about the things in your life that make you feel disorganized. If the first thing you write on your list is "everything," tear off that sheet of paper and try again! You need to focus on isolated problems so you can systematically work out solutions.

Emotions can be useful clues for identifying and isolating specific problems. Think about a typical day and run through it event by event in your mind. Stay tuned in to your emotional responses to various situations. If you begin to feel anxious just thinking about the milk that's still on the grocery store shelf instead of in your refrigerator, you've hit on a problem! Continue the process by writing down each problem as you think about it.

Put Limits on the Number of Problem Areas: Don't give up if you end up with pages of identified problems. Pare down your list by initially setting aside everything but the first four to six items. You might try to analyze your list by ranking the problems in a general way and focusing only on the most problematic issues. Your ranking can be based on the level of personal aggravation: drives me crazy, sort of bothers me and no sweat. Perhaps cleaning out the storage closet doesn't have to be done right now, but if the mess constantly grates on you, rank it close to the top of your list.

Work with Your Prioritized List: If you get this far and file it somewhere in your unmanageable file cabinet, you will accomplish nothing except to have wasted some time. Although you may have precious little down time, schedule some extra to deal with your problem-solving list. If you simply wait to get around to it, it will never happen. Make a conscious decision to meet with yourself at prearranged times to visit your list and develop solutions.

Organization experts focus on simplifying issues by breaking them down to smaller, more manageable parts. Consider the components of each problem area and individually list them on your paper. If your cluttered office is driving you crazy, think through the specifics of the problem. A cluttered office is a space problem with many sub-items. Is your desk messy? Are there too many papers tossed around carelessly? Are your garbage cans overflowing? Is your calendar still turned to the previous month?

This detailed list will help you get started with your personally designed organizational system. As you consider the discussion and ideas that follow, use your prioritized list as a framework. Think about your particular problems and individual style and try to match them to the ideas that appeal to you. Ignore the others and don't get distracted by things that aren't on your list. They may be important, but you can't fix everything at once.

General Mess Management

If you are like many ADD adults, your *What Drives Me the Craziest* list probably includes a variety of time and space problems. We'll save discussion of time management for later in this chapter and focus on space problems or mess management now.

Mess management has two components: clearing out and storing. Keeping track of the stuff of your world requires the same effort and planning as many other areas of your life. It really is a shame that planning—the thing most of us hate more than anything else—is the single most important thing we can do for ourselves! It's probably more accurate to say we're planning impaired than organizationally impaired.

You'll need to make a plan if you're going to have control over the stuff of your life. A logical way to start developing this plan is with an analysis of the clutter in your world. Take a house tour and make an inventory that focuses specifically on stuff. By using this *Stuff Inventory* and the *What Drives Me the Craziest Inventory*, you'll have a framework for your action plan.

Compile Your Stuff Inventory: Do you live in a house with large storage closets? They are great places for dumping the stuff you clear out from other places but have a particularly troublesome drawback. They are deep, black holes into which stuff falls, never to be seen again! When it's time to get out your winter boots, you may not be able to remember where you put them. You're probably already late for the sledding party and in too much of a hurry to find them. You may arrive home hours later with wet gym shoes and frostbitten toes!

As you do your inventory, make a note of how often you use various items. Divide your paper into three columns and categorize everything: the things you routinely use, occasionally use and haven't used anytime in recent memory. When your list is complete, schedule a time to come back and get to work clearing out the clutter in each room.

Arm Yourself with Three Big Boxes: Physically separate the objects in each room according to their frequency of use. For starters, put anything you access with great frequency in a *Use All the Time* box. Everything else should go in the garbage can or into one of two clearly labeled boxes: *Occasionally Use* and *Haven't Used in a Long Time*. If in doubt about whether to keep something, don't waste time thinking about it. For now, just put it in your Haven't Used in a Long Time box.

Work with your first box, putting these routinely used items in readily accessible places. If you need to buy a bookcase or hanging shelves to maximize storage, jot a reminder in your notebook. Tape contents lists on your other two boxes, put them in a closet or out of the way somewhere and schedule a time for their subsequent review. When you discover several months later that you still haven't used something, take the plunge and throw it away!

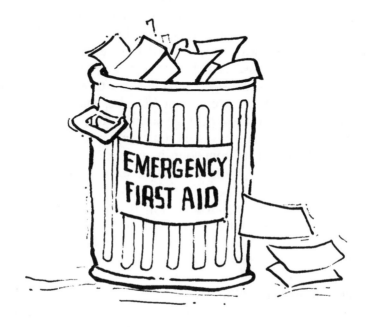

Make Liberal Use of a Trash Can: The trash can is an indispensable aid in the war on clutter. Each item you discard reduces the quantity of stuff you have to manage. Of course, some impulsive ADDers may use their trash cans to excess and end up rummaging through the debris to locate the tax refund check they hastily discarded by mistake!

Some of us, however, tend to keep everything. Perhaps we do this because we can't trust our memories or our organizational skills and are scared to death we'll discard something important. It seems easier to keep everything so we don't have to make any decisions. The more things you can clear out, however, the more comfortable you'll feel about managing the remaining stuff.

Schedule an Inventory Review: It is important to schedule review sessions to reassess organization decisions. During your inventory review, go through the contents of your stored boxes. Have you had to refer to your content's lists to find something you needed? If so, leave it where it is or move it to a more accessible location.

If your boxes remain untouched, it's probably time to make liberal use of your trash can. After several periodic checks, you'll probably end up with boxes considerably emptier than when you started. If you still can't bring yourself to throw out some of the unused items, consider moving them to a fourth, *Almost Ready to Discard* box. Remove it from the main part of your house and store it in your garage or attic. Keep your list handy in the unlikely event you need something in it. At least you'll remove these objects from your living space and perhaps convince yourself that you really won't ever use any of this stuff!

We'll leave it to the organization experts to help you with managing most of the stuff of your world. You can get ideas from a self-help book in your local bookstore. But let's look at just a few sources of household clutter.

Newspapers and Magazines
We bet that when you do your household inventory, you'll find miscellaneous magazines and newspapers in many places other than your magazine racks. The clearing out part of mess management is the most important part of dealing with the clutter of these reading materials, so get out your trash can and use it!

If you find more than two unread back issues of a particular subscription, don't send in the renewal notice when it arrives. Save a few issues if you really think there's a chance you'll have the time to read them; throw out the old ones and resist the temptation to buy any more.

What about the newspaper? Do you typically put a week's worth of unread issues in your recycle bin on garbage day? If this happens regularly, cancel your subscription and buy a newspaper at the corner stand only when you know you'll have time to sit and read it. It's amazing how available space grows when the piles of newspapers and magazines are discarded.

If you want to keep some articles for future reference, don't just stack them in the corner. Tear out the pages you want to save and put them somewhere you have a chance of finding them again! A labeled file folder might work. If you prefer keeping the entire issue, note the article and page number on the cover as a prompt. Otherwise, you'll repeat the cleaning process when you come across the issue later and wonder why you kept it.

Miscellaneous Stuff

You've read our suggestions, referred to organization self-help books and organized some of the household clutter. Now what do you do with your car keys, sunglasses, bike-lock key and miscellaneous puzzle pieces? They need permanent homes so you'll be able to find them easily.

If you have an assortment of keys, try hanging a key rack with labeled hooks right by the door. A key rack in the line of traffic is readily accessible and prompts family members to use it. Dropping your keys in your purse or belt pack is fine, assuming you can remember where you've tossed them! Purses and belt packs can be moved, but the key rack is always in the same place.

What about those puzzle pieces? Some children can manage to get the big toys put away but don't know how to handle the miscellaneous pieces. A labeled box in the corner of the bedroom or playroom can be a collection bin for these things. The child can drop them in her *Lost and Found* box for your help later in finding their rightful places. You can make a project out of painting the box or personalizing it in some way to encourage its use.

A box also works well for items that family members need to take with them. Your child's backpack or the dress that needs to go to the cleaner's can be dropped in this box. If people have to practically trip over the box to get out the door, there's a better chance they'll pick up the items in it.

General Office Management

If you take the time and effort to carefully design your Clearing Out and Storing Mess Management System, you'll begin to feel more in control over the disorganization in your world. Unfortunately, household stuff isn't the only source of organization problems.

We started with these general stuff issues because they're the easiest to manage. After you get some of these things under control, you need to think about some of the tougher issues of time and space management. These involve the daily handling, sorting and storing of a multitude of details—appointments, bills and "to do" lists. Time and space issues are tough because they change frequently and require persistent, ongoing attention.

You can think of these details as home-based work that doesn't pay any salary. The payoff comes in peace of mind. Let's take a look at these management issues and some strategies that may help you realize your personal payoff.

Design a Personal Work Space: When you're on the job, you have a work space. It might be an office, a construction site or the backseat of your car if you travel as a salesperson. Regardless of the parameters of this work space, it provides the framework for the tasks you perform. When you're at home, your work space is usually less well defined. Without a plan, it's easy to become disorganized.

Do you have a specific place where you handle paperwork? Or do you handle it wherever you happen to be at the moment? When you note an error in your utility bill, do you have to go to several different places before you have the pen, stationery, postage stamp and bill you need to write your inquiry letter? To avoid this waste of time and energy, you need to set up an office where you will handle the organizational details of your life.

This space will become a structured place for your work. Ideally, this space would be unused for anything else. If you don't have this luxury, set aside some space that will be exclusively yours at certain times. And it needs to be a place that makes you feel comfortable.

We were recently in a newly constructed business office that had virtually no exterior or interior walls. There were several large conference rooms with floor-to-ceiling windows and views of the rooms across the hall and the courtyard below. It was absolutely beautiful and totally useless for a distractible ADDer! Your office doesn't have to be big and beautiful. But it does need to be designed to match your style so you'll be more inclined to use it regularly and consistently.

So where will you set up your work area? Of course this depends on available space. Even if you don't have a house large enough to accommodate a separate room for your organizational chores, it's imperative that you find a space somewhere. Is there an unused corner in your attic? What about the garage? Don't forget one end of your living room, particularly if the family seldom uses it. With some ingenuity and an inexpensive freestanding screen, you can create your office within a room.

Organization experts emphasize the need to assess individual needs in determining the best place to work. Do you prefer having a good supply of light in your work space? When is the best time for you to work?

Do you need to be able to look out a window or is this too distracting? Are some colors more comforting to you than others? Is the space in the line of incoming traffic? Do you work better away from family activity or right in the middle of it? If the space doesn't have a telephone, can you add a phone jack?

What about storage space? Is there a place for a filing cabinet or drawers for your office supplies?

Think about these questions as you take a house tour with pencil and planning notebook in hand. Take a look at the spaces and note the pros and cons of each. If other family members use the space, how does the timing of their use correspond to your needs? The kitchen table may fit the bill for your work space. But if it's always in use during the early-morning hours you prefer to work, the space may not be a good choice. You might not come up with a place that perfectly matches your needs, but you can find one that fits your greatest needs.

Consider the Ergonomics of General Office Organization: "Ergonomics" is a fancy word with a simple meaning: a design for easy and comfortable access. It's a key component in organization. If your telephone is within reach but the phone directory is in the closet across the room, you may opt to ignore making the call. It's just too much trouble to walk across the room to find the number you need.

Do a personal office inventory in much the same way you inventoried the space and stuff in your house. Look around your space. Do you ever use the hole punch you keep in your pencil holder? If you use your stapler every day, do you keep it in the back of your drawer? Rearrange your space so the frequently used items are within easy reach. Store the hole punch in the closet and move the stapler to your desktop.

Note: If you're using shared space for your office, you'll need portable storage for your supplies. A rolling file cabinet or a box divided into sections may do the trick.

Practical Tools for Mess Management

As you design your work area, consider some of the tools and equipment you can use. Undoubtedly you'll equip your space with a desk or writing surface and some file folders, pens and pencils. But there are other, less obvious things you can use to make your life easier. You might want to add them to your supply basket.

Postage Scale: If you frequently mail more than just letters, consider buying a postage scale. Weighing your mail at home saves the time and trouble of driving to the post office. It also enables you to complete your task and get the extra paperwork immediately off your desk. Without a scale, your paperwork may end up on your desk a second time when the post office returns it for insufficient postage.

Assortment of Postage Stamps: To avoid wasting money on excess postage, keep a variety of stamps on hand for your special mailings.

Return Address Stamp: Along with these mailing supplies, have a stamp made with your return address and several others for people you correspond with frequently. Although a rubber stamp is more expensive than paper mailing labels, it reduces the quantity of materials you need to handle. It also eliminates the problem of remembering to mail the reorder form before you run out of labels.

Letter Opener: This might seem like a rather silly item to list as an important tool. Your fingers probably work just fine for this job. But it really is a useful contribution to the order in your office. Torn envelopes are messy and don't lie flat in a pile. The postage date or return address you need for your records might also be unreadable. Neatness isn't essential to a sense of order, but it doesn't hurt!

Staples: Why would we bother including this in our list? Of course you have staples in your supply basket. We're not trying to insult your intelligence! We bet, though, that when your stapler is empty, you might reach for a paper clip instead. In a word: don't! Paperwork clipped together has a mysterious way of becoming unclipped! Then you have to take the extra time and trouble to find the missing page and reattach it in its proper place. Always keep your stapler loaded so you have to do a task only once.

A Computer and Printer: This is an invaluable aid for the organizationally impaired! One advantage of a computer is the reduction of the sheer quantity of paperwork and files. Much of what typically has to be stored in files in a cabinet can be stored instead inside the magical electronics of the computer. The monthly chore of writing checks and reconciling your checkbook can easily be accomplished with accounting software. Better still, sign up for automatic debit bill paying.

As seasoned computer users we want to caution you about the limitations of computer magic! If your hard drive crashes and burns, you'll lose your data forever or at least until a data recovery expert charges a keen fee to retrieve it. Make sure you follow the suggestion of computer users everywhere: BACK UP YOUR DATA!

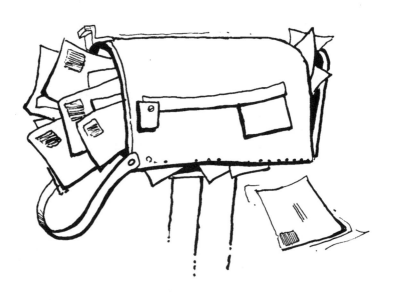

Paper Pile Management

As a child, do you remember longing for the mail carrier to deliver a letter with your name on it? We do. Were we nuts? Didn't we know that mail has the uncanny capability of multiplying when we're not looking? Well, at least that's how it feels.

Figuring out what to do with the paperwork is a source of aggravation and confusion. We can sort our belongings and cancel magazines and newspapers, but the paperwork keeps arriving in our mailboxes!

As soon as you order from one mail-order catalog, you're quickly deluged with catalogs from other companies who have purchased your name and address. Mail order can be a great way for an ADDer to shop. Eliminating the distractions of other shoppers and rows of items to choose among can be a relief. The disadvantage is finding a place to put the four or five catalogs that find their way to your house every day.

Mail isn't the only source of paperwork. After a day of errands, you may arrive home with a large pile of bank slips, store invoices and credit card receipts. You also accumulate miscellaneous reminders that you've written for yourself. It doesn't take more than a day or two for a mountain of papers to have grown on your counter. To deal with Paper Pile Management you need a plan.

Use Your Planning Notebook Again: Every day when the mail arrives, jot down the things you receive. For a week or so, put all accumulated receipts and pieces of paper in a box. At the end of the week, go through your pile and add each item to your list. At the end of this process, you should have a reasonable idea of your paperwork inventory.

Categorize Your Paper Pileup: Your next job is to divide your general list into small, more manageable parts. For now, you might want to start out with two large, relatively easy-to-use categories: *Trash* and *Things to Keep*.

Divide a second sheet of paper in half and put everything from your master list in one of these categories. You might prefer to dump out your box and physically put everything in the proper pile. If you agonize over trashing versus keeping, you might want to start a third pile for *Maybes.*

Whether or not you realize it, you've just begun to create order out of paperwork disorder. You're working with a plan and that's what organization is.

The only category you need to be concerned about is your Things to Keep. Things to trash should already be in your garbage can. If you can't do without your third category of Maybes, put that paperwork aside for now and don't use it during the next step of fine-tuning. Although your pile may not look much like a filing system yet, it will soon.

Sort your list into two smaller groups or make two piles on the floor: *Things to Do* and *Things to File.* Put anything that you need to act on, such as bills, in the "to do" category. Put everything else in the "file" category.

As you continue this sorting process, keep in mind your needs and lifestyle and those of your family. The book club mailing may interest you, but be honest: Is there any way you'll have time to read any of the books you might order? If the book club uses a system of automatically sending selections, are you prepared to keep track of the deadlines and deal with the extra paperwork? As you make decisions to discard some of these things, you can significantly reduce the quantity of paperwork.

Set aside your entire "to do" file for right now. To keep track of these current and pending items, you'll need to design a system for easy, automatic access. We'll talk later about managing these important "hot" folders. For now, focus only on your "to file" pile—the paperwork you seldom need to access. We'll start with this part of your filing system because it's more easily managed than your daily paperwork.

At this point, you should feel less anxious about the Paper Pile Management you've pared down in size. So, get out some file folders and sort the papers in your "to file" pile into subgroups. We can't tell you specifically how to organize these because it will depend on the kind of paperwork you handle. But you might try using general categories of *House and Financial,* plus *Personal* and *Spouse.* The key is to keep your groups simple and broad. Although there will be some overlap, sorting according to these categories will be fairly straightforward.

Cardinal Rule #1: Use Your Filing System Regularly and Consistently

Should you set up your files alphabetically or by type? Again, we can't tell you how to arrange them because there isn't a right or wrong way to do it. But we can offer two guidelines. First, regardless of the system you design, you must use it regularly and consistently. We know we've already said this, but it warrants repeating.

Cardinal Rule #2: Keep It Simple

Don't be tempted to be too organized. For example, you'll probably want to keep records of home improvements and related items in your Home/Financial file. You could keep separate folders for each item—carpeting, appliances, lawn care equipment, electronics, etcetera. If you fine-tune your divisions too much, though, your system will become too complicated. It would probably be better to group these related items in one or two folders. Since it's a good idea to keep records of home improvements for tax purposes when you sell your house, you might want to keep these separate. But keep other home-related records together in one folder.

Cardinal Rule #3: Meet with Your Paperwork at Scheduled Times

After you finish sorting, labeling folders and filing every piece of paper, immediately make a decision about *when* you will file your incoming mail and paperwork. Check your schedule and pencil in an appointment to *meet with your paperwork* on an ongoing basis. If you don't make a specific plan to do this, you'll experience the perplexing phenomenon of the Plague of Paperwork—it spreads and multiplies with astonishing speed and disastrous results!

Cardinal Rule #4: Always Handle Your Paperwork in the Same Place

Successful organization depends on thoughtful planning and a routine. Make a habit of always handling your paperwork in your office space. Avoid opening your mail on the kitchen counter, in the front hall or on the run. Take incoming mail and miscellaneous paperwork to the place you've chosen to work. If you flip through your mail when it arrives or open several pieces on your way out the door, you will be greeted by a messy pile when you get home. You'll begin to feel out of control again.

To-Do's and Paper Pile Mismanagement

Now that you've taken care of your permanent filing system, it's time to deal with the primary source of disorganization—your "to do" pile. This is where problems of time management intersect and often collide with those of Mess Management.

To deal with the confusion of this paperwork, assign an importance factor to every piece of paper. Use the degree of urgency to separate the paperwork in your "to do" file: important—must act on now; important—must act on sometime soon; important—pending a response; may be important; unimportant. If you've already made judicious use of your trash can, you shouldn't have many unimportant pieces of paper left.

As you do this sorting, use some kind of marking system to track how long and how many times you've been shuffling the same piece of paper. For example, you could date-stamp each piece of paper every time you handle it. This serves two purposes. First, it will document the date of receipt of the paper. Second, it will prompt you to make some decisions.

If your piece of paper becomes wallpapered in date stamps, it's been handled too much! Maybe it's time to schedule a special date to get the job finished and out of your "to do" pile. Maybe it's time to question whether the job should be on your list at all. Weeding your flower garden may be something you really need to do, but the weeds won't get any shorter as the days go by. Hire a neighborhood child to do the weeding for you so you can get the job off your list and onto hers!

Make a Decision About Storage and Access: Now you have to figure out where to put this important paperwork so you can quickly access it. Many organization experts say that you should put it in a "hot" folder in the file cabinet. We're not so sure this is a great idea for an ADDer. Putting something away in a file can be akin to burying it in the yard under eight feet of dirt! Once it's out of sight, it's out of mind. You can't take action on it and you can't retrieve it.

If you *need to see it to do it,* you may have to come up with some alternatives to the file cabinet. Perhaps one of these suggestions will work for you.

Bulletin Board: Consider hanging a bulletin board. Divide it in four sections to match your *importance* categories. Instead of residing in the depths of your file cabinet or taking up residence over the expanse of your desktop, your pending notes and messages can be readily seen and accessed. Hang your bulletin board at eye level to act as a visual prompt.

In/Out Baskets: If you have sufficient space on your desktop, try using four baskets. Use three as *In* baskets for your Important/Now, Important/Soon and Maybe Important paperwork. The fourth, your *Pending* basket, is for your Already Done/Waiting for Response paperwork. Put a label on each to remind you what the basket is for.

Desktop File: Without question, a file cabinet is useful. It efficiently stores a lot of paperwork and keeps office clutter to a minimum. It would be a great system if only it didn't *hide* everything!

Keeping papers sorted in piles might work—at least until a gust of wind sends them floating through the air. Since piles aren't particularly efficient, the next best thing is a desktop file. Although keeping files in plain view might not look neat, it can help you keep better track of your important and pending paperwork. It has the added advantage of being portable so you can move it off your desk to provide extra work space. If you don't have room on your desktop for a file box, buy one that hangs over the top of a drawer.

If your files are at your fingertips, you'll be more inclined to put your paperwork away before it accumulates. Having to walk across the room to a filing cabinet may be too much trouble!

Personal Yellow Pages: You might be using your permanent files for business cards or flyers of services or stores you'll need some time in the future. Although this kind of information shouldn't be with your "to do" paperwork, it probably shouldn't be stored in your filing cabinet either. A more useful system might be to set up a Personal Yellow Pages Directory. It might be a good idea to list your entries alphabetically by service rather than by name. When you need to call John Alverstraton, the carpenter who fixed your porch steps, you may not be able to remember his name. It's a lot easier to find him under "C" for carpenters.

Cues, Prompts, Memory and Mess/Paper Pile Management

Mess and Paper Pile Management is largely dependent on the components of attention and memory. To be better organized, you will need to work at your system and attend to the details of the task. Moreover, you need to REMEMBER what to do with the details. Do the following scenes look familiar?

You spend an entire afternoon clearing off, straightening up and filing away piles of paperwork. You look around your space and feel quite proud of yourself because you have efficiently filed everything in its proper place.

Fade to the same place, one week later

You confidently begin your scheduled chores of sorting and filing, secure in the knowledge that your great system will work again. You open the first letter and begin to feel uneasy. What should you do with this response to the inquiry you wrote last week? And just where did you put your copy of that inquiry? Did it go in the "to do" file or the "pending" file? With increasing anxiety, you scan your files trying to recapture the systematic process you designed last week. Much to your dismay, you realize that you don't have a clue how to begin . . .

Many ADDers find that this perplexing scenario repeats itself time and again. Our response to the dilemma is often to design yet *another* new system! We don't really need a better system—we need a better memory. Let's consider how Memory and Mess/Paper Pile Management can work together in our war on disorganization. In the following chapter, we'll look at other issues of memory management.

Regardless of the degree of your disorganization, when you want an ice cube, you go to the freezer and get one—assuming you remembered to refill the tray the last time you emptied it! When you want to put your hands on your car title, however, your search may be considerably more convoluted. Although you probably won't look in the freezer for it, you might look in many other places!

You know where the ice cubes are because you repeatedly access them from the same storage place. The car title is an entirely different matter because the possible storage places are innumerable. Did you file it alphabetically by name? Did you file it under your Personal file, Spouse file or in the Home file?

Did you file it in your "hot" file because you knew you would need it soon?

Put Your Planning Notebook to Work Again: To prevent the panic of filing system blackouts, you may need to keep a running list of the contents of both your current and permanent files. Make a dated outline of your files, jotting down the contents of every folder. Be sure to update your list anytime you make changes to your folders. If you need to see it to do it, your list will be the next best thing to having your files physically spread around you in plain view. If you'd rather take the time to sit and memorize the location of every paper, we suppose that would work! Somehow we think you probably have more pressing things to do with your time.

Your planning notebook also comes in handy when you need to stop working in the middle of a task. Use it to jot down some notes about what you're working on and what still needs to be finished. While the process of the particular job is still clear in your mind, write a short description of how to restart the job tomorrow. Otherwise, when you get back to work next time, you may have forgotten that the job wasn't finished. You may also waste time reconstructing what you were trying to accomplish and how you were doing it.

Use a System of Color Coding: Another prompt that might help you work more efficiently is color coding. Your color-coded system can vary according to the categories of paperwork you handle. You might use green labels or green folders for banking and financial information—green for Money items. If your house is yellow, you might want to put all house-related items—mortgage papers, warranties and renovation expense documentation—in yellow files.

Using the color prompts of a traffic light works well for the hot files you keep on your desktop. The green folders can store your get going/must do now files. The yellow folders can store your slow down/should think about doing files. And the red ones can store your stop/already done and waiting for response folders.

You can probably dream up many other color-coding systems. The rationale for using colors or similar ideas you come up with is that they support the memory part of organization. They prompt you to remember.

Use Post-it Notes: We're not sure what people did before the arrival of these wonderful things. They can't replace a filing system but they're great as reminders of important "to do" tasks. If you want to be really creative, you can use color-coded notes. Your *phone call reminders* could be on red notes, your *bills to pay reminders* on green and your *appointments* on yellow. If you want to make your own Post-it notes, you can buy a special adhesive stick that works on any paper.

Removable color tags are another useful prompt. The colored end hangs off whatever you stick it on and is easily seen. If you're working on something and are interrupted, mark your spot with a color tag. When you come back to the task, it will be easier to know where to start.

Keep an Ongoing "To Do" List: You can use several of the ideas we've suggested to keep track of the pending "to-do's" in your life. Regardless of the method you use, it's essential that you don't rely on your memory. Write things down in some fashion, and keep your reminders where you can see them. If you've ever participated in a meeting without an agenda, you know the importance of a plan. Your "to do" list is your personal agenda that keeps you focused and productive.

There are a variety of ways to organize your agenda. You can keep one running list or group things as timeline items—things to do today, tomorrow, by next week, etcetera. You might prefer to separate your agenda in categories of *Phone Calls to Make, Letters to Write, Appointments to Schedule,* and so forth.

285

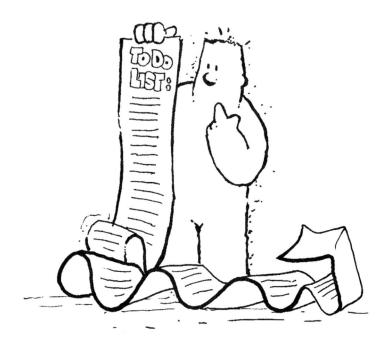

Keep your system up to date. It's a good idea to review your list every day, congratulate yourself on completed tasks and plan for the next day. It would probably also be helpful if you date-stamp your list as you did with your sorted paperwork.

One little trick that's great for the morale is to use the same "to do" list for a couple of days. Seeing the crossed-off tasks you've already completed is self-rewarding as you add new items to the list.

A final note is in order here. Don't get carried away with your daily "to do" list! As an ADDer, you probably overestimate the number of tasks you can accomplish in a given time. You will be frustrated and discouraged by an impossibly long list and might abandon your entire organizational system. Don't become a slave to your list, losing sleep and leisure time as you pursue the impossible goal of crossing everything off of it. Remember this axiom and learn to be content with keeping up with your list just enough to make your life manageable:

You will never get to the bottom of your list!

Time Management

As a framework for our discussion of organization, we arbitrarily began with space and stuff management. In the real world, of course, it doesn't work this way. Regardless of what you set out to do, it is framed within the element of time.

Many people have little problem handling the time details of their lives. Sometime around the middle of December every year, they make a trip to their local store and buy calendars for the coming year. Armed with their purchases and their pens, they're prepared for their Time Management for the next twelve months.

Calendars and their close relation, appointment organizers, are things an ADDer loves to hate. Everybody uses them. They are the basic, number one tool for time management in this busy world of ours. It's virtually impossible to get along without them. We bet that many ADD adults with shelves of organization self-help books also have numerous unused or partially used calendars and appointment organizers!

If calendars are such great organizers, why don't they work? It seems so simple. If you need to remember an appointment, you just note it on your calendar, right? Well, for an ADDer, it's a bit more complicated.

First, you have to remember to add items to your calendar. This presupposes that you can find your calendar! You could hang it on the wall or on the kitchen cabinet as your mother did, but then you'll be out of luck when you take a message in the TV room. During your trip to the kitchen, you're distracted by the doorbell or a crisis in the kids' room and completely forget to jot down the appointment with your boss.

Of course the problem isn't with the calendar per se. It's a problem of poor planning or a faulty time sense. Noting an appointment on the calendar may help you remember an event, but it doesn't help you plan what you'll need to do to get ready for it. Scheduling several activities in one day is fine as long as you have a realistic idea of how long each one will take.

If you've compiled the various inventories we've talked about, you've already started working on Time Management problems. At the heart of the discussion of balance were issues of simplifying the complexity of your life. The goal of the more practical inventories of the stuff in your life was to reduce the quantity of things you have to handle.

Many of us are too overwhelmed to manage all the details. Before you waste your time seeking the perfect daily organizer, you need to take a studied look at your lifestyle. Cut out everything you can, to make your life more manageable. Then start thinking about some of the strategies that follow. We can't promise that these ideas will work, but they may help you design others that will.

Keep a Daily Time Log: We know that the inventories you've been making are adding to your paperwork pile. But we're going to suggest that you do just one more. If your One-Rat Study or your inventory from Chapter 5 includes the details we'll mention, you can use them instead, adding anything that you haven't included.

For a day or two, keep a diary of how you use your time. Jot down everything you do, including eating lunch and taking a shower. Note starting and stopping times for anything that takes more than a minute or two. Keep your diary in a small pocket-size notebook you can carry throughout the day.

Your time log can provide information about productivity, wasted time and interruptions. You might spot time periods that seem to work better for you than others. You might be able to make some decisions about grouping certain jobs together in a time slot that affords you the most uninterrupted focus.

Electronic Stuff: Calendars and appointment organizers are the backbone of a time management system. Today, however, many of us have replaced the paper and pencil versions with electronic devices of various kinds. Computers and PDAs can keep your calendar and appointments handy, and even send an alarm when an important deadline looms. There are wonderful software programs available to help you manage and prioritize your "to do" list. Even our cell phones are beginning to take on the organizing function—for example, it is possible to record voice memos on your phone. Who knows what dazzling devices and programs will be available when this book has been on the shelves for a few years?

Personally, we are holding out for the ultimate in organizing tools—a robot, powered by artificial intelligence, who will organize our lives for us and just tell us what to do! Better still, little Jeeves can just do all the tedious and boring stuff for us.

We can pay our bills, send electronic mail and even shop online. All these things have the potential for saving time. Our time-saving devices, however, can also become time eaters. E-mail boxes fill up with spam, time disappears as we surf the Net and that computer requires maintenance. Electronic, human and ADD error can all bring down the complicated systems we use to keep ourselves organized.

PR: "Years ago, both of us had our ADD meds prescribed by a psychiatrist who also had ADD. On a routine visit, I was astonished when I walked into a waiting room filled wall-to-wall with people. An hour later, when I went into the consulting room for my appointment, the doctor sheepishly filled me in on the reason for the packed waiting room. A few months prior to my visit, he had obtained a new gadget—the Wizard, an early version of the PDA. He had happily booked several months' worth of appointments in his new toy, only to discover sometime later that his Wizard had two points of data entry and that he had double-booked all his time slots!"

We don't intend to try to talk you out of using helpful electronic organizing devices; just be cautious when you use them. We know this may be hard, but take time to get up to speed when you upgrade your electronic tools. Watch your impulsivity when you punch those buttons, and keep your system as simple as possible. The latest bells and whistles can be fun, but not if they add too much complexity to your life. Also, be aware that using multiple devices for tracking time and appointments can create problems if you don't take care to put *all* your critical information in *each* device.

KK: "The key to my system is a simple week-at-a-glance planner that I use to plan my weekly responsibilities. Of course, there are tasks that require longer preparation. I handle this problem by breaking the job into smaller, weekly segments that I pencil in as weekly tasks.

"I have trained myself to look at my planner several times a day but have also developed a system for reminding myself to look ahead to the next day. I pencil 'see AM' in my planner the day before any important event. Without a cue for upcoming events or deadlines, I would fail to plan for them.

"When I check my planner at the end of the day, my cue reminds me that my daughter has a field trip the next day. I avoid the inevitable morning scramble by organizing the night before. Before I go to bed, I pack her lunch, pull out the permission slip from the appropriate folder, sign it and put her money in an envelope. I leave everything on the kitchen counter so I'll see it, even in my early-morning foggy state.

"I use the same cuing system to keep track of birthdays and other important dates. Entering these reminders in your planner at the beginning of the year is a great idea, but it doesn't solve the whole problem. Without an advance reminder, I would regularly read the current day's entries and discover that TODAY is the big day. Unfortunately, it's too late to send a card or gift!

"A portable planner works best for me. I'm always on the go and need something I can take along on my travels. When I'm out shopping, I can remember to buy the cookies for the class-room party tomorrow."

Structure Your Planning with Daily Time Sheets: Time sheets are highly structured daily calendars that manage time by the hour rather than by the day and date. Many computer software programs offer preformatted daily calendars and time sheets. If you don't have access to these, you can make your own.

Although we suggest that you start with half-hour time seg-ments, you'll need to decide how much structure you need. Your time sheet can help you compensate for a faulty internal time clock.

Whenever you schedule something that involves preparation, get out your planning notebook and make a list of everything you'll need. Will you need to wear a particular outfit? Add it to your list. Will you need to make provisions for the family while you're gone? What about calling a babysitter? And how about the emergency numbers the babysitter will need? If you fre-quently hop into your car only to discover that the gas tank is empty, add a note to your list to get gas.

Put your reminder list in a logical order, estimate how long each item will take and double your estimate. If you tend to grossly underestimate preparation times, triple your estimate! Write the time of the event on your time sheet and work backward, entering each item on your list in an estimated block of time. When you've finished this process, you'll know precisely when you need to begin getting ready for your appointment.

An interesting experiment to evaluate your time sense is to jot down your "starting time" guess before you go through this process. After you make your list and complete your backward time entries, see how close you were to your guess. Our bet is that you'll discover you were pretty far off!

Compile Master Lists of Reminders: Consider making a master list for recurring appointments. Put the babysitter's emergency phone list in the kitchen cabinet so it will be there every time you need it. Keep a vacation checklist in your file so you don't have to start from scratch each time.

A lack of planning usually causes overwhelming feelings of disorganization. Although this preplanning may initially take extra time, it will ultimately save you time, aggravation and the wrath of a boss who impatiently sits in the conference room waiting for your late arrival. When you think things through and make detailed lists, the readiness steps become more automatic. Over time, you'll probably discover that you can accomplish the planning steps more quickly as they become habits.

Compile "Everyday Get Out the Door" Master Lists: How many times do you spend your car trip across town trying to remember whether you turned off the iron and turned on the porch light? Rather than relying on your memory, make a list and post it at your door. Include the things you need to do whenever you go out: put the dog in the basement, turn off the computer, turn on the porch light, leave a note for your son, and so on.

Taking the time to think through your routine and write it down will save much time and aggravation in the long run. You won't need to remember these details every time you get ready to leave. You won't need to waste time racing back home to save your computer from getting zapped by the thunderstorm and lightning that hits. A quick look at your list as you head out the door will shave precious minutes off your preparation time.

Prepare Duplicated "School" Master Forms: If you have school-age children, you undoubtedly write many notes for field trip permissions, absences, special after-school bus changes, and so forth. Make some master forms for as many of these activities as you can. A generic "please excuse Zachary's absence" can be made with spaces for name, date and reason. A quick fill-in-the-blank later, your task is finished sooner than if you had to compose a new note for every occasion. Your forms may not be personal, but they will save you time.

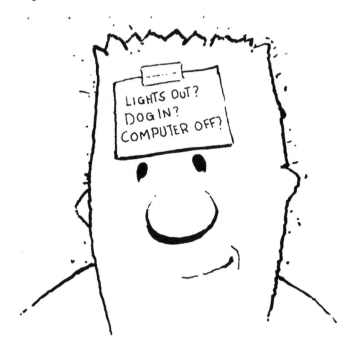

Buy a (Waterproof) Watch with an Alarm: Alarm watches are wonderful. Depending on the style, you can set alarms to ring every hour or at the same time every day. You can use an alarm watch as a reminder for appointments or to keep yourself on track.

Set it to ring in a reasonable amount of time and then make a decision to work at least until the alarm rings. Plan a break at that point and reset the alarm. You can accomplish the same thing with an alarm clock, but your watch is portable.

If your watch is waterproof, you won't have to take it off. It's one less thing you have to keep track of, and it can prevent cold showers. You know what happens—you hop in for a quick five-minute shower and emerge shivering thirty minutes later when your hot-water tank is empty!

Use Stenographer Pads and Large Index Cards: Aren't index cards the awful things we were instructed to use when we had to write a research paper? They were supposed to help us organize our ideas but often ended up being used as paper airplanes! In spite of any negative experiences you may have had using them, index cards can help with organization of thoughts and daily details.

Even the best system in the world is put to the test by distractibility. Many of us get sidetracked because ideas keep popping into our brains. With some ingenuity, one ADDer we know uses steno pads, index cards and his distractibility to accomplish wonderful things.

He keeps a supply of steno pads at his work site and also by every telephone and chair where he may sit. He uses one exclusively for the phone calls he receives. Whenever he makes or takes a call, he jots down the name and phone number, the time and date of the call and any notes that apply. He checks off each call after he returns it. He starts a new dated list every day. This steno book is a permanent record he can refer to whenever he needs to remember the details of a particular call. More than once, he has been able to access a phone number he would otherwise have lost.

He also uses steno pads for jotting down ideas. His work is only briefly interrupted as he captures the essence of his ideas on paper. At the end of a work session, he transfers his random thoughts to index cards, categorizing them as he goes. He files his index cards alphabetically until his next work session, when he adds new ideas to existing cards or creates new ones.

Our photographer friend's system may be helpful for you. The steno telephone record can act as a backup to your phone number directory and "to do" list. And the index card system can enable you to use distracting thoughts to your advantage without interfering with the task at hand.

The key in using steno pads, a planning notebook or Post-it notes is to use them to keep yourself on track and to regulate your impulsivity. In the middle of writing checks, don't stop to make the hair appointment you just remembered. Instead, jot yourself a note as a reminder and immediately get back to work.

Schedule Telephone Callback Times: Schedule specific times to make or return phone calls. If you don't have a secretary to screen your calls, you will have to come up with your own screening script. Tell the caller that you're in a meeting and will call him back. Don't worry about lying. You *are* in a meeting—a meeting with yourself! Better still, let voice mail pick up when you are busy.

Discover "Found" Time: Take another look at your time diary. Are there periods of lost time? What about the waiting room in the doctor's office? How about the commercials during the TV program you were watching? See how much time you can find.

We aren't suggesting that you schedule your life to excess. That could be quite depressing. You don't want to carry your pending file around with you to work on while you wait for the red light to turn green!

But what about the time you spend in the waiting room? You've been wanting to write a letter to your friend who moved out of town. It's been on your "to do" list for weeks. Rather than reading outdated magazines, why don't you write your letter while you wait? It's something you've been unable to find the time to do.

Structure Procrastination to Your Advantage: Procrastination is the number one enemy of Time Management. Although ADDers tend to procrastinate more than our non-ADD counterparts, no one is immune from the Peril of Procrastination! What if we make this enemy our friend? What if we make it an advantage rather than a disadvantage?

We really do need to preface this suggestion with a warning to use it at your own risk! It's possible to capitalize on procrastination, but it involves *very* careful planning.

The unfortunate reality is that many people work best when deadlines loom. As the deadline gets closer, the adrenaline starts flowing, energy goes into overdrive and tasks are cranked out at astonishing speed. If you know your limits and are fairly good at estimating time, you can structure your task by purposely waiting until the last minute.

This is contrary to conventional wisdom. It's usually better to plan extra time rather than less time to get things done. So you probably ought to try using structured procrastination for a job that won't yield disastrous results if it doesn't get finished!

This is how it works. Figure out the absolute shortest time you can reasonably expect to be able to accomplish a particular job. Get out whatever time organizer you're using and write down the deadline for your job. Then add a second deadline—the absolute latest time you can possibly start working on your task. You absolutely must have everything else cleared off your daily time sheet for the starting deadline you've established. Then be prepared to do nothing else but use your pumped-up energy to finish the job.

We've used many "absolutes" in this discussion of structured procrastination because this is a risky strategy. We would suggest that you try this only as a last-ditch effort. The safer strategies should be your first line of attack. Check out the meditation chapter for information on why adrenaline surges are not a great idea.

We've considered time and space as distinct organizational processes. If you recall from the diagram at the beginning of the chapter, you know that organization is dependent on memory and attention. They're all interrelated—organization strategies depend on your remembering. And to remember, you must be able to attend in the first place. In the next chapter, we'll continue our discussion by examining the other two parts of this interrelationship.

CHAPTER 12

Dynamics of ADD in Memory: Mechanics and Methods

Two hundred years ago, the English author Samuel Johnson wrote, *"The art of memory is the art of attention."* Does an impaired memory and its negative impact on organization skills result from an inability to focus?

Although debating this question would be interesting, we don't think we dare make this book any longer! Since we've already explored the organization piece of the puzzle, we'll focus now on the interrelationships of attention, memory and learning. In the first part of our discussion, we'll look at memory apart from associated learning problems. Later in the chapter, we'll consider the impact of specific learning disabilities.

Memory functions as the *starting pitcher* of a *learning team* that collectively processes language, organization, thinking, social interaction and *doing*. Models of both anatomy and neurochemical brain metabolism have been used to explain the process of memory. Since we can't control these aspects of memory, we won't examine them in this book. Instead, we'll consider memory as sensory information stored according to how well it is first acquired, or learned. Since we *can* control some aspects of learning, we can control some aspects of memory processes.

In Chapter 2, you learned that memory is a complex system of acquisition, registration, storage and consolidation, access and transfer. Since this isn't a textbook, let's put those terms into ordinary language.

Memory is the system for getting information in,
hanging on to it for a while
and getting it back out again when you need to use it.

In her book *Don't Forget!*, author Danielle Lapp explores the concept of memory as a *conscious* and *subconscious* process with a potential for breaks in its chain. This is an important idea. It means that you don't have a *bad* memory. It means that you have a break somewhere in your memory chain. And it means that by understanding how the process works, you can strengthen or bypass the broken link. The following chart, adapted from Lapp's book, illustrates the memory chain.

PROCESS OF MEMORY FORMATION: GETTING IT INTO MEMORY

sensory input – need/interest – motivation – attention – concentration – organization – depth of processing

TIME FRAMES OF MEMORY STORAGE

instant recall – working memory – short-term memory – long-term memory

PROCESS OF MEMORY STORAGE: GETTING IT BACK OUT AGAIN

memory access: subconscious, automatic, cued
active storage layer – passive storage layer – latent storage layer

---

Let's think about how the process works. When you tie your shoes, take a test, repeat your phone number, tell humorous vacation stories or follow the clerk's directions to the boys' department, you're using your memory. You probably don't have any trouble remembering how to tie your shoes. You go through the steps on automatic pilot. Memory traces of the steps of shoe tying are sharply and clearly etched in storage areas you can quickly access. The skill has become a subconscious memory because you worked hard to learn it years before.

You learned the skill as a young child *motivated* by the *need* for independence and being "grown-up." You *attended* to an adult tying his shoes and *concentrated* on repeating the steps he demonstrated. You *organized* the information in some fashion to learn the skill. You might have practiced the process by repeating the steps as you fumbled with your shoelaces. Maybe you learned a rhyme or visualized the steps as you repeated the skill again and again. All the links of the memory chain were in place. Over time, the skill was etched in your long-term memory so you didn't have to rely on cues any longer.

Many skills are stored below the level of consciousness, similar to shoe tying. You have practiced them so much that you can perform them without conscious effort. When you walk into a darkened room, you automatically remember to turn on the light switch. If you are like us, however, you might never know which of the three available switches is the one you want! Even though you use the switches daily, you may get the porch and hall light turned on before you finally flip the one for the overhead light.

Does that mean you have a bad memory? No, it means you never took the time to concentrate and organize your remembering for automatic recall. Your memory chain has a weak link. Remembering which switch to flip might not be important because trial and error work just fine.

The next time you find yourself announcing that you forgot something, stop and think about the memory chain. Did you truly forget, or were you unable to instantly recall the information? Did you forget, or did you decide that the information wasn't something you chose to remember?

Memory lapses occur when one or more links in the chain are weak. The specific social, emotional, learning or living circumstances in which the information was originally presented affects the individual links. The use of memory techniques can also affect individual links and the quality of the memory chain as a whole.

Memory Storage and Access

For our readers with "poor memories," we'll do a quick review of memory in case you can't remember what you learned about memory earlier in this book! Memories aren't useful if you can't *recall* them. When you acquire information, you put it in one of several different safe-deposit boxes, characterized by their time frames. When you talk of your great or terrible memory, you're talking about the *duration* of your remembering.

The shortest duration is that of *instant recall.* Closely related to instant recall storage is *immediate or working memory.* You use this storage capacity to hold in memory several different steps or combinations of data simultaneously as you work on something.

When you remember your license plate number long enough for your credit card purchase at the gas station, you're using *short-term storage.* Short-term memory has a maximum capacity of seven items and five seconds. Your so-called terrible memory is frequently a reference to this short-term memory.

Information that is remembered for a long time is stored in long-term memory. Many people complain of their terrible memories, yet recount in precise detail events that occurred ten years earlier.

Lapp, who has worked extensively with the memory problems of the elderly, uses another model of storage and access. She offers a visual representation of the brain as three layers of storage. The upper one is the active, busy layer close to consciousness; Lapp visualizes this layer in a clear, bright blue color. This layer contains the memories of information used daily: frequently used names and telephone numbers, recurring appointments, and so on. These memories are quickly and effortlessly recalled.

The middle layer contains the rusty, seldom-used memories that are more difficult to retrieve. You remember these through cues that prompt recall. The layer is rust-colored to represent the old, worn and passive quality of the stored memories.

Remote memories from long ago are stored deep in the brain in a large, gray-colored zone. Although these memories are seldom accessed, there are literally millions of memory traces available for recall. Memories no longer needed are stored in this layer. Memories of emotional trauma are also stored here. When someone talks about repressed memories, he's referring to these memory traces of traumatic experiences.

Remote memory traces are recalled through involuntary memory. A mood or sensory perception typically prompts recall of the stored memories. The smell of perfume triggers a memory of playing dress-up with a childhood friend you haven't thought of in fifty years.

PR: "I'm sure that readers have had the experience of suddenly remembering something they had long ago forgotten. Several years ago, I accompanied my husband to the funeral of a family friend. I completely fell apart as soon as I walked in. I couldn't stop crying and felt emotionally beaten up. My intense reaction wasn't caused by my feelings about the person who had died. I had never even met him. Instead, it was an involuntary reaction to the smell of all the flowers. The scent triggered powerful, repressed memories of my brother's funeral that I had refused to think about for twenty-eight years."

Organization and Registration:
The Key to Memory Access

Storage is just the first step of either organization or memory. The second step is accessing the data. The problem for many of us isn't that we can't remember the data, it's that we can't find where we put what we remember! In other words, we haven't lost the data *from* memory but *in* memory. It's floating around in there somewhere, but where?

Erratic storage results in slow and unpredictable retrieval. It's as if we head to our safe-deposit boxes with thousands of keys in our hands. Which box and which key should we use? By the time we finally figure it out, the teacher's question or the boss's comment has passed us by.

Although some memories find their way into storage with little effort, many require a conscious decision to remember. The key to storing and accessing the items in your home or the data in your memory is an efficient system of storage. This process involves coding and categorizing information in ways similar to the organization systems we talked about. If you can't find the medical receipts after you've filed them, you won't be able to submit a claim to your insurance company. If you've ever searched on every floor of a huge parking garage for your car, you understand the importance of memory registration!

Information Input

There is an aspect of memory we haven't mentioned yet. Although we've talked about the quality of memory, it's probably more useful to think about the quality of your *Memories*. We're not referring to pleasant or unpleasant memories but to your Auditory Memory, Visual Memory, and other senses. How well do you remember things you've seen, heard, smelled, touched or tasted? Think about the quality of your memory for the varied kinds of sensory information listed below and rate yourself on a sliding scale from 1 (excellent) to 6 (terrible):

REMEMBERING
Auditory—Things You Hear:
   oral multistep instructions
   oral one-step instructions
   the names of people you meet
   words—what you want to say in one-to-one situations
   words—what you want to say in group situations
Visual—Things You See:
   written one-step instructions
   written multistep instructions
   how and where to get started after an interruption
   the faces of people you meet
   words—details of things you read
Kinesthetic—Things You Do:
   episodic—personal experiences
   how to get to various places
   time details
   space—where you put belongings
Overall Memory
       (Adapted from a list in Lapp's *Don't Forget!*)

All human beings are born with unique memory differences. If we use the number of available memory training books as a measure, *many* people have problems with remembering! This list might help you better understand your own memory profile.

Memory problems aren't unique to ADDers, but they are compounded by the associated deficits. Systematic remembering requires concentrated effort, attention to detail, organized thinking and planning strategies. These tasks are difficult for many of us.

To remember, you need to figure out why you forgot! If you can determine where your memory chain breaks, you can work on the weak link. For instance, you can't change your attentional problems but you can take steps to minimize the distractions that interfere with focus. Further, if you know which of your memory types is the strongest, you can use it to develop memory tricks. Later in the chapter, we'll look at some ideas for doing this.

Memory and Learning—You Can't Have One Without the Other

If we enlarge the concept of memory to one of general learning, you can better understand how the interconnections play out in your daily life. If you've spent a lifetime with the label of underachiever, you may have a feeling of dread at the mere mention of the word "learning"! We hope you're using your new knowledge to understand the learning problems you may have had.

Knowledge and learning levels are typically assessed not by the storehouse of knowledge you carry inside your brain, but by your productivity—what you *do*, or *don't* do. When you were a child, your teachers often misinterpreted your failing test grades as a lack of learning. Now that you're an adult, your spouse and coworkers may attribute your inconsistent performance and slow reaction time to your lack of ability.

The difficulty for many of us is that we aren't always able to demonstrate what we know. Our problems are often not ones of learning per se, but rather of performance. We can't process our knowledge fast enough, maintain our focus long enough or perform consistently enough.

Learning is often equated with listening. Many of us "learned" through one-way teaching—our instructors talked and we were expected to acquire knowledge by listening. Unfortunately, one-way teaching isn't particularly effective for many learners, including those without specific deficits. It's not that learning by listening is totally ineffective. Some people remember and learn best in this mode. But it's ineffective for those who learn best by seeing or doing. The key is to improve the effectiveness of the *learning team* by matching the mode of learning to the individual learning style.

Learning Styles

We want to expand our earlier discussion of learning styles to help you analyze your individual mode of learning. What is your particular learning style? What skills and information do you easily acquire? How do you learn best and in what setting? Understanding your preferred mode of learning is important not only in school but in life. Learning is intertwined with memory and organization. The tips and tricks you use to tame your time and space monsters will be effective only if you match them to your preferred learning style.

Let's review what learning styles are. How do you figure out the one(s) that work best for you? We all learn through our five senses: by seeing (visual channel), hearing (auditory channel), touching (tactile/kinesthetic channel), tasting and smelling. Most learning takes place through visual, auditory and/or kinesthetic channels. The sense of smell and taste do provide important information but are less important in *higher-order* thinking and processing—unless the other channels are impaired in some way.

Learning styles aren't mutually exclusive. You may learn best through one channel or a combination of two channels. Or you may be a multisensory learner who uses all three channels—many ADDers learn best this way. In their book *Unlocking Potential*, Barbara Scheiber and Jeanne Talpers explore the mechanisms of learning styles. The following list, adapted from their book for learning-disabled adolescents and adults, offers some clues you can use to determine your preferred learning mode.

The Visual Learner . . .
has a strong color sense
follows written directions well
has difficulty following lectures
processes auditory input slowly
"translates" verbal input into pictures
needs to closely watch the speaker's facial expression and
body language

is particularly distracted by noise or people talking in the
background
uses visualization to remember things
takes notes with visual representations: pictures, diagrams,
graphs, etc.
knows something by seeing it

The Auditory Learner . . .

effectively sorts out multiple word and sound inputs
follows verbal directions well
learns best in a lecture format
processes visual input slowly
has to vocalize written information to anchor it in memory
"translates" pictures into spoken words
is distracted by visual stimuli
ignores the speaker's body language to focus on the spoken
words
knows something by hearing it

The Tactile/Kinesthetic Learner . . .

has an excellent sense of direction
is well coordinated in sports and physical activities
uses his body sense and "hands-on" performance to anchor
information in memory
has difficulty processing both visual and auditory input
"translates" pictures and words into movement
uses imprecise words: "talks" with his hands
follows directions best by watching and *doing*
learns best through physical activity
needs a lot of movement
knows something by doing it

You will undoubtedly identify with certain parts of this list. You
probably notice similarities between this list and that of memory skills, which was roughly divided into sensory modes. Since
memory and learning are integrally connected, it isn't surprising
that the quality of your memory is directly related to the mode
of input. If your preferred learning style is auditory, you proba-

bly identified memory problems with visual tasks. In school, you may have had problems in reading and in subject areas like geometry that require a visual orientation.

If you're primarily a visual learner, you probably identified memory problems with verbal input. You may be a good reader who picks up social cues well but who has difficulty responding to the verbal interactions in those settings. Unlike your auditory learner counterpart, you may have encountered particular difficulty when lectures became the teaching vehicle in junior and senior high school.

If you're a kinesthetic learner, you may be an excellent navigator, athlete and "fixer-upper" with your tactile, body-sense memory. But you may have memory problems when input is visual or auditory without having any action connected to it. School probably worked best for you when you were actively involved in learning groups or physically manipulating instructional tasks.

Of course learning and memory are more complex than this overly simplistic framework. Individual aptitudes for math, language and mechanical skills factor in to the equation. For example, you may learn best through auditory input of numerical data rather than language. Your unique ADD deficits are also part of the puzzle. You may be a visual learner who doesn't read well owing to specific problems with cognitive fatigue or inattention to detail. Or you may be unable to clearly define your preferred learning style because you use them all. You may be a multisensory learner who needs to hear it, see it *and* do it to anchor information for learning.

Learning/memory styles are further defined by individualized systems of information processing. You may be a detailed, sequential learner who learns through step-by-step, logical, structured thinking. You may be a realistic, practical, concrete learner who prefers hands-on learning. Or you may be a perceptive, intuitive learner who begins with the big picture, learns through abstractions and loves fantasy and humor.

Tuning Up Memory Techniques

This framework doesn't provide clear-cut definitions and tidy boxes you can use to categorize your learning/memory modes. But it can help you customize the tips and tricks you use to by-pass weak areas and maximize the strong ones. Consistently writing things down is helpful for many ADDers. But if you aren't a visual learner it may not work for you. You may do much better with tape-recorded reminders. So, as you read some of the suggestions that follow, keep your learning style(s) in mind.

Analyze the Circumstances: Are you trying to remember something in a noisy, distraction-filled environment? Can you change the circumstances under which you're trying to remember? Can you find a time and place that enhances your memory power?

Relax: How are you feeling? Are you stressed or depressed? Mood and emotions impact your ability to remember. If your thoughts are preoccupied by worry and various life stresses, you can't concentrate and remember.

Get in the habit of using various relaxation techniques. The techniques of progressive muscle relaxation, deep breathing or visualization can free your mind and body from preoccupation with thoughts that interfere with concentration.

Various kinds of relaxation training courses are offered in recreation and community learning centers and are outlined in a number of books and tapes on the subject. Try to find a system that works well for you and use it regularly. Make it a part of your daily schedule to improve your memory and also your general emotional well-being.

Minimize the Anxiety That Interferes with Memory: How many times have you started your sales presentation only to "blank out"? Your hands are shaking, your stomach is churning and your heart is pounding. As you begin getting the words out of your mouth, your brain is filling with words of its own: "You're going to blow it! You know you always forget what you're going to say."

Lots of people approach public speaking with a sense of dread. But an ADDer can experience a paralyzing degree of stage fright. He's terrified that his erratic memory won't work. He'll blank out at the wrong time and history will repeat itself. He'll fail miserably—again.

There isn't a simple solution to this problem, but understanding that anxiety interferes with memory can provide a place to start. Use the anticipation to work for you instead of against you. In the comfort of your home, sit back and allow yourself to imagine all the details of the situation you dread.

Think about your physical reactions: your palms sweating and your heart racing. What does it feel like? Use the mirror as your audience and practice. Do you remember what to say? Is it firmly anchored in your memory? What questions might someone ask about your presentation? Are you prepared to answer them?

Consider a worst-case scenario. What do you fear about the situation? Are your fears realistic or only remote possibilities? After you visualize the situation at its worst, visualize it at its best. Positive thinking puts you in control and gives you a useful frame of reference when you're talking to an audience instead of your mirror or spouse.

By thinking realistically about some of these things, you increase your focus on task performance. You have less time to focus on your fears and worries when your mind is constructively occupied. If you can decrease your anxiety, you can free up your energies for remembering instead of worrying.

When it's time to make your presentation, choose a neutral focal point such as a light fixture and gaze at it to ground yourself. Although you'll need to gauge audience reaction, you can use your focal point as your cue to relax. This can increase your attention to memory and distract you from focusing too much on the faces and reactions of individual audience participants.

You can also use an actor's trick to conquer stage fright. Imagine your audience sitting in their underwear or in the nude. In your mind's eye, they will appear rather silly and much less threatening. Just don't indulge too much in this fantasy or you may burst out with uncontrollable giggling!

Make the Choice to Remember: To remember anything, it is important to be mentally present. Stimuli from the environment will make their way to your sensory organs whether or not you want them to. But you can't properly store anything until you make a conscious effort to file it somewhere.

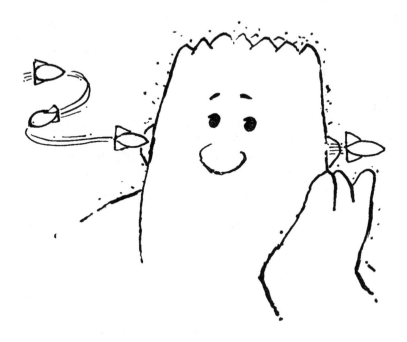

When you were growing up you may have frequently heard the words, "I tell you what to do and it goes in one ear and right out the other." Wasn't it great when you were punished for not listening and got sent to your room? You had uninterrupted time to conjure up a wonderful mental picture of hundreds of tiny word rocket ships zooming into your right ear, traveling through the twists and turns of your brain and shooting out your left ear! Seriously, that visualization is an accurate representation of what happens when you don't work at remembering.

You need to slow down the velocity of those *data input* rocket ships to make use of the cargo they carry. It isn't easy but you need to make a conscious decision to remember or you will lose the information.

Train Yourself to Be a Better Observer: Simply seeing or hearing something doesn't provide an anchor to secure the data in memory. But careful observation does. When you meet someone new, say his name several times to yourself and make mental notes of cues that set him apart from someone else. Is there anything unique about his appearance? Does he wear a pocket watch that is his personal trademark? Does he continually re-adjust his belt?

Use planned practice sessions to improve your powers of observation. Years ago there was a TV game show that used visual memory as its format. Contestants examined a photograph and reported all the remembered details when the picture was removed. You can do the same kind of visual memory exercise by using a magazine photograph. Try allotting shorter periods of "study" time as your recall improves, and keep track of the number of accurately remembered details.

Reduce Your Use of Rote Memorization: Simple repetition of information may be helpful for short-term memory. It can help you remember which parking garage you parked in—at least long enough to write it down. But if you don't anchor that data in another way, you may end up calling a taxi to drive you home and a detective to find your missing car!

Understand What You're Trying to Memorize: If you try to remember information of a complex nature simply by regurgitating it, you won't be able to permanently store it in long-term memory. Make sure that you clearly understand the meaning of what you're trying to memorize. Ask questions and anchor the new information to something you already know.

Put Information in a Larger Context: Struggling with "It's right on the tip of my tongue" is extremely frustrating! The next time you find yourself hoping that you'll somehow miraculously remember where you left your raincoat last week, go in to your memory files and activate associations. What day did it rain? Wasn't it the day you got soaking wet running through a downpour with your briefcase and three bags of groceries? If you were carrying your briefcase, were you on your way to or from work during the rainstorm? If you were running, had you already lost your raincoat?

Through these side associations, you may be able to find both the memory and the raincoat you left on a shelf in the garage before you headed out to the grocery store. Finding the missing memory piece is easier if you can put the rest of the connected puzzle pieces together.

Use Your Senses—Visual Memory: The expression "Do you see what I mean?" is an example of the use of imagery in thinking. Many people remember best through visual memory. Incoming information, feelings and experiences are rather effortlessly translated into concrete mental pictures.

An ability to design mental images and "play" with them in the mind is the basis for imagination and creativity and is a good anchor for remembering. You can use visualization and mental imagery to improve the initial registration of information and to prompt its recall when you need it. If you routinely misplace your car keys, try using the following technique the next time you start to put them down somewhere.

As you drop your keys on the bathroom sink where you've stopped to wash your hands, look at them and the faucet and create an imaginative mental image—visualize your keys tossing about as they are swept over Niagara Falls! Taking a moment to create the image may be enough to stop yourself from breezing out of the room without them. But even if you do leave them behind, chances are that an image of the falls will pop up in your mind when you start searching for them later.

Mental imagery works well for remembering names. If you need to remember the name of your new client, Stuart Carpman, you might create a mental image of a giant fish (*carp*). Your giant fish is covered with mounds of red hair because this is the real Mr. Carpman's most significant feature. Unlike ordinary fish, your carp is swimming in a huge bowl of *stew* which is, of course, your visualized connection to his first name. The more outrageous the connections and visualization, the more effective the image will be in prompting your memory.

Use Your Senses—Auditory Memory: Verbal learners can use their word, rhyme and sound sensitivity to prompt memory recall. Try putting your shopping list in a rhyme or inserting the things you need to remember into the lyrics of a well-known song. Record your speech or list of errands on a tape recorder and repeat it as you play back your tape.

Use Your Senses—Kinesthetic Memory: If your preferred learning mode is kinesthetic, borrow from the actor's repertoire and use your body sense to memorize. Think about what you need to remember, visualize yourself doing it and then act it out. If you frequently leave the iron on, exaggerate the motion of turning it off and think about how wonderful it will feel not to wonder later whether you turned it off. The action can physically trace the memory in your mind.

Try sitting in your rocking chair and memorizing to the rhythm of the rocking. Use your restlessness as a memory aid. Instead of simply spinning in your desk chair or pacing around your office, practice remembering at the same time. On each spin or stroll across the room, repeat the names of your new clients or the things you need to do before you leave for vacation. Memorize to the rhythm of your movement.

Use Multisensory Strategies—Don't Just "Try to Remember": We know we probably don't really need to say this again, but always write down your appointment if you want to arrive at the right place at the right time! You probably already have notes written and posted in a variety of places throughout your house. But don't stop at simply writing down your reminders. Notes are great prompts for short-term memory but don't really help you store information for subsequent recall unless you actively use them as memory tools.

To do this, you need to write things down and practice them. Read your note, close your eyes, visualize it and say it aloud. Check the accuracy of your visual memory by looking at your note and then practice it again. By using your kinesthetic channel (writing it down), your visual channel (reading it and mentally seeing it) and your auditory channel (saying and hearing it), you'll have a more secure anchor for later recall.

Mental image associations are useful for folks with good visual memory and can be combined with other kinds of sensory awareness to improve the quality of remembering. Try memorizing your company's product specifications list, for example, by seeing and speaking the words, writing them down and pointing to them in your catalog as a metronome beats. If you're trying to remember to turn on your security system before you leave your house, visualize the control box and the room sensors. Move around your house to each sensor and imagine yourself flipping a switch at each location. This will help you see and feel yourself proceeding through the activity and will help to fix the process in your conscious memory.

315

Use Visualization Combined with Associations: Much of what we learn is accomplished through various associations. One idea naturally flows into another and creative thinking is born. Sometimes the associations occur logically and effortlessly—you associate the sound of the teakettle whistling with the action of turning off the burner. The memory is called up automatically. When less obvious associations are required, your creativity gets a workout.

When you say "That reminds me of . . . ," you're using an association to prompt a memory. Your ability to accurately recall memories largely depends on how you initially organize the associations of input.

When you call your local animal pound to report the ferocious animal who just took a bite out of your leg, you quickly identify your assailant as a large brown dog. You don't have to describe the beast as a fur-covered animal with four legs, two ears and eyes, one tail and a snout resting over a powerful jaw of two rows of very large teeth! You know it's a dog because you have previously categorized the information in your memory bank. You rely on a mental outline.

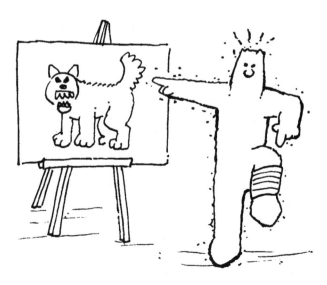

Whether you're remembering dogs, history events or a current project at work, you need to put the multiple pieces of data into a mental outline. There are far too many details to remember if you attempt to do it piece by piece. Work at identifying common threads or logical ways of grouping the pieces under main headings so you have fewer things to remember. Your main headings become flags that guide you to the other items you need to remember.

When you use a comb on your hair or a glass for your drink, you're using the simplest kind of *paired* or *grouped* association. When you use *analogical thinking* to remember things, you associate them by similarity. You remember your friend's birthday because it is the same as your child's. The converse is *differential thinking*, which uses comparison and differences to form associations. You remember that your doctor's office is on the east side of the street because his name is Dr. West.

Organizing your memory by using categories is particularly useful for lists. For instance, if you have to remember to go to the butcher shop and fill the gas tank for your grill, the two items are logically connected. With little more than a quick mental image of steaks on the grill, you will probably remember your two errands.

Sometimes, you have to be a bit more creative with your associations and mental images. If you have to remember to call the vet and go to the dentist, you can try visualizing your Great Dane lying back in a dental chair with cotton stuck in his jaws! By pairing the two items and visualizing them in a humorous way, you have a much better chance of committing them to memory.

It might seem that these techniques complicate things by adding extras to the memory burden. But they actually reduce the complexity by providing cues to remember things that would otherwise have no intrinsic reason to be remembered. Of course, if you're suffering from a terrible toothache and your dog has just broken its leg, you probably won't need any additional reminders!

Invent Your Own Mnemonic Tricks: Developing useful mnemonic tricks (memory techniques) is limited only by your imagination. Many tricks for remembering can be devised using letter codes. One well-known one is using the word "HOMES" to recall the five Great Lakes: Huron, Ontario, Michigan, Erie and Superior. The five-letter code calls up the names more precisely and quickly than your trying to remember them without any cues.

How can you remember that the boss of the school is the principal instead of the principle? One trick might be to think of the ending—pal. A pal is a person so the correct spelling of the school's boss must be principal. Now, it may be hard for some of us to think of our principals as our buddies, but we think you get the idea!

What about the spelling of the container we use to keep our drinks hot or cold? It sounds like it should be spelled thermis, but it's not, because a thermos has a circular opening, like an "o." Thus, the correct spelling is thermos.

Tricks are also effective for remembering a series of numbers that are random or may not immediately suggest any mental image. One way to remember a series of numbers is to make the information familiar by designing a clever storage framework. The combination for your lock—14, 27, 30—might be difficult to remember without a memory trick. But if you remind yourself that the first digit in each number increases by one, and the second by three, you'll improve your chances of remembering them.

Chunking is another trick that many of us use. Remembering a seven-digit telephone number becomes much easier when you break it into smaller groups of two or three digits. If the smaller parts happen to contain your age or house number, it's even easier to remember.

A coding system combined with a visual association is another good way to remember numbers. Try setting up a list of numbers using either rhymes or visual cues: one=run, two=moo, three=bee, four=shore, five=hive. If you prefer visual cues set up your list slightly differently: one=long stick, two=kids on a seesaw, three=a triangle, four=the tires on your car, five=fingers on one hand.

When you need to remember that your car is parked in space 134, you can translate it to run–bee–shore and visualize yourself running from a bee that is dive-bombing at you on your beach blanket at the shore. At first glance this may seem complicated. With practice, you may discover that it can really work. Numbers don't have any intrinsic meaning—this trick assigns meaning to them.

Rehearse, Rehearse, Rehearse! Without planned rehearsal, the best memory techniques in the world won't work very well. When it's time to recall something, review the strategy you used to store it. And then practice, practice, practice the strategy—again and again and again!

Cram sessions won't work! Your teachers were right when they repeatedly warned you not to wait until the last minute to study. Information is retained best if it's practiced over time. This enables you to practice informally in between and build on the partially learned information from earlier sessions. Educators refer to this as *overlearning*.

General Learning Tips

Use Music or Background Noise: When you were a child doing your homework, were you continually amazed at the seemingly magical power of the radio or television set you turned on? Within *milliseconds* after you hit the power button, did your parents arrive at your door with dire threats of the consequences that would follow if you didn't turn it off? How did they get there so fast?

Although parents and teachers alike have preached for years that learning must take place in a quiet area with no distractions, their sermons may have missed the mark. In reality, quiet can be excruciatingly distracting for some of us! Quiet can foster wonderful mind trips and excursions to places much more exciting than the desks in our rooms.

Background noise, particularly music, can be an effective tool for blocking out the expanse of quiet that permits your mind to roam. It also helps to ground you on the task at hand by blocking out the extraneous noises in your environment. Although studies have suggested that Baroque music is a particularly effective backdrop for some kinds of learning, you'll need to figure out what music, if any, works well for you.

Television typically creates more distractions than it prevents because of the story line and the message created by accompanying music. But if you're careful about the specific program you watch, TV can be a useful learning aid. Reruns are probably best because you'll be less inclined to become distracted by the plot. Some ADDers report using the TV for the dual purposes of intermittent self-reward and a refocus of wandering attention. They report that periodic glances at the screen interrupts the wandering and grounds them on their work.

Schedule Learning Times: Try to become aware of the cycles of your internal clock. This isn't necessarily a simple task, because ADDers typically have fairly unpredictable cycles of arousal and fatigue. But you may find that you are generally more efficient during one part of your day than another. You need to schedule intense learning during these peak times and leave the car washing for the other times.

Use Color to Maximize Learning: This is another tip primarily for the visual learner. Adding color to your work space can make use of your strong visual channel. Use a large piece of brightly colored poster board under your paperwork. The color can *pull* in your focus. Placing a color transparency over a page

320

in your policy handbook can improve the rate of your reading and the level of comprehension. The transparency makes the text appear sharper and clearer and therefore easier to read.

Walk, Juggle or Ride an Exercise Bike: Many of us can have extremely small mental fuel storage tanks. As we use up our meager resources of brain fuel, we become increasingly under-aroused and just plain tired. Sitting down to read anything more complex than a comic book can be an instant sleeping pill! To keep our storage tanks filled, we need to continuously pump in additional fuel. We can often do this by moving.

What about reading while you pedal your exercise bike, or taking a brisk walk with your upcoming meeting notes playing on your tape recorder? Can you watch a learning video while you do your floor exercises? Any physical activity paired with data input can be helpful for visual, auditory and kinesthetic learners.

Get Comfortable! There is no right or wrong way to learn de-spite what you may have been told about sitting up straight and quiet at your desk. If you like to twirl in your desk chair, go ahead and do it. If you prefer standing up or leaning against the wall, go for it. If you need to chew on toothpicks while you work, that's okay too.

Go with your instincts and do whatever it takes to facilitate your learning. You know better than anyone else what works for you, so erase the teacher and parent learning advice tapes from your memory bank. Orchestrate your personal learning envi-ronment so it works for you.

A Final Word: Learning Disabilities and ADD

Estimates of the number of learning-disabled individuals vary. The U.S. Office of Education estimated in 1978 that there were under two million learning-disabled children. But most special-ists disagree, some estimating that there are at least eight mil-lion learning-disabled children.

A specific learning disorder is described by the U.S. Department of Education as "a disorder in one or more of the basic psychological processes involved in understanding and using language, spoken or written, which may manifest itself in an imperfect ability to listen, think, speak, read, write, spell and do mathematical calculations."

All learning has four components: input, processing, memory and output. A learning disability is a disruption in the learning process within or between these components. The following chart from the book *The Misunderstood Child*, by Larry Silver, M.D., provides a summary of specific learning disabilities.

Input/Perceptual: A disability in the brain's interpretation of sensory impulses

    visual perceptual disabilities
    auditory perceptual disabilities
    smell, taste and touch disabilities

Integration: An inability to understand the information registered by the brain

    visual sequencing disability
    auditory sequencing disability
    visual abstraction disabilities
    auditory abstraction disabilities

Memory:

    visual short-term memory disability
    auditory short-term memory disability
    visual long-term memory disability
    auditory long-term memory disability

Output: An inability to get information back out of the brain

    spontaneous language disability
    demand language disability
    gross motor disability
    fine motor disability

The following was written by a learning-disabled nineteen-year-old and illustrates written expression/output disabilities:

> *Dear Mother—Started the Store several weeks, I have growed considerably I don't liik much like a Boy now—Hows all the folk did you receive a Box of Books from Memphis that he promised to send them—languages. Your son Al.*

Al was Thomas Alva Edison. He certainly went on to prove his teachers wrong about how *slow* he was!

Since this book is about ADD in adults, you may wonder why we're including this discussion. The primary reason is that some ADDers also have associated specific learning disabilities. In fact, some experts believe that the *majority* of ADDers have associated learning disabilities.

Probably the most common is a receptive or expressive language disability. In simple terms, this is an impaired ability to receive oral or written language and/or to process language for oral or written expression. A difficulty with written language may in fact result from an associated learning disability.

Attentional problems can mimic learning disabilities and learning disabilities can mimic ADD. It isn't easy to tease out the reasons for an individual's learning problems. Is it a specific learning disability, ADD or both? One could argue against the sometimes arbitrary divisions of ADD and learning disabilities because there are many overlapping symptoms. Despite the overlap, having a learning disability is different from having ADD.

Having ADD means having trouble initially getting information into the brain because of attention problems. If you are present in body only, with your brain out on the golf course, you won't process incoming information very well.

Having a learning disability means having trouble processing information because of a specific impairment in the components of learning: input, integration, memory and output. A learning-disabled brain flips letters and numbers around, puts data in the wrong order and confuses the meaning of incoming sounds, among other things. Medicine is useless for treating learning disabilities because it can't correct errors in the brain's interpretation and output of data.

The issue of ADD versus learning disabilities comes down to definitions and descriptions. At this point in research and understanding, the two are considered separate entities. Although we don't want to get hung up on labels, we think it's important for you to consider the possibility that you are also learning disabled. It may be the missing puzzle piece in your recovery. If your medicine is working and you're making progress with your ADD issues but still have inexplicable problems, you may have an undiagnosed learning disability.

This possibility underscores the importance of having a complete psychoeducational evaluation. We encourage you to have additional testing if your diagnosis was based solely on history and observable symptoms. Unless you were in school after the 1975 passage of Public Law 94-142, the Education for All Handicapped Children Act, it is unlikely that your learning disabilities were diagnosed.

If your evaluation uncovers a learning disability, seek help for your LD as well as your ADD. Don't assume that educational remediation is just for children. There are tutors who work exclusively with adults. The Orton Dyslexia Society and the Association for Children with Learning Disabilities are two resources you can contact for a referral in your area. Both are national organizations with branches all over the United States. The Orton Dyslexia Society in Cincinnati, for example, has support groups specifically for adults with LD and uses local tutors who specialize in working with adults.

Paralleling the current interest in adulthood ADD, learning specialists are increasingly focusing on LD in adults. Special tutoring in the areas of specific learning disabilities can reap wonderful rewards. Whether you're twenty or fifty, it's never too late to learn strategies for dealing with learning disabilities.

Many colleges and vocational schools are developing programs specifically for learning-disabled students. In fact, these programs are often found in institutions for graduate education. The University of Cincinnati College of Medicine, for instance, has an excellent support service for LD medical students. Discovering an underlying learning disability can help you reevaluate educational goals you've been unable to attain. With your newfound knowledge of your ADD and LD, you may decide to try the higher education route again. Chances are, with some research and planning, you'll find a college that can meet your needs.

We hope you don't feel overwhelmed at the prospect of another problem to deal with! But *not* dealing with it is the worst thing you can do. Accepting the reality of your ADD opens doors to understanding and gaining control. Dealing with the possibility of your LD can accomplish the same thing.

In the next four chapters, you may notice a shift in style as compared with the rest of the book. With the exception of the gender and sexuality chapter, the earlier part of this book was written thirteen or more years ago, when we were newly diagnosed. From this point forward you will find that we put our coaching hats on, speaking as professionals with more than ten years of ADD coaching experience.

The cornerstones of ADD recovery are summed up in the next four chapters. We call them the M & M's—short for meditation, medication, mental hygiene and moving forward. In the first of these chapters, "Meditations on Meditation," we will explore ADD-friendly ways to calm and soothe your adrenalized system.

CHAPTER 13

Meditations on Meditation

Meditation? You Must Be Kidding . . .

If you came to us as a coaching client, sooner or later we would start mentioning the "M" word. Meditation. Most ADDers we have encountered are allergic to that word, to a greater or lesser extent. So were we, until we had calmed down enough with the aid of medication and other self-care techniques. When you have spent an entire lifetime feeling as if there were a pinball machine in your brain, it is hard to imagine yourself peacefully sitting in the lotus position. The big secret that nobody seems to clue us in on, is that you don't have to sit in the lotus position at all . . . you don't even have to sit down or (thank God!) stop moving. You don't have to have a fancy mantra, a guru or extensive notes from your trek to India in order to do this meditation thing correctly. There is no one true path to calming down the mind.

As ADDers, we have extensive experience with "failure," or what we think is failure. Often, we never get far enough along in a particular direction to actually fail. We don't even make it out of the starting gate. We get distracted by something that seems more interesting or more important or glittery than the thing we are supposed to be engaged in. Or, we might push the start button on that old familiar tape—you know, it's the "I f—ed up, I always f—k up, it will never be any different—I might as well quit right now" self-flagellation tape.

We submit that the problem with meditation is our image, our belief that it is a hairy scary thing that no ordinary human being could possibly accomplish. It's hard to begin if we hold in our minds that picture of some accomplished Tibetan monk who sits in absolute stillness and who, by the way, has been practicing meditation an entire lifetime (or many lifetimes). We don't see his learning curve or any struggle on the way to mastery. So we think we can't measure up.

You Can Do It . . . Really!

The key is to allow yourself to take those baby steps, to make "mistakes" and make room for a certain amount of fumbling around. No one ever learned anything without missing the mark quite a bit at the beginning. Did you know that the ancient definition of "sin" is simply "missing the mark"? Oh boy, and all along we thought it meant bad-bad, punishable by death or something. It's possible to take meditation a bit at a time and get more comfortable with it, just as we might do when learning to dance, play tennis, draw sketches or write poetry.

We promise you that it's not possible to "fail" at meditation. It is astonishing how many of our clients have told us that they tried meditation and found it an exercise in frustration. The problem was that nobody told them a critical piece of information: how it actually works. These clients thought that if there was a lot of activity going on in their brains, they were just not doing this meditation thing right. In fact, everybody has a lot of stuff going on in their brain most of the time. The Buddhists refer to this as "monkey chatter." If you are anxious about all the noise in your brain, there is a tendency to try to get rid of the chatter, to literally push it out of your mind somehow. In fact, pushing, pulling, talking back to or otherwise engaging with the contents of your mind keeps the whole show going. Meditation begins by just observing. Then we can practice detaching from that jumble of thoughts—to let the mind do its thing without interfering. Eventually those thoughts get tired of trying to push your buttons. They get bored and go away . . . find something more exciting to do. Well, we don't really know if thoughts actually have a mind of their own, but we both have had the experience of the noise fading to the background. And sometimes, when we remember to keep meditation at the center of our lives, as a daily practice, the noise gives up the ghost and goes away.

It is possible to have a peaceful, still mind. We have been there and are taking steps to spend more and more of our time in that pleasant place of being. You can go there too, and we will give you a road map and tools for the journey.

The following is a list of helpful guidelines for meditation. Please, please don't think of them as rules. The "R" word is an automatic signal to our inner adolescent, which is committed to breaking, ignoring or otherwise circumventing anything that smacks of authority. Also, we know from experience that our creative ADDult readers will come up with new, improved versions of our ideas, tailored to their unique brain style.

An ADD-Friendly Guide to Meditation

1. Repeat to yourselves a thousand times (or as often as necessary): Meditation is a practice. I intend to enjoy and learn from the experience. There are no wrong ways to do it and I will refrain from grading myself.

2. Get comfortable. Many meditation books and teachers will warn you to avoid getting too comfortable, because then you might fall asleep. Our thought on that is that if you fall asleep, you probably need it. You got relaxed enough to fall asleep . . . terrific! It is unlikely that you will fall asleep every time in any case. If you are concerned that you will then sleep the day away and miss work or something, set an alarm.

3. "Comfortable" for you might involve standing on your head or lying in your bed—you are the best judge of what works

for you. No meditator needs the additional distraction of physical discomfort.

4. Take slow, even breaths. Don't worry if you begin in out-of-breath mode. As you relax, your breathing will slow naturally.

5. A word about relaxation: If you are in full high-speed adrenaline mode, you won't be able to stop on a dime, change gears and get into meditation mode instantly. One might think that particular piece of wisdom is perfectly obvious, but we have personal experience with the hazards of frantic mode . . . how it seems to suck out your functional brain cells like a vampire.

6. When you have calmed your system down through meditation, and a more meditative approach to life, accessing that deep state of relaxation will not involve such a major transition. In the meantime, honor your need to take the time to settle down before you meditate. A hot bath might do the trick, or listening to soothing music. Set a timer for a wind-down ritual. Put your planner and your "to do" list away; get into comfortable clothing. Any activity that is simple and points to your intention to enter a meditative frame of mind will do.

7. Sensory cues are excellent ways to help you transition from one mental state to another.

KK: "One of my clients worked at home and devised a system to help him transition in and out of work mode. He had a special hat, special chair, scented candle and certain kinds of music that he only wore/smelled/listened to when he was at 'work.'"

You might use this technique to facilitate your transition to meditation mode. The sensory cues help you "remember" how you felt during previous sessions and thus enhance your ability to return to that familiar place.

8. Choose a single focus for yourself, something to listen to or watch while you meditate. Some people pay attention to their breath, while others repeat a word or phrase in their minds. That repeated phrase is a mantra. It does not have to be a fancy code thing given to you by your guru, who has received the magic words from his illustrious teachers. You can just make it up. Kate's favorite is "let go." You can also use a visual focus, such as a candle flame. Experiment . . . find what works for you.

9. So, the single-focus "thing" could be one of several choices. (Choosing a visual focus is a common childbirth technique that is also a form of meditation.) Obviously, if you are using a visual focus like a flower, a flame or some other object, you will need to keep your eyes open. With an auditory focus, closing your eyes will block out any visual distractions. With ADD, some of us are more visually distractible, others are more distracted by sounds. We suggest that you try out different "points of focus" to find what works best for you.

10. You can also use music as your focus. Steven Halpern's tapes are especially good for meditation. We recommend that any music you choose be free of words—it is too easy to get caught up in lyrics.

Take a break . . . This is a long list.

11. Okay, you are now seated on your favorite super-duper meditation pillow, or on your bed or whatever position is comfortable for you. Your breathing is slowing down and you are repeating your mantra, listening to your music or watching that candle flame. Are you bored yet?

12. Some people do just fine sitting or lying down, but many of us get unbearably restless when we are required to be physically still for any length of time. Don't "should" all over yourself if you have a higher need for activity than someone else. Just work with it. Allow yourself to have *your* experience; there's no need to judge or compare yourself with others here. We promised you that you did not necessarily have to sit down to meditate.

13. Moving meditation is just as good as the sitting/lying variety. It is actually a better choice for the active ADDer. You don't need the additional distraction of an antsy body when your goal is to calm the mind. We recommend that the activity you choose for meditation be something simple and repetitive. Something you can do on autopilot. Walking is a moving meditation that works well for many people. You can use awareness of your feet moving on the ground as your focus. This would be a good one for people who are strongly tactile/kinesthetic.

14. You are now sitting or moving and it is time to meditate. You notice all the thoughts in your head clamoring for your attention. They may be annoying or irritating. What do you do? When you notice your attention drifting in the direction of that thought salad, gently disengage your attention. Bring your attention back to your focus. At first, and on those bad brain days, you will be repeating this process quite a lot.

15. Stay with it. We promise it will get easier as you go along. The key to success in this case (as with any new challenge) is to take it in very small bites.

KK: "As I write this I am sitting at Peggy's computer with a jumble of random papers scattered in front of me. There is one with a paragraph entitled 'taking little steps.' It says to think about how you eat a hamburger. If you jam the whole thing in your mouth and try to swallow it, you will have little pieces falling out all over your shirt! It works much better if you take smaller bites."

16. The smaller bites in this case involve time. Start your meditation practice in small increments. Meditate for five minutes a few times a day. As you become more comfortable in

the practice, you will likely increase the length of your sessions because they have become so enjoyable. And you will begin to see benefits spreading out to encompass the rest of your life.

17. When you have gotten into the meditation groove, you will be able to get into a state of deep relaxation more quickly. Sometimes a few deep breaths will do the trick. When the workplace or a social situation is getting you into a tizzy, you can retire to the men's or the ladies' room and "take five" to get recentered.

18. Remember, the purpose is not to actively clear your mind but to step back from the noise, to put your attention on your chosen focus. This practice will help you to begin choosing your focus in everyday situations. Imagine that— your attention under your control. And this gets stronger with practice!

19. Of course, the results are not instantaneous. Many, if not most, ADDers are unable to successfully practice meditation without the benefit of medication. An optimal dose of stimulant medicine can turn the noise down to acceptable levels.

20. What about the regular practice part of meditation? Don't we ADDers have a lot of trouble sticking to any routine? Well, it is true that we struggle with structure and routine, but there are ways around it. Get yourself a coach to help you stay on track. A good ADD coach will help you with accountability for your goals without making you wrong. Accountability in this case is not about guilt or failure. It *is* about you and your coach not letting the goal drop, staying in the conversation about how to accomplish it, and celebrating the little steps as well as the big ones. Finding out what works for you as an individual is a trial-and-error process. If you forget to practice for days or even weeks, you can always get back on the horse.

Why Do We Have to Read So Much About Meditation?

Some of you are probably wondering why we are spending so much time on meditation in an ADD book. There are all kinds of books out there on meditation—how to do it, why to do it, and so on. Those books can be helpful, but they don't speak directly to the ADD experience—namely, that the brain noise is so much louder and the restlessness several notches more intense than for those without the ADD challenge. They also don't address the reasons for apparent "failure" in the past.

The other reason for including this material is that we believe it is absolutely critical for ADDers to develop some form of accessing a meditative state of mind. We pick up some habits in the course of compensating for ADD that serve us poorly in the long run. One of the most common and the most deadly is the habit of running on adrenaline. This is how the pattern begins: Early on, we discover that excitement wakes up our sleepy brains. We then, generally without conscious thought or choice, arrange our lives in such a way that there is a fair amount of drama and crisis happening on a regular basis.

Now, we know you may be reacting to what we said in the previous paragraph. Your experience is that the drama and crisis happen because ADD makes you foggy about details, or forgetful. The drama is the result of dropped balls and missed deadlines, right?

The answer is: yes and no. Of course the fogginess of ADD is a major player in the less than tidy experience of living with the disorder. The question to ask is not which explanation for the resulting mess is true, but how do the contributing factors work together. At this point in time we don't really know the answer to the chicken or egg question when it comes to ADD. We do, however, have an inkling about how the sleepy brain phenomenon and the adrenaline habit interact.

The Stimulus Junkie

Let's start with the core symptom of ADD . . . a brain that is not awake and alert enough to function at an optimal level. The owner of said brain (we'll call her Carol) discovers that she can improve matters by feeding it more stimulation. Adding more activities to her busy schedule is one method, so is waiting until the very last minute, creating a fear-based deadline crisis. Short term, these strategies solve the snoozing brain problem. There is an immediate rush of neurotransmitters available to help Carol push through the tasks at hand.

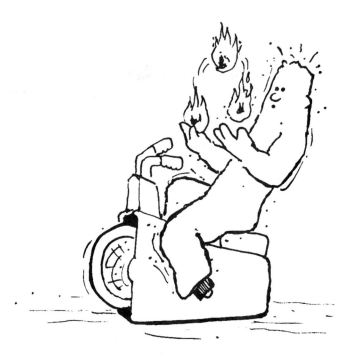

Carol learned to be a stimulus junkie in her teens. She didn't find out she had ADD until she was thirty-seven years old. She had no medication or information about how her brain worked when she was forming her life habits. Those habits have been practiced so many times they are like second nature. The grooves of those habit patterns are deeply etched in Carol's mind at this point.

Carol hires one of us as an ADD coach. She has been on medication for several months and is wondering why her life is still chaotic. She has a schedule that would break the back of most human beings. There is no room for the kind of personal time that would allow her to rest and rejuvenate. Carol is wondering if she needs to be on a higher dose of medicine.

Maybe, maybe not. This is where the chicken and egg problem gets tricky. In some cases, having a little medicine is worse than none at all. You have enough stimulant on board to be more aware that your functioning is not optimal, but not enough to solve the problems. So sometimes the answer is to increase the dose of stimulant. However, it is never the final solution. The only thing medicine does for you is to turn down the noise and thus help you become available for the learning. We are not talking about formal school at this point but the life classroom in which we are all enrolled.

Coaching Carol

Carol is not exactly flunking at the moment, but she is on probation. She gets sick a lot, is often angry and impatient with friends and family and still has difficulty making progress on the goals she has set for herself. As coaches, how do we help Carol get off probation and onto the track of steady growth and progress?

Our initial-session homework has three parts. First, we would give Carol a prescription to begin some form of meditative practice. She might have an interest in yoga, tai chi, knitting or walking. It doesn't matter which . . . they all work. Next, we would request that she read our chapter on balance and begin to look at ways she can eliminate some of the tasks on that massive "to do" list she has going. Finally, we would ask Carol to put a time space between any request and her response. For the next week she is to answer any requests for help with "I will consider your request and get back to you" . . . in an hour, the next day or next week—whichever time frame seems appropriate. Of course, if one of her children has fallen out of a tree and is hollering for help because he has a broken leg, Carol has permission to respond immediately. Anything other than a true medical emergency, however, can handle a delay in response.

You may have guessed where we are going with Carol's coaching homework. Our intention is to help Carol take the first baby steps toward awareness of the need for personal breathing space. Note that we used the word "awareness." We don't expect Carol to report back in a week's time having started a daily meditation practice and tossed out all the extraneous busyness in her life in one fell swoop. Often, the first week, or even the first several weeks, of ADD coaching are spent dealing with the ADDults' guilt because—oh gosh, oh golly—the dog seems to have eaten their homework! Our job as coaches in this case is to normalize the clients' experience. To reassure them that it takes time to form new habits and that our many successful clients also generally started out in a hit-or-miss fashion.

So Carol comes to next week's coaching call apologizing profusely because she didn't have time to read the book chapter, only remembered to put the time space in once and missed the tai chi class she intended to take. We then congratulate Carol for taking the first steps—she thought about reading the chapter, remembered at least once to delay her response to a request and found a class for herself. Great! Even more important, Carol had a big aha about the impact of her frantic style on her ability to function. She observed herself in motion as a result of our initial conversation and noticed that she made more mistakes and snapped at her children on days packed with back-to-back activity.

Now Carol is ready to own the problem. She recognizes the need to slow down, even if she isn't sure yet how to make that happen. Over time, we will help Carol take the steps necessary to "deadrenalize" her mind, her body and her life.

The following is a list of principles we would work with in the initial weeks and months coaching Carol:

1. Much of the speed involved in an adrenalized lifestyle is self-induced.

2. It is possible to resist the hurry-up entreaties of others.

3. Nothing is worth compromising your mental, physical and spiritual health.

4. It's okay to clear your schedule of everything other than basic survival activities.

5. The time you free up by doing #4 is to be used only for self-care until you have calmed yourself down.

6. If you get caught up in your responsibilities to your children, spouse, relatives, coworkers . . . remember this handy dandy rule from the airlines: "Put your oxygen mask on first, and then assist your child."

7. To our knowledge, no family ever died from eating pizza seven days in a row.

8. Never underestimate the importance of a full night's sleep. Running on empty in the sleep department will definitely lead to more stress and difficulties in the typical ADDer's life.

Most of the resistance to following these principles comes from the belief that you will turn into Rip Van Winkle and snooze for all eternity if you get off the frantic treadmill. If you don't push yourself, this thinking goes, the whole show will just stop. You will never be a functional member of society again.

We promise that if you take the time to slow down and make real choices about your life, your functioning will eventually far exceed your performance (even on your very best brain days) in hurry-up mode.

In true ADD style, we just took a somewhat meandering path from our statement about the interaction between the sleepy brain and the adrenaline habit. So be it. There really was a point to the apparent detour. We needed to cover some background before we proceeded with this discussion.

Carol's Brain Boosting Methods

Let's go back to Carol. Because she has lived her life with a brain that is not consistently alert, she has learned various means to give it a jump-start:

1. Scaring herself—this is what she is doing when she waits till the last minute.

2. Creating excitement—drama, too many things to do.

3. Mentally beating herself up (this is what she is doing when she makes herself wrong for failing to do her "homework" properly). S&M folks say that they engage in certain practices because it is stimulating. The mental version can produce similar results.

Of course, this is a very short list. There are a gazillion ways to stimulate, or overstimulate, yourself. High-risk activities such as speeding come to mind. But we won't get into all the ways and means in this discussion.

Earlier, we stated that an adrenalized lifestyle was deadly. This is both literally and figuratively true, but we will address that a bit later.

The immediate problem for Carol is that the temporary methods she uses to pump up those brain chemicals act much like the junkie's fix. There is a short-term rush of increased functioning, followed by a crash. The crash may involve complete shutdown, with the need for a nap, or a day spent in bed. Often, the crashee doesn't actually stop in his or her tracks but continues to limp along in a shuffling imitation of their daily routine. This phenomenon is a variation on the out-of-body experience . . . one's body goes through the motions, but the mind is on some other planet somewhere.

The symptoms of ADD are magnified during a postadrenaline crash. Yes indeed, the adrenaline solution creates the very problem it is intended to solve. In addition, the crash and recovery time take longer than the time spent functioning in adrenaline mode. We know this because we have observed the results of a stimulus junkie pattern in ourselves and in over a hundred clients. This brings us back to the interaction of the "not alert enough" brain and stimulus addiction. Which comes first is almost impossible to tease out in ADDulthood. They feed upon and magnify each other. It is essential to address both problems in order to stop the vicious cycle of adrenalization and crash.

Working with the M & Ms

In this part of the book, what was formerly (in the first edition) a series of chapters on treatment has become a section labeled The "M & M & M & Ms"—short and catchy for meditation, medication, mental hygiene and moving forward. In our experience, both as ADDults and ADD coaches, these four areas of focus are essential components of a successful recovery plan.

All the "Ms" work together in concert to help you clear away the mental debris that interferes with your optimal functioning.

Here is a little story that illustrates how the M & M & M & Ms can interact to break up a stimulus junkie pattern:

Dave is an ADDult in his fifties who originally hired Kate as an ADD coach. He hoped that coaching would help, because medication had been a disaster for him—or so he thought at the time. Dave described himself as sensitive to medications in general. He said that taking medication caused unbearable anxiety. He tried some herbal remedies and found that St. John's wort helped him a little bit with depression.

Since medication was not an option, Kate and Dave focused on meditation and mental hygiene in their sessions. Dave learned to put a space between requests and his response to the request. Over time, he was able to be more mindful about how he spent his days, and got rid of a lot of unnecessary stress/activity in his life. They worked on Dave's self-talk (mental hygiene), helping him to relanguage old, self-defeating beliefs about himself. It became apparent that much of Dave's frantic lifestyle was a result of his sense that he wasn't good enough, that he had always been "behind" and therefore had to run like hell to play catch-up. Dave also began a practice of moving meditation, gradually making it an integral part of his daily routine. Eventually, Dave expanded the mindful mind-set from his meditation practice to situations in his everyday life. As he describes it, he settled his system down. He was no longer addicted to adrenaline. At this point, Dave decided to give stimulant medication another try. This time, the medication trials were successful. He found an optimal dose and kind of stimulant that increased his alertness without increasing his anxiety. The interesting part of this story is that the medicine that finally worked for Dave was one of the ones he had tried before he began coaching. When Dave had done the readiness work that enabled him to be more relaxed and aware, he then was able to move forward, to take the steps needed to design a life that was a better fit.

What Happened Here?
Here is Dave and Kate's sense of what happened to Dave to cause this seemingly miraculous change in medication response. Initially, Dave was not tuned in to himself enough to realize that he had an adrenaline addiction going. He had little or no awareness of how his habit patterns and his thoughts contributed to a frantic lifestyle. Fight-or-flight

neurochemicals flooded his body/mind system almost constantly.

The fight-or-flight response was not designated for chronic, heavy use. It works best for dealing with brief, concrete threats, such as revving up to kill a woolly mammoth. When the body's mechanism for dealing with threats is overused, its stress response is kicked into overdrive. What Dave originally thought were medication side effects were nothing more than his response to chronic stress. The stimulants did not cause his anxiety, he was just tuning in to his body's sensations, perhaps for the first time in his life.

By the way, Dave is now an ADD coach and the "meet and greet" person on our Web site—addcoaching.com. His warmth and caring are a wonderful welcome home for ADDers coming to us for help and direction. Dave made a successful transition from a management job that was a poor fit to the world of self-employment.

Not everyone is like Dave . . . one size definitely does not fit all ADDults. Many of the clients we have worked with have been unable to meditate or work effectively in coaching until they experienced the benefits of stimulant medication. In our personal experience with ADD recovery, neither of us did very well with the meditation/mental hygiene part until we were more calm and awake . . . on stimulants.

Upping the Ante

Recovery is a complex process with a number of passages and stages. One of the stages it is important to mention here is what we call the "up the ante" phase. You get diagnosed and begin medication, after all those years of living in the fog. At first there is a sense of relief, calm and often delight. Wow, this is what it feels like to be normal. You cruise along for a while, functioning at a higher level than you have in the past. Life seems a lot easier.

If only it stayed that way . . .

Most of us are not content with the status quo . . . we start pushing the envelope. We wonder what we are really capable of now that the ADD is under control. In truth, we have an infinite capacity to grow and change. The sky is the limit—ultimately. We forget (or never knew) that it can't all happen *now*. So without taking time to monitor the effects of small changes, we start piling more and more stuff on our plates. In short order, we are right back where we started. Remember, an overload of stress equals more ADD symptoms.

Basically, this chapter has been one long commercial for the benefits of meditation . . . essentially taking a more meditative approach to life. We are not real big on the hard sell, but we decided to push a little bit more than we normally would because we think it is so important. Correction: We know it is absolutely critical to your recovery.

General Health and ADD

ADD symptoms are only part of the picture. Did you know that your general health is affected by the stress of living with ADD? Four years after our own initial diagnoses, we consulted a physician who had extensive experience treating ADD adults and children. He had worked with thousands of patients by the time we connected with him. It is unfortunate that his research findings have not been published or widely disseminated, because the implications of his observations are stunning.

This doctor has collected all kinds of data on the effect of ADD treatment on general health issues. He is a primary care physician by background who happened to end up specializing in ADD. He has found that all kinds of general health issues improve or resolve when ADD is effectively treated. The following is a partial list of the health challenges he has found can improve with ADD treatment:

Hypertension
Irritable bowel syndrome
Asthma
Allergies
Arthritis
Fibromyalgia
Ear infections

It is important to note that the treatment in this case is multi-modal, involving coaching/counseling around lifestyle and self-care, as well as a prescription for meditation. It involves much more than "sprinkle a little medicine on" and see if that works.

Some of the disorders on the list may make intuitive sense to you. Most of us are now aware of the impact of generalized stress on health. I don't think any reader who lives with ADD would disagree with us when we state that trying to cope with an unpredictable brain is extremely stressful. Irritable bowel and hypertension, for example, are known to be stress related. What about allergies and asthma, though? Well, the jury is out on those health issues . . . scientists are still doing the research to attempt to tease out the complicated interactions of mind and body. What we do know, however, is that the nervous system, endocrine system and immune system are intricately interconnected. It makes sense that a brain somewhat out of whack would interact with other body systems in a less than optimal fashion. Allergies and asthma are primarily disorders of the immune system.

Kate's former husband and founder of a large group practice treating ADD states that he also sees improvement, over time, of general health issues with ADD treatment. The most striking improvements, in his experience, are seen with autoimmune disorders. (The immune system again.) Stress is known to be a major culprit in the cause and severity of autoimmune issues.

The endocrine system is also involved in the ADD + stress equation. In the chapter on women with ADD, we went into a bit more detail about the impact of falling estrogen levels on ADD symptoms.

Paying for Focus at High Interest Rates

In our stories about Carol and Dave, we talked about addiction to adrenaline, but we did not go into the physiological reasons for why ADDers might tend to get addicted to adrenaline and how it may lead to health problems.

In the central nervous system, the stress response heightens levels of arousal, alertness and vigilance. It also focuses attention and enhances cognitive processes. In the body, blood pressure increases, as do breathing and heart rate. Blood sugar is raised and the immune system is suppressed. All of these changes are designed to increase the ability to problem-solve and take action, while temporarily shutting down the functions that we don't need immediately. When we have adapted to the stressful situation, the brain (and more specifically, the hypothalamus) gets messages to turn down the system . . . just like a home thermostat.

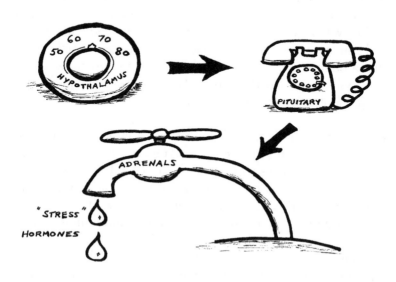

The HPA Axis: The human stress response is designed to ready us to deal with the immediate source of stress and then return our brains and bodies to a balanced state. In the brain, the hypothalamus sends action messages to the pituitary, which in turn sends the message "downstream" to the adrenal glands. The job of the hypothalamus is to keep the body on an even keel, while the pituitary is the master gland of the body, directing the various glands to produce more or less of their particular hormones. The adrenal glands produce the hormones most important to the stress response, including adrenaline and norepinephrine. These hormones communicate both with the central nervous system and the body, producing the changes needed to ready us for action. The hypothalamus-pituitary-adrenal connection is known in scientific circles as the HPA axis.

You may already have had some "aha's" while reading this little lecture on the HPA axis and the stress response. Hopefully, it has helped to answer the question of why on earth we ADDers would want to create crises and chaos in our lives. If you trip the stress response circuit, you get arousal, attention, alertness, vigilance . . . all the tools you need to complete that project you have procrastinated on right up to the drop-dead line. Cool . . . sign me up!

Sounds like a pretty nifty strategy at first glance. Our effort to solve the sluggish brain problem with an injection of stress, however, has consequences for the body. Recall what those adrenal hormones do to the body—they raise your heart rate, blood pressure and blood sugar. They also dampen your immune system. The stress response was not designed to handle constant, chronic stress. It evolved to deal with the needs of our ancestors (150,000 years ago) in a world where change was the exception rather than the rule. The ADD adrenaline junkie is, in effect, paying for focus at high interest rates. Yes, you get a few hours of higher performance, but you pay on the back end with the impact of stress on your brain and body.

What happens when the stress response system (HPA axis) is overused and abused?

From ADD to Stress to Illness

Research on the mind/body connection and ADD is in its infancy. A number of health professionals who work with ADD have noted and written about the apparent connection between chronic fatigue syndrome (CFS), fibromyalgia (FMS) and ADD. It has been observed that there is a higher incidence of CFS and FMS among ADD women, but the studies to back up this observation are only just beginning. Other ADD specialists have found that a number of general health problems are more common in their ADD patients, particularly stress-related and autoimmune disorders. These specialists, unfortunately, have not published their data as of this writing. In a chapter on FMS/CFS in *Gender Issues and AD/HD*, the authors—Kathleen Nadeau and Patricia Quinn—propose a model for explaining how the stress of ADD may lead to physical illness. Bear in mind that a model is not proven fact—it is a working hypothesis, or educated guess, about what might be causing an observed pattern.

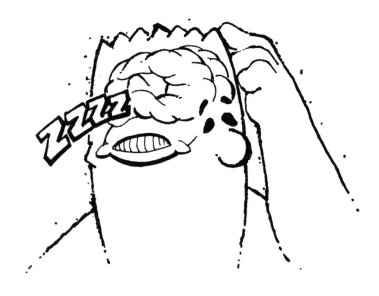

Warning . . . Warning! The next paragraph contains scientific information that may temporarily boggle the ADD brain. If this occurs, discontinue reading that one and skip to the next paragraph.

Many studies indicate that an imbalance of the neurotransmitters dopamine and norepinephrine underlies the symptoms of ADD. There is too much neurotransmitter activity in the brain's limbic system and not enough in the frontal lobes. As a result, the frontal lobes don't have enough fuel to carry out important executive functions, while the limbic system is hyperreactive. The limbic system is the seat of the emotions. One of its important roles is to evaluate input from the brain/body and the external world. It takes this input, compares it with previous experience and labels it with appropriate emotional coloration. The resulting information is then sent to the frontal lobes and to the body (via the HPA axis). It is the job of the frontal lobes to provide guidance to the body's "support services." These support services (endocrine, immune and autonomic nervous systems) allow the body to take action.

Here is the "lowdown" on the "ADD to stress to illness" model. While it has not been "proven" it makes a lot of sense.

The person with ADD encounters a stressor or a problem to be solved. His or her limbic system sends messages "downstream" (to body systems via the HPA axis) to get ready for action. So the heart rate and blood pressure go up, along with the other changes activated in the stress response. The frontal lobes of the brain also get an action message. If you recall, it is the job of the frontal lobes to provide guidance, to tell the rest of the brain and body *what* exactly they are supposed to do. In the ADD brain, however, the frontal lobes are often caught napping. They don't respond to the action message and the task goes undone. When nothing much happens, the limbic system keeps sending its request for action and support. It's as if the limbic system is shouting, and the HPA axis is overreacting,

347

while the frontal lobes are still snoozing with the headphones on and don't hear the shouting.

Of course, it is also emotionally stressful to experience this pattern of sluggish or absent response over and over. When you add the negative self-talk about being dumb or lazy, it piles more stress onto an already overloaded system. There is evidence that stress can actually cause changes in the way the brain and body function. The HPA axis can "burn out" under a barrage of stress, leading to abnormal functioning and stress-related physical illness. The immune system may also give way under an onslaught of stress, increasing the chance of infections, autoimmune disorders and acquired sensitivities.

We don't mean to scare you. Life with ADD can be scary enough without adding more stuff to worry about. There are countless ways in which ADD causes stress in our lives. We have touched on only a few in this chapter. The reason we have raised the issue of the ADD-stress-illness connection is that there is something you can do about it. We want you to take self-care seriously. You are worth it.

The first step is to take some time to become aware of the impact of stress on your mind and body. For a few days, make an effort to focus on your body sensations. What patterns of stress show up in your body?

When you are aware of your stress patterns, you can use your meditative activity to relax the body. You can also decide to retreat from stressful situations until you are ready to deal with them.

Here's a piece of homework for you, should you choose to accept it. The next time you go on an adrenalized productivity binge, make a few notes to yourself. Rate your functioning every hour or so during the binge on a scale of one to ten, with ten being peak performance. Note how long your enhanced performance lasts. Then rate your functioning for several days

to a week after the binge. How long does it take for you to recover? Is your period of focus worth the price or are the interest
rates just too high?

This chapter has been about finding ways to slow down and become more mindful about the effects of your lifestyle on your
brain and body. Putting the meditation chapter *before* the chapter on medication was intentional. Without putting in those
pauses to check in with ourselves, it is all to easy to use medication as a tool for pushing ourselves harder than we already do.
In the next chapter we will explore medications and a few alternative methods for waking up the brain.

CHAPTER 14

Medication
and a Few Alternatives

Running Away from Ritalin,
a New Book by Dr. Knowitall

This new addition to the ADD bookshelf tells you
everything you need to know in order to make the decision to run as fast as you can away from anyone who
dares to breathe a word about how you might want to
consider medicating your ADD. It does a terrific job of
presenting the horrors of the evil stimulant drugs in full
living color and gory, graphic detail. You will find out
how Ritalin (and other stimulants) will turn you into a
character from *The Night of the Living Dead*, among
other things. This sequel to *Reefer Madness* is a warning
of the dangers awaiting you if you stray from the path of
clean, wholesome, stimulant-free living. Ritalin and its
evil twins can turn you into an instant junkie, lead to
incurable madness and even make your hair fall out!
Thank God for the author of this groundbreaking
book—he has saved us from the fiery pit of stimulant
Hell. Read it . . . before it's too late—ARGhhhh!

—I. M. Wrong, *Fear* magazine

We bet that you have never seen a book review quite like this one, but really, it is only an exaggerated version of common fear-based thinking about stimulant medication. All right, we know it's a rant, but you have probably run across Internet postings, books, radio shows and other highly negative communications about the first-line medications used to treat ADD.

We are not here to make the decision on medication for you. As good coaches, our job is to offer information and help guide you through the process of making a sound decision for yourself. As writers, however, we feel a responsibility to make a recommendation based on our personal and professional experience. Stimulant medication is the most powerful treatment currently available for waking up the ADD brain. It has been a lifesaver for many people. We have had positive personal and professional experiences with stimulant medication. Do yourself a favor and at least consider exploring this option. When you make your personal decision, you can consider that opinion along with the other pro and con factors on your list. Medicine, of course, is only one part of the solution to ADD recovery. It helps you to be available for all the learning and changing you will need to do in order to create the life that you deserve.

There Are No Right or Wrong Answers to the Question of Medication
To Be or Not to Be Medicated?

Contrary to the sensationalized reports of doctors passing out stimulant prescriptions like candy, our experience is that most ADDults are initially very reluctant to consider medication for themselves. They think long and hard before they take the step of seeking medical treatment for their ADD. The following are common questions and issues ADDers ponder when they are making the decision about medication. We will address each area of concern. In this section we are specifically discussing stimulant medication, such as Ritalin, Adderall, Dexedrine and related pharmaceuticals.

1. *Will the medicine control me?*

The right dose of stimulant medicine does not control you . . . it allows you to have better control of yourself. Rather than being at the mercy of a brain that is going off in a million directions at once, you will be able to steer your attention in the direction you want to go. A good analogy is that medication helps you to drive your own brain, rather than having it drive you.

2. *Will I become boring?*

3. *I am not sure I really want to be normal—will medicine take away my uniqueness?*

4. *Will medicine take away my creativity?*

We are answering these questions together because they are related. Most people have heard stories about children, in particular, acting like zombies on Ritalin or other stimulant meds. What these stories fail to mention is what, if anything, was done to carefully adjust the kind of medicine and the dose. One size does not fit all when it comes to stimulants. Some people have a bad experience with Ritalin and a positive response to Adderall, for example. For other people, the situation is reversed. In addition, the specific dosage can have a profound effect. At certain dosages, people can indeed become sleepy or dull. The solution to this problem, of course, is to talk to your doctor about adjusting the type or dose of medication. We have worked with a number of folks who were dismayed because they felt their uniqueness, their sparkle or their creativity was dampened by taking stimulants. Some did decide to go off medication. Others compromised by taking medicine for tasks requiring attention to detail, while giving themselves periods of unmedicated time for a more freewheeling thinking style. Many ADDults, however, seem to go through a phase of stifling themselves. It has nothing to do with the chemical action of the drug and a lot to do with their newfound ability to observe themselves. For the first time in their lives, the brain noise has calmed down enough to allow them to watch themselves in action, and they are judging what they see. Until they become more self-accepting, they are hampered by self-consciousness. It doesn't help to stop taking the medicine. You don't forget what you observed about your own behavior. The solution is to hang in there . . . it is indeed just a phase. (Take a look at the chapters on mental hygiene and meditation in this book for more about this.)

5. *What kind of side effects can I expect?*

The most common side effects are disturbed sleep and appetite, headaches, stomach upset, cardiovascular changes and anxiety. Another common effect is rebound symptoms, which occur when the medicine is wearing off. For a time, the symptoms return in a magnified form. Generally, with the longer-acting forms of medicine available today, rebound is not as big an issue as it was in the past. Rebound can be minimized by carefully timing the dose. A bit later in this chapter we will discuss side effects in more detail, offering practical solutions for dealing with them.

6. *What are the long-term effects of taking these medicines?*

There is no evidence of negative long-term effects from taking stimulant medication.

7. *Is taking medicine just a crutch? Maybe I just need to try harder.*

This one is a big stopper for a lot of ADDults. Many people still view mental or emotional challenges as diseases of the will. In some ways, it may be easier to view the symptoms as something you can control—none of us like to feel out of control, after all. And there are old, outdated notions still hanging around about being, well, weak, if you can't solve all your problems on your own. When we imagine a crutch, in this sense, the picture is of someone leaning very heavily on it. Imagine instead that your medicine is not a crutch but a ladder. It is not something you lean on because you are helpless, but a tool that helps you rise in life, rung by rung. Are your glasses a crutch? What about your blood pressure medicine? Trying harder does not work to lower your blood pressure, and it doesn't usually make things better for your ADD (in fact, it can often make things worse). Yes, it is important to take steps that will make your life more manageable, but trying to force your brain to do something it is not capable of at a given moment will only result in shutting it down.

8. *I am functional . . . I have a responsible job. Medicine is for people who are really sick.*

It is a mind trap to think that you have to be practically on skid row before you accept help. There are ADDers who struggle ferociously just to keep the basics in place . . . or are dependent on others for financial help. Many of us, however, manage to function, at times on a very high level. We are so used to the effort of keeping all those balls in the air that we don't register the level of stress and strain involved in doing it. Are we doing ourselves, our loved ones or anyone else a favor by continuing to live this way?

9. *I don't even like taking aspirin . . . aren't there some herbal remedies that can help?*

Of course, if you are generally opposed to taking medicine for any reason, pharmaceuticals for ADD may not be an option for you. Toward the end of this chapter we will include some alternatives for your consideration.

10. *Will I jeopardize my job or career by taking medicine?*

Good question. There are some positions that do not allow workers to take stimulant medication on the job—pilots, for example. For most people, however, there is no clear information about the impact of taking stimulants on your career. If you are not willing to disclose your diagnosis and treatment to your employer, there is also the issue of drug testing to consider.

It may help to know that methylphenidate (generic for Ritalin) and Dexedrine are detectable in a standard urine test for only one or two days. We were unable to find any specific information about Adderall and drug testing.

Actually, we found an interesting tidbit when we did a Google search for "pilots and stimulant medication." Apparently, the army and the navy have approved the use of stimulants (called the "go-pill") for fighter and bomber crew members in combat. The name of the article we turned up was entitled "Fatigue Kills."

11. Can I afford it?

Do your homework before you make this decision. Find out what it will cost for a diagnostic assessment prior to scheduling your appointment. Ask your potential prescribing physician how often you will need to see him or her once you are on a regular dose of medication. Factor in the cost of office visits as well as the cost of the medicine itself. Check with your insurance company to find out how much they will cover. Get on the phone and do some comparison shopping about the price of medication. Ask a number of pharmacists for information on the best deals. For example, you may save some money by getting a prescription for a higher dosage than you need and then cutting the pills in half. Make sure you check with your doctor on this one, however, as the longer-acting stimulants are not generally designed to be broken up. Our own research turned up some substantial bargains at Sam's Club and Costco, for example.

Of course, the answer to this question is not strictly about dollars and cents. How do you assign a monetary value to your ability to function and your quality of life? If your children get a parent who is more available, isn't that more important than providing certain nonessential material items? Do you wonder if you are worth all the trouble and expense? We, of course, are convinced that you are worth it, and that you deserve whatever it takes to get the help you need.

12. *Taking medicine makes me feel defective.*

Many of us are ashamed about needing to take medication, especially at first. We often go through some pretty funny "cloak and dagger" stuff to ensure that we are not caught taking those telltale pills. Well, it's funny later on, when we are more self-accepting. In the moment, that feeling of shame is painful and nothing to laugh at. The most effective antidote to this particular pain is to seek out the company of other ADDults. Together we create a forgiving subculture that nurtures all of us. In fact, that culture already exists. Spend your next vacation at the ADDA conference or one of the other ADD conferences to experience the warm, wonderful feeling of coming home. There is nothing quite like the experience of taking out your pill bottle and seeing everyone around you suddenly remembering to take their medication too. It's kind of a spiritual experience, like taking communion.

13. *I am very sensitive to any kind of medicine . . . I am afraid of having a negative experience.*

If you have fears, respect them. It does no good to try to frog-march yourself toward something that really scares you. Beliefs are very powerful. The placebo effect can actually work in a negative way—your fears can produce unpleasant effects. Be aware, however, that some adults with ADD have had the experience that they are not so sensitive once they have calmed themselves down through meditation, coaching and other strategies. Dave's story in the meditation chapter is a good example of this.

14. *I don't want to be dependent on a drug.*

Do you mean you don't want to realize that your functioning/dysfunctioning has a biological basis? This one can be a tough hurdle. Acknowledging that we can't do everything all by ourselves through sheer force of will can be a bitter pill to swallow. Ask anyone who has worked the Twelve Steps and they will tell you that the surrender part is the most challenging. Not the surrender itself, but allowing oneself to get out of the way so a Higher Power can take over. Have you ever considered that your Higher Power might just be offering to take the burden off your shoulders in the form of a medicine? Most of us have trouble accepting help in any form. We have been programmed to believe that we must be independent at all costs. This belief does not serve us.

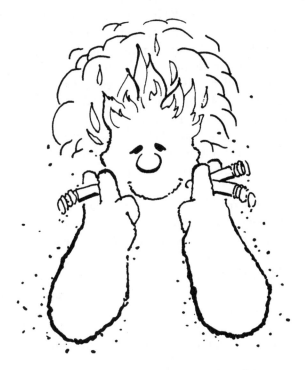

15. *Will I have to take medicine for the rest of my life?*

Maybe, maybe not. Of course, the choice to take medicine is always yours. It is not a "have to" but a decision based on what serves you at a given time. In general, ADDults seem to need less medication over time—we have taken an informal poll of a number of professionals who have treated adults with ADD for a decade or more. There is no research available that would give us clues as to why this would be so, but we have a few theories:

- When you are medicated you work more effectively—this includes psychological work as well as the work of putting supportive systems in place. When you are anxious or disturbed, the ADD symptoms get worse. The medication often allows us to get our lives running more smoothly, thus there is less need for a higher dose.

- Does taking medication over time actually foster positive changes in the brain? **KK:** "For example, I have not taken stimulants for the past ten years. Ten years ago I noticed that my baseline brain functioning had changed. I no longer experienced the same level of mental fog that had plagued me all my life . . . this was off medication. I discussed this surprising development with a neuroscientist friend. He said that there was evidence that some antidepressants might actually reset the brain. He didn't know of any similar findings on stimulants but stated that it was not out of the realm of possibility.

  "Over the years, I have noticed that my ADD symptoms appear in specific situations—my baseline functioning is pretty good, but when I am dealing with psychological issues or certain performance challenges the symptoms come back. The more I face those challenges and deal with them the less the symptoms interfere. However, please don't take this information as a recommendation to say no to medication. I was on stimulants for five years, and I don't think I could have gotten where I am today without that jump-start."

Don't forget that we carry a lot of baggage as a result of living our lives with an unidentified neurological difference. We have skill deficits and life messes to clean up, as well as emotional fallout that needs to be processed. These challenges add to our mental processing load. When we get farther along on the path of recovery, the need for medication is likely to change.

In the realm of possibility . . . what would happen if every ADD child was totally accepted for who they were from the very beginning? What if our schools and other institutions didn't make us wrong, but worked with our differences? What if we never had to be institutionalized at all? It used to be thought that ADD was a disorder of childhood, that we matured out of it at some point. The growing number of diagnosed adults blows that theory out of the water. But what if we never heard the message that we were defective? Without the overlay of guilt and shame and fear, might we have outgrown our ADD?

16. *I heard that some people get psychotic from taking stimulant medication. Is this true?*

If you also have bipolar disorder, taking stimulant medicine for your ADD may trigger a manic episode. It is important to let your doctor know if you or any close family members have a bipolar history. He or she may prescribe a mood stabilizer (such as Lamictal or Depakote), and then add medication to treat your ADD.

17. *I took Ritalin before and it didn't help me (or I had a bad experience with it).*

All stimulant medications are not the same. You may have uncomfortable side effects on Ritalin, for example, but do very well on Dexedrine or Adderall. Or the situation can be reversed. Side effects are not the only issue. Many people find that there is a dramatic difference in effectiveness between different stimulants. Doug Pentz, Ph.D, is codirector of The Affinity Center, a Cincinnati clinic specializing in ADD and related disorders. His advice is to keep trying. In his experience, 95 percent of the adults treated at The Affinity Center eventually find a medication or combination of medications that work for them.

18. *Will I get addicted?*

There is no evidence that taking stimulants in therapeutic doses leads to dependence or abuse. In fact, there is evidence that successful treatment of ADD with stimulants lowers the chances of substance abuse. Think about it: Impulsivity is one

of the hallmark symptoms of ADD. If your stimulant medication gives you the ability to stop and think, you will be less
likely to make choices that don't serve you. In the book *When
Too Much Is Not Enough*, author Wendy Richardson says that
"some professionals believe that ADHD medication has a high
potential for abuse. If this were true, why do so many with
ADHD forget to take it? Those with ADHD who are addicted
to sugar, alcohol, or street drugs sure don't forget to use them."

19. *I am an alcoholic/addict in recovery . . . doesn't that mean I
can't take these drugs?*

No. It means that you need to be more cautious than the average
ADDer. We recommend that you read Wendy Richardson's books
for more detailed information, but we will include a few highlights
here. The stage of recovery is very important. The following information is from *When Too Much Is Not Enough* by Wendy Richardson, who adapted recovery stages from the work of Terence T.
Gorski and Merlene Miller (*Counseling for Relapse Prevention* [In-
dependence, Mo.: Herald House-Independence, 1982]).

Pretreatment: This is the stage before alcoholics or addicts
enter treatment. When the addiction is out of control, it is
not the time to treat ADD with medication.

Stabilization: This is a time of physical and emotional
detox. Treatment for ADD is also not recommended during
this stage.

Early Recovery: This is not the ideal time to begin medical
treatment for ADD. The commitment to recovery is not as
solid as it needs to be. There are people, however, who are
affected by ADD to such an extent that they can't focus
enough to participate in recovery programs. In those cases,
it may be necessary to treat the ADD with medication. Of
course, it is important that these individuals be highly motivated and monitored closely. They need to be involved in
an active recovery program.

Middle Recovery: This is the stage of creating a life based on recovery. It is now time to begin the process of evaluating and treating ADD. It can help you stay sober and increase the quality of your life.

Ongoing Recovery: This may be a stage when untreated ADDers are challenged by feelings of frustration, anger, shame and confusion. They have been working hard at recovery—doing all the right things—but don't seem to be getting anywhere. The problems with jobs, relationships and concentration are still there. Treatment with medication can support further recovery and prevent relapse.

What Do I Do Next?

I want to try medicine.

Do some comparison doctor shopping. Ask other adults with ADD who live in your area for referrals. If you don't know any, go to the CHADD Web site (www.chadd.org) and click on Support. There is a locator function that will provide information on CHADD chapters in your state. Go to a meeting and ask other ADDults for suggestions on physicians who are experienced with ADD. Another option is to go to addconsults.com. For a fee, you can hire someone to do the legwork and find ADD-savvy professionals in your area.

Get an Official Diagnosis

Avoid bursting into your doctor's office with guns blazing, demanding an immediate prescription for the ADD you have self-diagnosed. We are only partly joking . . . this has actually happened more than once. Well, not the guns part, but the attitude. It's important to form a partnership with your prescribing physician, and it certainly doesn't help to create an atmosphere of attack and defense on the very first encounter.

Remember, You Are the Customer

It is important to work with your doctor, so what should you do if your doctor is not a good fit for you? For example, if you are a person with years of sobriety, who has come to realize that treating your ADD is now a priority, it doesn't help to have a physician who believes that stimulants should never be used by recovering individuals. Look for a doctor who has some experience treating people with ADD and addictions. If your doctor always seems in a rush and doesn't seem to listen to you or have time for your concerns, let him know that this is not working for you. If your attempts to communicate aren't getting through, go shopping again.

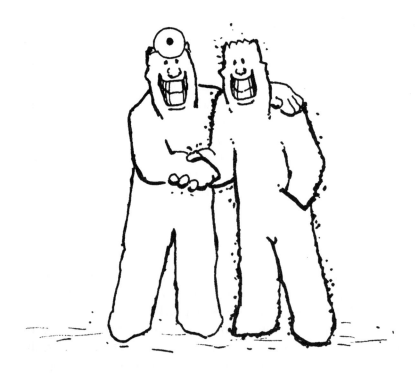

Finding a Doctor

The Doctor Test
Most of the advice given on how to evaluate a physician's experience with ADD is pretty general. You are told to ask a prospective doctor questions like:

How many ADD patients do you have?

Have you had specialized training in ADD?

What's your philosophy about treating ADD?

These are not bad questions, and we encourage you to ask them. However, they are not specific enough. Read this chapter and ask the following additional questions when you are interviewing a prospective physician:

Can you explain rebound to me?

Can you tell me about extended release versus regular stimulant medication?

Can you tell me a little about how a stimulant can settle my brain down?

Please tell me about the difference between Strattera and Ritalin.

No One Local?
You may not be able to find an ADD expert right in your backyard. If this is the case, you have a few options. You can travel. Many ADDults end up pursuing the long-distance option. A number of specialty practices are willing to set up a concentrated ADD evaluation and medication trial package for out-of-towners. Unless you are willing to travel every three months or so after the initial evaluation, you will also need to find a local doctor who is

willing to work with you and the long-distance folks. In fact, most of the centers who do this insist that you have a local doctor to monitor your progress more closely. If travel is not an attractive option, seek out someone who has at least some experience treating ADD. When you are doctor shopping, look for someone who can admit that they don't know it all, and who is open to input from others with more expertise. It is possible to arrange for your doctor to have a phone consultation with an expert of your choice. You, of course, would be responsible for the payment, but this option is less expensive than travel.

A Trial-and-Error Process

Many of the adults who come to us for coaching are dismayed to find that it takes time and patience to find the right dose of the right medication. Nobody told them what to expect, and so they often feel that their doctor doesn't know what he or she is doing when they encounter the "let's try this" approach. Expect that it will take weeks, months or even as long as a year to get stabilized on a steady dose that works for you. We know it is hard for ADDers to wait, and we confess that we were not exactly models of calm patience when we went through all those medication trials. At times it seemed as if they were trials of a different sort—trials and tribulations! You are still allowed to fuss and fume if that helps, but perhaps it will help to know something about the "whys" of this seemingly endless process.

Getting treatment for your ADD is not like going to the doctor for your flu shot or an antibiotic. It is just not that straightforward. Your doctor can't take blood levels to determine how much stimulant medicine you need, because blood levels don't tell anything useful. There are no guidelines for what particular stimulant medicine will work for you as an individual. Dosage and the timing of the dose are also very individualized. What is known is that (1) stimulants are the first-line (and generally most effective) treatment for ADD; (2) there is a generally accepted dosage range for stimulants (1 to 2 mg/kg for methylphenidate, 0.5 to 1 mg/kg for Focalin and amphetamines, including Adderall); (3) it is standard to start with the lowest dose and gradually increase it.

Exceptions to the Rules

We stated that stimulants are the first-line treatment for ADD, but there are always exceptions. Some people cannot tolerate stimulants for various reasons. For example, people with high blood pressure or heart conditions may need to avoid these medications. An increase in heart rate or blood pressure is a possible side effect. This is not a hard-and-fast rule either, as some people with these conditions can take stimulants along with their blood pressure or heart medicine without ill effects. If you have either of these conditions, treatment would need to be closely monitored by your doctor, or doctors.

There are also exceptions to the dosage guidelines. Scientists and prescribing professionals are still trying to figure out the appropriate stimulant doses for adults with ADD. More research is needed, and physicians are understandably cautious about prescribing controlled substances. However, in the current CHADD resource sheet for medication management, it is stated that underdosing stimulant medication in adults can lead to decreased effectiveness. Although we stated earlier that adults seemed to need less medication over time, it is also true that the commonly prescribed doses for adults are higher than they were when we first wrote this book. By the time this revised edition is published and has been on the shelves for a couple of years, the guidelines for dosage range may have changed again. There are a number of physicians who treat adults successfully using higher doses than those recommended by CHADD. It seems that the jury is still out on the optimal dosage range for adults with ADD.

In addition, the weight guidelines for stimulant dosage are being questioned. There is no scientific evidence that weight is useful in predicting the dosage needed for an individual. You will see weight-based guidelines in print in a number of places, but they are the results of an educated guess about how to make dosing decisions. Stay tuned, as these guidelines are likely to change as more research is done.

More on Medication

How Do the Stimulant Medications Work? They affect the neurotransmitters norepinephrine and dopamine. If you recall from the neurology lesson in an earlier chapter, the neurotransmitters are messengers for the brain's postal system. No one knows yet *exactly how* the stimulants alter neurotransmitter functioning, we just know that they do.

Off Label: Did you know that Adderall XR is currently the only one of the stimulants that is FDA approved for treating adults with ADD? This is due to the long and arduous process of getting FDA approval. It doesn't mean that other stimulants are not safe or effective for ADDults, just that research needed for approval is not complete. It is standard medical practice at this point to prescribe drugs *off label* for a variety of medical conditions. For example, aspirin is FDA approved as a painkiller but has been used to prevent heart attacks for a number of years. With the exception of Adderall XR, the stimulants are approved only for treating children with ADD and adults with narcolepsy. This information is current as of August 2005, however. By the time you actually buy and read this book, the information may well have changed.

Medication and the Wake-Up Call: For most ADDults, the process of accepting that we have ADD and getting the right treatment seems to move at glacial speed. As hard as it is to wait, this state of affairs can actually be helpful. It gives us a chance to prepare ourselves for the life-altering experience of being awake for the first time in our lives.

The experience of having a good response to stimulant medication can be mind-blowing. Before, perhaps you had an intellectual understanding of ADD and its impact on your life. Now it is *right in your face.* You can *feel* the difference. Many people have compared the experience of being on stimulant medication for the first time with being reborn. The world is sharper and clearer, and that mind chatter has faded or even gone away. You may feel relaxed in a way that you never have before. Some people say they had their first good night's sleep ever when they started taking stimulants. Others express that they feel truly alive and truly themselves for the first time in their lives.

This, of course, is heady stuff. Be prepared for a mixed bag of emotions. You may feel joyful, sad, angry and confused all at the same time. Joyful that you are having a wonderful experience, sad and angry that you had to spend so many years in a dark, foggy place, and confused as you try to integrate a profound shift in your relationship to the world and yourself.

Do yourself a favor. Clear your planner of nonessentials for at least a week after you are scheduled for your first medication trial. If you can take a few days off, that would be optimal. This is not small potatoes—it is a *Big Deal.* You will need time and space to process the changes you will be going through.

Of course, some of you will be disappointed, at least the first time around. As we said, it can take time to find the right medicine and dose. If the earth doesn't move for you, so to speak, don't despair. Keep trying, and you will eventually join the vast majority of ADD adults who find the right medicine or combination for them as individuals.

Caution: Take That Lead Foot Off the Accelerator! It would be ideal if we used the marvels of modern pharmacology to settle down, to clean up the messes in our lives and to get well enough organized. The reality for many of us is quite a bit different from the orderly plan we just proposed. This is how it goes . . .

Janet has just started Adderall and has had a good response to the medicine. Yee hah! She gets excited about all the things she can now do that she was never able to do before. She starts out with the greatest of intentions. On her "things I want to do" list are:

1. Get rid of piles and find an organizational system that works

2. Set up a daily routine with a reasonable bedtime

3. Get into an exercise routine

4. Balance my checkbook

Her list then segues into somewhat more grandiose goals, like:

67. Write the great American novel [she has always avoided writing]

68. Remodel the entire house by myself

69. Learn Chinese

70. Master the violin

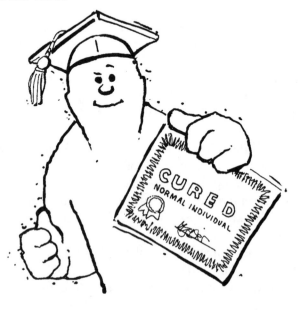

What actually happens is that Janet joins a writers group, signs up for the violin and Chinese lessons and then starts ripping up carpet and tearing down wallpaper. Pretty soon she is up to her ears in chaos, skimping on sleep and wondering why the medicine has stopped working. We know there is at least one other similar story in this book, but it bears repeating. You *know* that we ADDers never get it right the first time around.

You have been duly warned. It is likely, however, that you will forget these words of wisdom when you are caught up in the excitement of having a more functional brain. This is where having a coach comes in handy to help keep you grounded. We are not saying that you can't write the great American novel or master Chinese . . . only that you can't do it all *today*. Take the steps to get your life in balance and you *will* be able to move forward toward your loftier goals.

Two Categories of Stimulants— Methylphenidate and Amphetamine

Methylphenidate (MPH) and amphetamine (AMP) are the two general types of stimulant medication. Both of them increase the levels of dopamine and norepinephrine in the gap between nerve cells. However, they achieve this goal through slightly different processes, so the effect on individuals tends to vary. There are no guidelines as to which type of stimulant is best to try first. If you have a close blood relative who has had a good response to one or the other, you may want to mention this to your physician.

Methylphenidate
This is the generic name for Ritalin, the stimulant that has received the most coverage in the media. Ritalin is not better or worse than any other stimulant, it just happens to be the one that was used most frequently for many years, and thus more people are familiar with it. Many physicians prefer it because they have more experience prescribing and monitoring the drug. There are two types of methylphenidate preparations: immediate release and extended release.

369

Immediate Release: These are the short-acting medications and this category includes Ritalin, Metadate, Methylin and generic methylphenidate. They are supposed to last for three or four hours, although many ADDults have found that they last only two or two and a half hours. Methylphenidate is a mixture of two mirror-image molecules (d and l isomers) in a one-to-one ratio. The d isomer (which is the active methylphenidate isomer) has been isolated and manufactured as Focalin. The doses for this drug are half of the standard methylphenidate preparation, the result of taking out the inert molecule. The idea behind the development of Focalin is the hope that there will be fewer side effects.

Extended or Sustained Release: The older-generation preparations of longer-acting MPH are disappointing. They contain a wax matrix, which does not have an immediate-release portion. The release of the drug over time is also irregular. These medications include Ritalin SR, Metadate ER and Methylin ER.

Extended Release—the Next Generation: The newer generation of extended-release MPH medications are generally more consistent in their effects over time. The delivery systems for releasing MPH during the course of a day are better than the old wax matrix method. The medications in this category are Concerta, Metadate CD and Ritalin LA. There are the following differences between these drugs:

- The way the MPH is released and how it is used in the body

- The amount (or percentage) of stimulant that is released immediately and the amount (percent) that is in the extended-release portion

- Whether the extended-release portion is released all at once or gradually (and continuously) over a period of time

- How long the drug lasts—the range is from five to twelve hours

What this means for you is that one extended-release medication can have a more gradual onset and last longer than others, while another may have a stronger effect at first but not last as long. Which one will work best for you is an individual matter. Again, it is a matter of working with your doctor in a trial-and-error process.

Amphetamine

One difference between MPH and amphetamine is that the mirror-image d and 1 isomers are both active in amphetamines but have different effects. Dexedrine and Dextrostat are amphetamines that contain only the d isomer. Adderall (or mixed amphetamine salts) contains both the d and 1 isomers. Therefore, it is likely that Adderall will have different effects than Dexedrine/Dextrostat.

Immediate Release: In this category are Dexedrine, Dextrostat and Adderall.

Extended Release: Dexedrine Spansules (dextroamphetamine sulfate sustained-release capsules) are the only older-generation sustained-release preparations. Adderall XR is in the second generation and thus has a more reliable delivery system.

Long or Short Acting—Which Is Better?

The answer is: it depends. In the old days, before there were more reliable longer-acting stimulants, we complained about the need to take medicine every few hours. Rebound was a major issue, as was remembering to take those "middle of the day" doses. Many people do very well on extended-release preparations, but others have a better response to short-acting stimulants. Still others need to be on a combination of long- and short-acting stimulant medication. Again, it is a trial-and-error process that also needs to take into consideration your particular needs for focus during the course of a day.

Medication for Work or Medication for Life?

Your life doesn't stop when you leave the office. Your home life, your friendships and leisure-time activities will benefit if you are more present as a result of taking your medication. Factor this in as you work with your physician on dosage and timing.

Managing Side Effects

As we mentioned before, the most common side effects of stimulants are appetite and sleep disturbance, rebound, anxiety, cardiovascular changes, stomach upset and headaches. It is important to inform your doctor of any health changes, of course, and to work closely together on side-effect management. We are, however, offering some words of wisdom, tips and strategies for dealing with the most common problems.

Appetite Disturbance: This one does not tend to be a big problem for adults. On the contrary, many people are rather disappointed when the hoped-for side effect of weight loss fails to materialize. Generally, a loss of appetite is temporary and short-lived. If you do experience a diminished desire to eat, don't panic. Continue to drink ample fluids, with the addition of protein shakes. You can also eat a hearty meal in the morning, before your medicine kicks in, or when your medicine wears off.

Sleep Disturbance: For most people, this effect is also temporary. The remedy is similar to that for appetite disturbance: ride it out until your system adjusts. Of course, you are allowed to whine and complain in the meantime—sleep deprivation is no fun! Often, changing the timing of your medication will solve the problem. There is an optimal time window for getting to sleep when you are taking stimulant medication. Most people can get to sleep when they have enough stimulant in their systems, and also when the medicine has worn off. The problems come when you try to get to sleep during that in-between period, when the medicine is in the process of wearing off. The solution for this is to work with your doctor on timing so that your medicine has either worn off or is still onboard at your regular bedtime. Sometimes a small evening dose will do the trick.

In the realm of the strange but interesting, we know an ADDult who has had severe sleep difficulties all her life. Her body clock appeared to be on something like a twenty-six-hour cycle. Well, since there are only twenty-four hours in a day (contrary to what many of us wish to believe), her sleep and wake patterns moved around the real time clock constantly. She could not keep appointments or do anything consistently at a given time. Finally, she found someone who was willing to experiment with her hunch that taking twenty-four-hour stimulant medication would help. She now takes a bedtime dose of a long-acting stimulant medication and has regular sleep and wake patterns for the very first time in her life. Go figure.

Rebound: This is perhaps the most annoying of the side effects. When your medicine is wearing off, your symptoms come back in a temporarily exaggerated fashion. You are more antsy, distracted, edgy, than you are when off meds. The solution is careful timing of dosages so the level of stimulant doesn't fall too much during your waking hours. Some people, however, still experience some rebound. If this happens to you, you will need to manage your life so that your symptoms don't get you into trouble. Take a break from work, people or general stimulation when rebound hits. You don't even have to invoke the ADD word; just tell your boss or coworkers that you are dealing with afternoon slump. If a total break is not possible, downshift to tasks that require less mental power.

Other Side Effects: Work with your doctor if you experience anxiety, stomach upset or headaches. Sometimes these are also just temporary changes as your body adjusts to the medicine. Cardiovascular changes can be more serious, so it is important to immediately report any changes in heart rate or blood pressure to your physician. Anxiety may be alleviated by switching to a different medication or adding another medication. Strattera, for example, is often helpful to those with anxiety.

Is It Really a Side Effect or Just the Experience of Tuning In?
Sometimes a side effect is not really a change at all but the result

of getting feedback from your body that you never paid attention to in the past. When your brain is more awake it is more tuned in to the signals from your body, as well as the data coming in from the outside world. That muscle tension or clenched stomach may have been there all along, but you failed to notice the stress signals your body was sending you. Try some stress-busting techniques like exercise and/or meditation.

Nonstimulant Medications

Generally, these medications are considered to be second-line treatments for ADD. In other words, they are used when the stimulants don't work, don't work well enough or produce intolerable side effects. They are also used for some people with additional psychiatric problems or medical conditions.

Strattera (atomoxetine): This is currently the one exception. It is basically an antidepressant that increases the availability of the neurotransmitter norepinephrine. It has been approved by the FDA for treating ADD in children and adults. One advantage of Strattera is that it is not a controlled substance. Therefore, it is possible to get refills and a prescription over the phone. This is a definite advantage for ADDers who have trouble keeping track of the monthly prescription routine. Strattera does take longer to take effect than the stimulants do—several weeks versus an hour. A major disadvantage of Strattera is that it may not be as effective as the stimulants. Limited studies suggest that Strattera and the stimulants are similar in effect, but a number of professionals who specialize in treating ADD are not convinced that this is the case. In our experience (admittedly limited, as Strattera has been on the market for less than three years as of this writing), Strattera alone has not been as helpful to our clients as Strattera plus a stimulant. We have a concern that inexperienced physicians may lean too much in the direction of Strattera with their ADD patients. It is tempting, as the hassles and concerns of prescribing a controlled substance are not an issue. Another concern is that Strattera can interfere with sexual functioning.

PROS
Not a controlled substance
Prescriptions can be refilled over the phone
Another option for people who have not had a good response to stimulants
Works continuously, contrasted to 3–12 hours for the stimulants
Preliminary evidence shows it may be helpful for ADDults who experience anxiety

CONS
May not be as effective as stimulant medication
Takes longer to take effect—weeks versus an hour or less for stimulants
Can cause sexual dysfunction

Second-Line Medications

These preparations are not as effective as the stimulants, but they are useful when stimulant medication cannot be used for some reason. If your physician prescribes a second-line drug first, ask (respectfully) to be told the rationale for doing so. There may be sound medical reasons for the decision, and you need to be informed. In some cases, however, the physician is inexperienced or generally reluctant to prescribe stimulants.

Bupropion (Wellbutrin): Bupropion is an atypical antidepressant that increases both dopamine and norepinephrine levels. It is helpful in relieving the symptoms of ADD but is not as powerful as the stimulants. A major advantage of this medication is that is does not cause sexual dysfunction, which is a side effect of the other antidepressants currently available. If you have a history of seizures, this drug is not a good choice, as it lowers the seizure threshold.

Tricyclic Antidepressants: Desipramine and nortriptyline both significantly increase the availability of the neurotransmitter norepinephrine. They can reduce the core symptoms of ADD but not as effectively as the stimulants. One advantage of the tricyclics is that they provide twenty-four-hour coverage. They take several weeks to take effect, however, and include some potentially serious side effects, such as cardiac problems.

Monoamine Oxidase Inhibitors: This category of antidepressants increases the availability of the neurotransmitters norepinephrine and dopamine. They are rarely used to treat ADD since a special diet is needed to avoid serious side effects (hypertensive crisis). Not a great option for those who tend to be impulsive.

Venlafaxine (Effexor): This antidepressant increases the availability of norepinephrine and serotonin. Currently, a few non-controlled studies have indicated that it may be helpful for treating ADD adults. Please note that it is important to taper off this medication gradually—stopping abruptly can cause very uncomfortable side effects. In any case, it is important to work with your physician when making any medication changes.

Modafinil (Provigil): Currently approved by the FDA for treating narcolepsy. Its main effect seems to be indirect activation of the frontal cortex. There is some evidence that it may be helpful for ADD adults, particularly for improving sleep cycles.

SSRIs: This is not a specific medication but a category of medications—the selective serotonin reuptake inhibitors. The net effect of these drugs is to increase the amount of serotonin available in the brain. They do not help wake up the brain like stimulant medication, but they do decrease impulsivity and alleviate depression. They are often used in combination with stimulants to manage the symptoms of ADD. Medications in this category include, but are not limited to, Prozac, Paxil, Celexa and Lexapro.

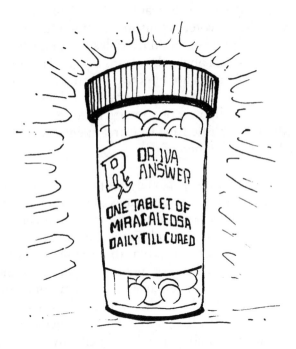

Caution: Labels can be misleading—medicine is not for everyone, and is never the whole answer.

Mood Stabilizers: These medicines are first-line treatments for bipolar disorder. Some ADDults have a combination of ADD and bipolar disorder. As mentioned before, taking stimulant medication alone can be risky if you have or someone in your family has a history of bipolar disorder. In this case, your physician will prescribe a mood stabilizer before adding a stimulant. Medications in this category include, but are not limited to, lithium, Depakote, Lamictal and Tegretol.

Alternatives for Waking Up the Brain

For those of you who can't or prefer not to take medication for your ADD, we are including some alternatives. This is by no means an inclusive list. Do a Google search for "ADD and natural remedies" if you really want to be confused. There are scads of Web sites devoted to nutritional and other nonmedical solutions for the problem of ADD. Folks in the medical establishment are skeptical about the claims that herbal remedies or nutritional supplements are effective for treating ADD. They want to know about the scientific studies done to back up those claims. We choose not to participate in that particular debate. Many established medical treatments have not been studied all that well either.

On the other hand, our personal and professional experience has been disappointing when it comes to nutritional/herbal interventions for ADD. Both of us went through a period of experimenting with herbals and supplements. Some of them seemed to help, but not as much as the stimulant medications. Our clients who started out on natural preparations and later switched to stimulants experienced a profound difference between them. The natural remedies were much weaker in effect. Peggy's experience was that some of the supplements worked well for a time, and then stopped being effective. She has not had that experience with stimulant medication.

That said, we are aware that this is just our experience, and certainly not the whole story. In the interests of conserving space, we will discuss a few alternatives, and refer you to *Delivered from Distraction*, by Edward Hallowell and John Ratey, for a balanced discussion of nutrition and ADD. In particular, they have included an entire chapter on the omega-3 fatty acids, a promising form of dietary supplementation for people with ADD.

Neurofeedback
This interesting and controversial treatment for ADD is based on the idea that we can retrain our brains. Meditators have long known that this is possible, but did you know that scientists are beginning to look for evidence by studying the brain images of Buddhist monks? One such preliminary study used EEGs and MRIs to observe the brain effects when six monks meditated on compassion. These monks had greater activity in the left frontal cortex of the brain than research subjects who were not practiced in meditation.

What, however, is available for the ADDult who has not been meditating for umpteen years? Neurofeedback is a technique that uses EEG readings to help clients shape their brain wave patterns in a positive direction so they can pay attention, rather than daydreaming, for example.

How Does Neurofeedback Work?
There are five major types of brain wave patterns. Multiple patterns are present in the brain at any given time, but each area of the brain has a predominant pattern that reflects the person's current mental state. These patterns can be measured and recorded by an electroencephalogram (EEG). The EEG can be used to make a map of the person's mental function.

The five types of brain wave patterns are:

Beta waves: These are the fastest waves. When a person is attentive, the brain has a lot of beta waves.

SMR waves: A subcategory of beta waves, they occur when a person is quietly focused to prepare for a physical challenge.

379

Alpha waves: These waves are slower. They are the brain waves of relaxation.

Theta waves: Even slower than the alpha waves, this is the brain wave pattern a person has when daydreaming or almost at the point of falling asleep.

Delta waves: The slowest brain waves, they are the brain waves of deep sleep.

When a person without ADD tries to engage in an activity requiring concentration, he or she activates beta waves in certain parts of the brain. When confronting a task that requires focus, children and adults with ADD increase theta waves instead (the daydreaming brain wave).

By showing the client what their brain waves are doing at a given time and rewarding them for shifting to helpful brain wave patterns, the neurofeedback therapist helps the client to gain control over her wandering brain. Essentially, it is behavior modification for the unruly mind.

Now, we mentioned that this therapy is controversial. For a long time, the scientific folks pointed out that there were no good controlled studies supporting the effectiveness of neurofeedback. Of course, what they fail to mention is that these types of studies are expensive and it is harder to get funding for them. In the past few years, some research has been done that suggests it may be time to give neurofeedback a second look.

We have heard mixed reviews from colleagues and clients. Some have found the treatment very beneficial, while others have been disappointed. There are no guarantees, but we have collected enough testimonials to warrant including neurofeedback in our listing of alternative treatment strategies.

PROS
A noninvasive alternative to medication If taking medicine feels too much like an alien force taking control of your brain, you may be more open to a therapy that helps you to retrain your own thought processes. No physical side effects

CONS
Expensive Can be time consuming—2 to 3 visits per week for 6 to 12 months required. (Time factor may be reduced with newer, in-home systems becoming available.) Currently not as much scientific evidence that it is effective compared to stimulant medication.

Madelyn Griffith-Haynie, the founder of the Optimal Functioning Institute for ADD Coach Training, has found that a combination of stimulant medication and neurofeedback has been the most helpful in managing her ADD. She points out that six months to a year is a long time to wait while you are failing at school, work or in relationships.

Workouts

Cerebellar Stimulation: In *Delivered from Distraction*, Dr. Hallowell tells a story about his son Jack, who hated reading until he started a program of exercises designed to stimulate his cerebellum. Until fairly recently, it was thought that this part of the brain was mainly involved in balance and physical coordination. Now it is known that the cerebellum is also involved in general brain functioning. For example, brain-scan studies have shown that there are connections between the cerebellum and the frontal lobes, as well as other areas of the brain that are involved in ADD and dyslexia.

Occupational therapists have long known about the connection between ADD and cerebellar functioning. They treat the symptoms of both ADD and learning disabilities using a variety of exercises that involve balance and coordination. More controlled research needs to be done, but the results of the existing studies are promising. For more information about this topic, we refer you to the chapter on cerebellar stimulation in *Delivered from Distraction*. In brief, a few of the specific programs mentioned are the Dore method, Brain Gym and Interactive Metronome.

Some examples of cerebellar exercises are balancing on a wobble board, juggling and standing on one leg. Basically the exercises involve balancing, coordinating alternating movements and activities that cross the midline of the brain and back again. One of Kate's clients is an extremely bright young woman who is a doctoral candidate at one of the world's most prestigious universities. Intelligence is not a problem in her case, but staying focused long enough to write her dissertation is a big challenge. She has found that alternating ten minutes of writing with ten minutes of juggling helps her to stay the course. She says that her juggling really stinks, but that isn't the point. Perhaps you might want to consider playing around with juggling, or walking a straight line to improve your balance. Experiment to see if these activities improve your ability to focus and concentrate.

Exercise: Of course, we all know about the recommendations to do aerobic exercise three times a week for your heart. But have you ever considered looking at exercise as a brain-boosting strategy? It promotes mental focus and sustained attention, as well as providing a buffer against stress. Consider conducting an exercise trial to determine a routine that provides the most benefit to you. Do you need daily exercise? How about several shorter periods of exercise throughout the day, whenever your focus is flagging?

Fidget to Focus: Do you wonder why you do the following things?

- Pace and doodle when you are on the phone

- Concentrate better when you are chewing gum

- Study with the radio and television on

- Retain the information from a lecture better when you are playing a video game or jiggling your foot

One of the biggest problems with staying alert and focused is that so many of the activities we are required to do are painfully boring—sitting in class, for example, or in those endless meetings at work. The problem is that snoozing is not an option. Loud snoring might earn you a pink slip or reverse brownie points toward a failing grade. Our brains need an optimal level of stimulation, and you can "feed" your brain using multiple sensory pathways. Check out the book *Fidget to Focus*, by Roland Rotz and Sarah Wright, for tips on sensory strategies you can use to boost your brain's attentional power. You can even buy some nifty fidget toys in the store at ADDconsults.com.

Blues Busters: Consider replacing all your lightbulbs with full-spectrum ones. Full-spectrum light is used as a treatment for seasonal affective disorder, otherwise known as the winter blues. While it is not a specific remedy for ADD, many of us also suffer from seasonal depression and can benefit from the additional boost provided by full-spectrum light. You can get these at your local chain hardware store. While they are more expensive than ordinary bulbs, they last much longer.

Get Your Thyroid Checked: A thyroid condition may mimic the symptoms of ADD. You may not have ADD at all, or your ADD symptoms may be increased by a hidden thyroid problem.

Food Allergies: Food allergies can cause ADD-like symptoms. Peggy had a client whose son had an allergy to corn. His physician was reluctant to consider that a food might be at the root of this child's "ADD." In desperation, the mom took her son to an appointment with a bag of microwave popcorn in hand, marched into the office and insisted on popping the bag of corn and then feeding it to her son in the doctor's presence. Right before the doctor's eyes, this woman's well-behaved son morphed into a "bouncing off the walls" terror. Needless to say, the doctor became a true believer in the power of food allergies to wreak behavioral havoc.

In this chapter we have reviewed the major medications used to treat ADD, as well as a few alternatives for waking up the brain. Of course, medication is never the whole answer to the puzzle of ADD. When it works well, it serves to help us to be available for learning. A huge piece of our learning, of course, is actually *unlearning* all the inaccurate thoughts and beliefs we accumulated when we didn't know that ADD was the problem. In the next chapter, Mental Hygiene, we will explore ways to get rid of that mental debris from the past.

CHAPTER 15

Mental Hygiene

"She was recycling the raw sewage of poor mental hygiene."

—Neil Anderson, LMT, subgenius, barroom philosopher

Our friend Neil uttered these words after spending an evening with a female friend, attempting to console her after a breakup with her boyfriend. We know you can imagine the scene . . . we have all been there at least once. The poor girl (we'll call her Karen) is an hour into her rant/crying jag. Karen has now moved beyond the specifics of the breakup and the horrible things her boyfriend did to her. She has segued into a painful litany of the reasons why, of course, no one in their right mind would want to be seen with or (God forbid!) date a worm like her. She is fat (or scrawny), ugly, stupid, needy, selfish, boring . . . you pick the adjectives. Any attempts to steer her into cleaner waters, so to speak, are met with resistance and a renewed outpouring of self-directed venom. Eventually, Karen cries herself into an exhausted sleep.

Karen has taken a big hit to her sense of self. Generally it takes more than a few repetitions of this cycle of self-loathing before the "hittee" is ready to pick herself up and move on. The length of time needed varies with the importance of the relationship, the current self-esteem level, what is going on in the rest of the person's life and other such factors. There are ways of moving through the process more quickly, and we will share these with you a bit later in the chapter.

It is easy to see the dynamics of lousy mental hygiene when you are sitting outside, watching a friend flail around in their personal mental sewer. You know that the person they are describing is nothing like the person you know and love. When we are the ones in that dark place, however, the nasty mental landscape seems as real and vivid as anything we have ever experienced.

It is as if our brain is buried under layers of dirt. And the dirt consists of all the mean, derogatory things we have ever said about ourselves or had others say about us.

KK: "Let me give you an example from my own life that has nothing to do with ADD. A few months after my former husband and I separated, I gained forty pounds in about six weeks. It seemed like a miracle in reverse . . . or a reversal of the Sleeping Beauty tale. My experience was that I (mostly) went to sleep for a few weeks and woke up in this bloated, alien body. Nobody kissed the princess and so she turned into a big fat ugly frog. In real life I took to my bed in the throes of depression.

"Our appearance has a lot to do with how we feel about ourselves. I believe that the weight was a physical manifestation of how I felt inside. The breakup of my marriage cracked my defensive shell and exposed a host of unhealed emotional wounds, bringing them to the surface.

"That weight stuck around for years—in fact, I am still carrying it. I know that it will come off soon, because I now like myself enough to feel that I deserve to be fit. One of the gifts of having this experience is that I got to see, in real time, that a certain kind of appearance has nothing to do with my lovability. I have a wonderful life partner now who tells me I am beautiful and sexy just the way I am! He is also not the only one who expresses admiration and interest. I now get more validation than I did when I was young and slender.

"For years postseparation, I couldn't get a date or anything approximating one. Like Karen, the girl who broke up with her boyfriend, I recycled that raw sewage over and over. I told my-self I was fat, ugly, unwanted. Four years ago I met a man in a drumming class and was attracted to him. After class one day we had a great conversation, but I was disappointed when he told me he had a girlfriend. I thought, 'Oh well, guess this one isn't a possibility.' It would have been fine if I had left it at that, but of course I didn't. I instantly went into he-wouldn't-want-me-anyway-I-am-so-old-fat-and-ugly (add stupid, untalented, dull . . . I probably used them all). 'Fat' was the dirtiest word, the one that hurt the most.

"Two years later I ran into the same man, only this time he was with his girlfriend. To my utter astonishment, I found that she was bigger than me! Of course, I rationalized; she was taller, more statuesque. She carried the weight better than I did. Still, I could not deny that the stories I told myself had been called into question. Maybe my appearance was not the problem I thought it was.

"I came to see that it's not the weight but the way you carry it that counts. I began to notice that I didn't feel heavy at all on those days when I felt good about myself. Like my beloved aunt Mary, who carried a lot of pounds but was light on her feet, I could dance through life. On days when I was riddled with self-doubt, it was as if someone had drastically turned up the 'G fac-tor' in gravity.

"Recently, I was chatting with a group of friends and found my-self patting my five months' gestation stomach (not pregnant— I am past that stage of life) and making a crack about getting in touch with my inner whale. In that moment, I realized I was home free. I could talk about my weight openly. I no longer felt ashamed.

"You may be wondering why I included this fairly long disserta-tion on weight problems in a book on ADD. This is not merely a useless tangent. Problems with poundage are a pretty good metaphor for all the heavy, useless, negative thoughts we allow to reside in our brains, rent free. If we can visualize those poisonous clumps of 'stinkin' thinkin'' as physical mass dragging us down, we might be more likely to pay attention to their presence. It doesn't help to chant positive affirmations all day long, trying to slap up a paint job over mildewed walls. We need to do the cleaning and prep work before laying on a shiny new surface."

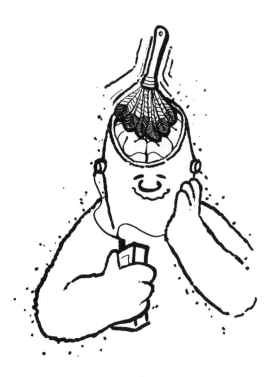

In this chapter, we will share some mental hygiene techniques designed to help you begin the process of cleansing your brain of the negative thoughts you accumulated before you knew about ADD. This book, of course, is a self-help book. But we don't recommend that your process of recovery be a do-it-yourself operation. A coach, a counselor or both can be the charge-neutral people on your team who reach in to offer a way out when you are swimming around in the nasty waters of a mental cesspool. You are worth whatever it takes to feel better about yourself.

In Times of Crisis . . . All Bets Are Off

Before giving you some helpful tools—the things that serve as soft cloths, scrub brushes and mild-but-effective "brain soap" in our mental hygiene toolkit—we suggest checking in with yourself a bit. Look at what is going on in your life right now. Has something got your situation spinning out of control so fast that you will need help in taming it first? In that case, "all bets are off." You need to have a nonslippery surface to stand on before you can tackle the mental hygiene tasks on your own. What sorts of things do we mean?

You have lost your job, your spouse, your home or custody of your kids. You have a DUI, other legal trouble or have been expelled from school. Maybe you have been hit by more than one disaster at once. Sometimes the trouble may seem milder, such as missing a deadline or bouncing a series of checks. You feel that you are at the end of your rope. The specifics don't matter. If it is a crisis for you, it is a genuine crisis. You are overwhelmed by emotions. Perhaps there is a barrage of nasty self-talk coming from a judgmental voice in your head, drowning out everything else much of the time. You can't function. We are not talking about the standard ADD baseline level of dysfunction that you have learned to live with, after a fashion.

This is not the time to go it alone. If you have a therapist, call for assistance in dealing with the crisis. A trip to the hospital may be in order if you are severely depressed or have other serious psychiatric symptoms. Many communities have psychiatric emergency rooms or crisis intervention teams that may even come to your home. In most cases, people in crisis do not need hospitalization. Emergency or crisis intervention personnel will make a plan to help you recover from the immediate crisis.

Staying with a supportive friend or family member can be very helpful. They can act as temporary caretakers. There is nothing wrong with letting someone else take charge for a while, until your ability to address problems resurfaces.

Something that we have probably all experienced at one time or another is a state of "emotional boggle," a difficult situation where we are overwhelmed by our emotions, unable to think clearly or act decisively. We can tend to forget that the emotional overwhelm leads to mental overwhelm. Quite simply, strong emotions can really mess with cognitive functioning; the problem-solving functions can even shut down entirely in such a situation, leaving us temporarily "boggled." If you could borrow another brain just long enough for you to move around or through the difficulty, things might look more doable. When you find yourself boggled, we recommend seeking out such a brain to borrow. This brain could belong to your coach, or even a trusted friend in a pinch (but take care you don't get into the habit of using friends for counseling—the friendship could really suffer!).

So, what do we do when an attack of self-loathing hits? How do we talk to ourselves differently so we don't accumulate more mental sewage? We will get to the answers to those questions, but first we need a brief vocabulary lesson.

Definitions

The following are terms that we will be using in this chapter.

The Witness—This is the part of us that watches and observes our thoughts, experiences and activities. It merely notes and records experiential data; it does not categorize, comment or judge. It is an aspect of our higher selves (we all have one).

The Judge—We know you are all too familiar with this character. The Judge is the aspect of yourself that makes judgments about the desirability of your thoughts, feelings, beliefs and actions. Most ADDers get a heavy dose of negative evaluations from their Judge.

Reframing—Or viewing within a different frame. Just as a painting can look very different if we change its frame, our experiences can look different if reframed.

Emotional release—A conscious, intentional release of emotions.

Let's take a moment to talk about The Witness and The Judge in a bit more detail, since working with them will be a major key to your mental hygiene program. If you skipped the meditation chapter you might want to go back and read it at this point. A main purpose of meditation is to practice being The Witness—the observer that doesn't make negative or positive comments about your thoughts, feelings, beliefs or actions. When we meditate, we take a step back from all the mental chatter and let it go on without our involvement or interference.

The goal is to operate as much as possible as The Witness, to separate ourselves from The Judge. Aside from meditation, how do we practice being The Witness? Well, one trick is to visualize yourself as an alien, a visitor from outer space. This one may come naturally to many ADDults—after all, we have felt like aliens for most of our lives. As an alien you are observing the behaviors of the people you meet—the customs on this new planet are so strange, you have no way of judging them. You could also imagine that you are a scientist and your job is to collect data without forming an opinion about what you are observing. Another scenario is to picture yourself as a witness in court where you are supposed to report the facts, without adding any guesswork or your interpretation of what happened. An extreme version of witnessing is found in Robert Heinlein's novel *Stranger in a Strange Land.* In this science fiction tale there is a new group of professionals called Fair Witnesses. When Fair Witnesses are asked to describe the color of a barn, for example, they say, "It is red—on this side."

Of course, what you are witnessing in this case is not alien planet customs, experimental data or the scene of a crime. You are witnessing your own internal landscape, your self-talk. The first step is awareness.

For the purposes of good mental hygiene, the goal is to be The Witness and separate from The Judge. The Judge is a part of ourselves that is not our friend. It hurls nasty criticisms that get in the way of our progress. When we suggest that you separate yourself from The Judge, we are not recommending that you throw out the concept of "good judgment." Good judgment is making a choice that serves you and is in alignment with your personal value system. We will talk about personal value systems a bit later, but we want to emphasize here that it is important to examine your beliefs and take out the components that are an unwanted legacy from your mom or your uncle Charlie.

It helps to visualize The Judge as a separate entity. Yours could be a person, an animal that talks, an animated figure or a monster of some kind. For example, Peggy imagines her critical Judge as a sardonic guy who sits in a lawn chair smoking cigarettes and commenting on her behavior.

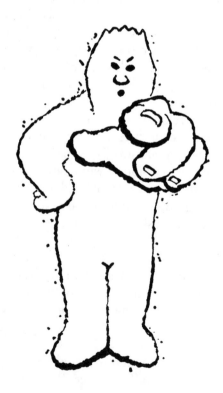

The Judge is never right. He/she/it offers a nasty dose of negative criticism designed to keep you in your place—whatever that is. Don't let anyone try to convince you that there is a certain kind of "constructive" criticism that is helpful. We never learned anything from criticism except to avoid it at all costs. Rather than a steady dose of criticism, we need an enthusiastic cheerleader in our corner who praises every baby step on the way to change. The better we feel, the more likely we are to make changes that serve us and those around us.

So Just What DO You Mean by "Mental Hygiene"? Mental hygiene consists of examining your thoughts and beliefs and eliminating those that don't serve you. The self-talk we keep going on about is where the most damaging of these thoughts and beliefs reside. Also, finding and using safe ways of releasing emotion is another important part of mental hygiene.

Initially, most of your efforts will go toward clearing the backlog of mental debris that was built up before you knew about ADD. But after much of that has been "washed away," the attention shifts to maintaining what you have gained.

So, we are not talking about a once-and-for-all binge of spring brain cleaning, but a program of regular maintenance.

In the next section, we will explore more about what the mental hygiene techniques are designed to address.

Recognizable Bits of Mental Debris

What are the common bits of mental debris that float around in the brains of ADDers? Everyone is unique and will have their own particular way of languaging their self-talk, but there are common themes and threads that most of our clients express. Some of these were mentioned in earlier sections of this book; we bring them up again in order to work with them in more depth. The following is a list of phrases we have heard over and over again.

I want to do (fill in the blank), but . . .

I never follow through with anything

I am afraid to have anyone come over to my house . . . it is such a mess

I am weird

I will never get it right

I'm ditsy

I am hopeless with money

I have no discipline

I did it again

I can't screw up one more time

I am so thoughtless and insensitive

I never get anything done on time

I will never grow up

I am irresponsible

I am a lousy husband (or wife)

I can't control myself

I am too slow

I am too fast

I have to do it all by myself

If either of us got up in the morning to face a list like that one, we would go promptly back to bed. In fact, we have done just that on more than one occasion. We are not the all-powerful and perfect experts, making pronouncements from on high. We have been working on our own mental hygiene for a long time.

Now, let's go back to that list of negative self-talk for a closer look. Generally, we don't say just one mean thing to ourselves, but a whole string of them. In fact, we can construct such a string from that list of phrases. Let's start with

"I Am Irresponsible"

Has anyone ever told you this? Ever uttered these words in the privacy of your own mind? How many times a day? An hour? Per minute? If someone offered you a dollar for each time you invoked this statement, would you be fabulously wealthy?

If this little phrase is an all-too-familiar litany in your everyday life, read on.

Okay, the number one step involved in good mental hygiene is to examine your language, your self-talk. At first, the goal is awareness—to simply notice what you are saying to yourself. Pretend that your job is to be an impartial witness. A witness notes and reports only the facts, without interpreting or judging. So the only thing you need to do is notice that you told yourself "I am irresponsible." If you find yourself going off on a tangent such as "I can't believe I said that . . . I am so negative . . . I am my own worst enemy," remind yourself to "be The Witness." Essentially, this is a practice that will reduce your judgment about the things you say to yourself. It is one layer of brain crud.

Next, set aside some time to dissect "I am irresponsible." Have a notebook handy to assist you in the process. What do these words mean to you? Where did the idea that you were irresponsible come from?

395

Being ADDers, we will take the backwards approach and address the second question first. Reach into your memory banks and pull out your earliest memory of hearing the words "you are irresponsible." Even if you can't retrieve a specific memory, chances are good that either a teacher or family member labeled you in that way.

Go back into those memory banks again to answer the question: What were you doing or not doing when they called you "irresponsible"? Since we are not currently standing at your shoulder, we don't know the answer to that question, but we can offer a few possibilities based on experience.

- You did not do your chores

- You did not have your assignment in on time

- You were playing when you were supposed to be working

Looking at these possibilities through the lens of our awareness of ADD (reframing them), we can provide an explanation for those behaviors that had nothing to do with a "moral" choice to be responsible or irresponsible. You did not do your chores because you forgot or got distracted by something else. You did not have your assignment completed because you were overwhelmed by the task and ashamed to ask for help. You were playing when you were supposed to be cleaning your room because you were overwhelmed by the job and didn't know where to start. Now you know how ADD works, but back then you didn't have a clue and neither did the people who were judging your behavior.

Let's get back to the first question: What do these words mean to you? Of course, we learned that the word "irresponsible" meant "bad" long before we knew anything else about what it meant. Let's see what the dictionary (in Appleworks) says about the word.

Irresponsible: (1) Not having or showing any care for the consequences of personal actions. (2) Not capable of assuming responsibility. (3) Not answerable to a higher authority.

A statement that you don't care about the consequences of your actions can be seen in more than one way. It could mean all of the following:

- You don't care about the consequences of your actions, because you don't care about anybody else.

- You don't care about the consequences of your actions, because you are too overwhelmed to even consider thinking about one more thing.

- You don't care about the consequences of your actions, because you are convinced that your course of action is correct.

Let's take an eraser to this series of statements so we can begin to take the punch out of them. Just erase the first one—unless you are a sociopath, it is not true that you don't care about others. We can keep the second one—it is a simple statement of "what's so." At least some of the time, we aren't thinking about others because we can't think—period. The last statement requires a bit more analysis.

In this case, you have decided that your actions are correct based on your value system—never mind the personal values of someone who is standing on the outside judging your behavior. For example, you may have been taught that it is irresponsible to leave a mess in the kitchen when you go to bed. Just before bedtime, your child comes to you wanting to talk about the friend who was mean to him on the playground. You decide that it is more important to nurture your child than it is to clean up the kitchen. Your mom might have lived by the rule "cleanliness is next to godliness," but you live by "kindness is more important than order."

In our second book, *The ADDed Dimension*, there are many more examples of how the "symptoms" of ADD can work for us or against us. This is an excellent resource for reframing the experience of ADD.

More on Thoughts, Feelings and Beliefs

Thoughts are just one component of mental hygiene. We also need to grapple with feelings and beliefs. Feelings emerge as a result of the stories we tell ourselves. They are triggered by the interpretations we make about events that happen to us. For example, let's go back to the story at the beginning of this chapter. Karen is upset because her boyfriend broke up with her. She took the fact of his desire to end the relationship and added her own interpretation. She could have just said to herself, "This relationship is not a good fit for either of us; he just recognized it before I did." Instead, she told herself, "I am not good enough for him." She then expanded her story to include all past and possible future rejections until she was telling herself she was just no good. Her intense feelings of grief and despair are based upon a faulty interpretation of events. At some point she needs to go back and correct the faulty logic.

Feelings, however, do not operate on the basis of logic. When you have just taken a big hit to your self-esteem, it does not help to have someone point out your errors in thinking. Or for you to point them out to yourself. Your need at this point is to experience your feelings, to get them up and out, so to speak. And you hope that you don't do any damage during the emotional storm. As ADDers, our feelings can be a big, scary monster. For one thing, we often feel things very intensely. For another, our ability to inhibit ourselves is erratic. Many of us have problems with rage. In *Emotional Intelligence*, Daniel Goleman coined the phrase "amygdala hijacking." This refers to the ability of the primitive parts of the brain to overwhelm the cortex, or thinking brain. When powerful emotions take over, there is no thinking going on. Trying to hold it all in or stuff the feelings back down does not work.

One of our most powerful life lessons came in the person of an ADDer (Ursula) who was off the charts when it came to "disinhibition." Everything that goes on in Ursula's head comes directly out of her mouth. She, however, has an interesting combination of high intelligence and high self-awareness, along with the lack of censorship. When Ursula takes a hit to her self-esteem, which she does often because she is so sensitive, she blasts her feelings out in a childish temper tantrum. However, she also has the capacity to observe herself and comment on the action in the moment. In the middle of cussing up a blue streak, Ursula makes a side comment like "this isn't personal—it has nothing to do with you. It's just my lower selves speaking. I can't work up to my higher selves unless I deal with the lower ones."

Hmmm. Makes you wonder about the "ADD as disorder" theory. We firmly believe that everything we humans experience is useful, and that even disorders have something to teach us, on a higher level. Ursula just can't be appropriate because of her neurological makeup. As a result, people who come in contact with her get to see her emotional process in its raw form. Her process is no different from that of people with a prettier social mask. Those of us who can manage to appear together have primitive feelings too. Her task is to manage those feelings so she doesn't attack others. She does this by narrating her rants. Those of us who are able to paste an adult mask over feelings we consider inappropriate have a different task. We need to find some way to acknowledge, express and process our feelings—without judging them.

Emotional Release

Most ADDults have some difficulty with emotional expression. Some of us have learned to stuff our feelings down, because we think they are unacceptable. Unexpressed emotion, however, always finds a way to let us know it is there. Sometimes it comes out as physical symptoms, like a headache or an upset stomach. In other cases, it manifests as a mental health problem, such as depression.

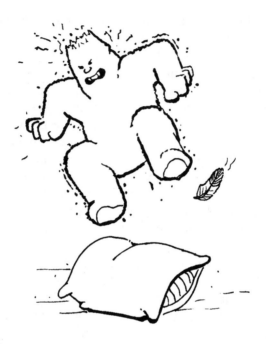

Other folks with ADD (like Ursula) don't seem to have a problem with emotional expression at all. They are unable to inhibit themselves, and so the anger blasts out or the tears come without regard for the situation. The problem in this case is not a lack of emotional expression but the inability to manage feelings in a way that doesn't create more problems than it solves. It is not a good idea, for example, to make a regular habit of blasting your boss.

The remedy for both stuffers and blasters is essentially the same. You need to set aside time and space for regular emotional expression. We do not recommend that you take a do-it-yourself approach to managing powerful feelings. Find a therapist or counselor to help you. Your therapist, however, will not be with you 24/7, coaching you through the inevitable life situations you will encounter. Our mental hygiene tips are practical solutions to help you deal with troublesome thoughts and feelings in everyday life.

Let's take a page out of Ursula's book to begin constructing the "feelings" aspect of our mental hygiene toolkit. Ursula has learned that it is important to let herself have her feelings, no matter how childish or inappropriate. She had no choice, but the value in her situation is that she has learned that expressing them helps her make a faster recovery. When you take a hit to your "sense of self," you can do the following:

1. Find a way to be alone. If you are at work, take a break and go sit in your car. If that is not possible, scope out a private place nearby—it could be the broom closet.

2. Allow yourself to cry, rant, rave, cuss people out.

3. Do not make yourself the target of your rant—find another focus and someone else to blame. It doesn't matter that your adult self knows this other person is not really the villain. The purpose here is to flush out those emotions.

Here are some tips for how to get the most out of your emotional release:

• You may need to give yourself permission to express your feelings. Remind yourself that it's okay to be angry. It's okay to be afraid.

• Do not censor yourself. We all have a part of ourselves—The Judge—that delights in criticizing. You can talk back to that Judge or even make it one of the targets for your rant.

• You may be aware, in the moment, that what you are feeling or ranting about is ridiculous, from a mature perspective. Remember that your job right now is not to be mature, it is to allow that unhealed part of yourself to have its say.

- You can be as mean, nasty or unfair as you want to be—the sky is the limit. Nobody is listening except The Judge, the part of you that is self-critical.

- If you really allow yourself to have a tantrum, you will naturally wind down in a fairly short amount of time. If you are concerned that you will go on and on and never stop, set a timer.

- Take a brief period of meditation before you reenter the world of other people.

- Try this at home first. You will feel more secure once you have done it a time or two and have found that it works.

But what if you can't find a way to be alone? You can rant on paper or in your own mind. Some people write raving e-mails and then never send them. Also, is it really true that you can't find a way to be alone? It may be that you don't know how to excuse yourself, or feel embarrassed that you require ranting space. One of Kate's clients has struggled with an anger management problem and has used her need for time-outs as a teachable moment for her family. She explains why she needs to go to her room now, and assures her husband and children that she will be in a better mood when she comes out. They get to see that her program actually works, and also get a lesson in how to deal with their own emotions.

Productivity, or "What Am I Here for Anyway?"

Did you know that in the United States people work longer hours than people in most other developed countries in the world? Something to be proud of . . . or is it? Sometimes it seems that we worship the god of productivity above all other gods. The workplace is leaner and meaner, with a "take no prisoners" attitude. Downsizing results in fewer people working much harder to get the job done. If you can't keep up, they downsize your sense of self by firing you. Nice.

The reality is that people without disabilities are having a tough time staying afloat. As ADDers, we are more vulnerable to the stress of overload than others. We are saying this not to scare you but to acknowledge the reality of the environment we live in. In short, at this point in time, there are aspects of our culture that are totally insane.

Think about it. What is gained by pushing people to the breaking point? Stress-related illnesses are on the rise, as are repetitive stress injuries. Of course, we know that cognitive performance also suffers. The question of why there seems to be so much ADD around these days may be partially answered by looking at the stresses and strains people are subjected to in our postmillennium world. We submit that anyone can show symptoms of ADD if they are pushed hard enough.

So, the culture holds up the gold standard of productivity and more productivity . . . productivity at all costs. The short-term results are similar to what we get as ADDers when we habitually use adrenaline to kick ourselves into high performance mode (you can revisit the end of the chapter on meditation for more on the downside of that). We get a period of higher functioning followed by a longer recovery time. In an environment that values productivity over human needs, the workers initially strive to produce harder and faster, generally coming from fear that they will lose their jobs. After a while, the strain begins to erode performance—the pace slows down and/or more mistakes are made. Eventually the situation deteriorates as employee turnover skyrockets and people go out on disability. Lack of concern over this kind of scenario comes from the notion that workers are replaceable. This notion is downright silly, even if you are considering only the bottom line. High turnover is costly.

The insane working conditions in our culture today are the result of placing a value on productivity that is way out of balance. In this distorted view, people are just cogs in a machine that is geared up to produce at all cost.

When we have talked to our clients about the craziness of our cultural values around work, they frequently respond with, "Yes, but . . . I am not going to be able to change things single-handedly. If the workplace does change so that it is fit for human beings, it certainly won't happen overnight. This is the reality I have to deal with."

And they are correct. We have to deal with "what is," even as we work and dream to create a better future. The better future might be starting your own business or becoming a freelancer, but it takes time to make that transition. In the meantime, you need to deal with what is in front of you. And what is in front of you may be a ridiculous "to do" list.

The most important focus in this situation is to refuse to own the value that says you are only as good as what you produce. In an environment of more-better-faster it is a game you can't win. As soon as you have completed one task, there are a thousand right behind it on that endless "to do" list. Chances are nobody is patting you on the back for the job that was well done. You need to do it for yourself. Or, better still, add the voice of a supportive coach to the mix.

Good mental hygiene in this case involves refusing to take on "their" values. You may not be living up to "their" standards—that's "what is." But you don't have to make yourself wrong for it. In our experience, the tasks are not as big a problem as the self-talk about how bad we are for not doing them sooner, faster or better.

Toxic Mental Debris: The Vicious Cycle of Shame, Perfectionism and Procrastination

Shame is the granddaddy of all toxic mental filth. In contrast to guilt, which is a painful response to one's less than optimal actions, shame is the emotion we feel when we think that we are just not good enough. We are compelled to hide our faces in shame when in the grip of that powerful feeling, because we think that no one would want to gaze upon the ugly, flawed creatures we believe we are.

Two of the biggest ADD bugaboos, perfectionism and procrastination, interact in a circular fashion to produce and reinforce a state of stuckness.

First, you have a sense that who you *are* (with all your ADD quirks) is not good enough. Next, you begin to set overly high standards for yourself to "make up" for the "fact" that your very being is deficient. Perfectionism then begins to rear its head, because no amount of "doing" will make up for your fatal flaws, or so you believe. You try harder and harder and get nowhere. In the state of procrastination, the following things may be going on: (1) You are fiddling around a task, trying to figure out how to make the results brilliant enough to compensate for the fatal flaw (and everything you have left undone or done poorly in the past), and (2) You are avoiding the task, because the process is miserable and doomed to failure the way you have it set up.

The deadline is missed or the completed job is not what it could be . . . and, once again, you feel that you have failed. You then dump another generous helping of toxic shame onto your beleaguered brain, and the cycle continues. With enough repetitions of this cycle, all forward motion stops.

In the next chapter, we will introduce more tools to use when you find yourself going in circles.

CHAPTER 16

Moving Forward

"Would you tell me, please, which way I ought to go from here?"
"That depends a good deal on where you want to get to."
"I don't much care where as long as I get somewhere."
"Then it doesn't matter which way you go."

—Alice and the Cheshire Cat from *Alice in Wonderland*

This final chapter is about moving forward. The "where to" is entirely up to you. That said, we think we have a general idea of the goals you are shooting for. You want peace in your life, and a sense of purpose. You want to feel that you are in the driver's seat, rather than having your frazzled brain driving you. You want to be master of those paper piles, rather than their slave. You want to stop going in circles and feel that you are actually getting somewhere.

It is possible to reach all these goals. We have walked the road of ADD recovery for a long time, and can see the positive results from all the little and big steps we have taken on the way. We are privileged to witness the transformation in our coaching clients, as they learn to take charge of their lives.

The process, of course, consists of making many small and larger changes over a period of time. Getting those dreams out of your head and translating them into manageable action steps. Working with an ADD coach is the best thing you can do for yourself if you want to lay the groundwork and then begin designing and implementing a life that is user-friendly for *you*.

There is not enough space in a single chapter to fully walk you through the coaching process (and your interaction with your coach is a critical part of the process; it's all customized specifically for you). The focus here is on how to keep moving forward when the inevitable obstacles present themselves.

In the previous chapter, we included a section called "In Times of Crisis . . . All Bets Are Off," which is about what you need to do when you are in crisis—when you have been hit with so many things you can't even put one foot in front of the other. Divorce, a string of DUIs, getting fired . . . when you are in crisis, you need someone who can tell you how to put one foot in front of the other until you have recovered the ability to do that for yourself. On your own, you can't even decide which foot to move first.

In our daily ADDult lives, however, we often find ourselves in a minicrisis mode several times a day. We are not even sure how we got there. We just know that we are overwhelmed and there is not much to be had in the way of problem solving at that moment. You can call it overwhelm, boggle, stuckness or shutdown—the problem is that all the circuits are jammed.

Later, we will talk about the kinds of things that get us boggled in the first place. But for now, it is enough to say that we are overwhelmed. We can't see what the real problem is, we can't decide between competing choices and we can't focus on anything long enough to do something about it. Help!

Your Basic First-Aid Plan for Overwhelm

Let's start with the most basic guide for moving through overwhelm and into action. The next time you find yourself spinning your wheels, try these steps:

1. Don't push through it. Take a step "backward" and institute self-care measures. (This could be a breathing break, a mini exercise break or moving to a calmer location where it's quieter and less hectic.)

2. Check in with yourself. Can you think clearly yet? If not, go back to #1.

3. If you are less frazzled but still not in clear-thinking mode, try doing some very routine, repetitive task that doesn't stress your brain but helps you to feel some forward motion.

4. Check in with yourself. Are you ready to do what you set out to do when you became overwhelmed? If not, go back to #3.

You may find that this first-aid process will be all you need to break through that aggravating place of being stuck, immobile and unable to get started. Let's look at these steps in more detail:

1. Don't Push Through It

The caption "The harder you try, the dumber you look" in the Despair.com poster "Humiliation," accompanies a picture of some would-be hot-dog skier who is taking a ridiculous and spectacular fall out of his aborted flashy maneuver. We can envision a slightly different poster, aimed at the ADDer, that says *"The harder you try, the dumber you get."* This may sound a bit harsh, but it is true. Persistence is not the same as attempting to squeeze the last drop of juice from your beleaguered brain.

In the chapter on differences, we talked about what the brain does when it is on overload—it shuts down. Pushing yourself too hard is a guaranteed way of tilting your brain in that direction. Of course, if you want a little mental health holiday, by all means keep up the pressure. Our experiences with the results of that sort of maneuver, however, left a lot to be desired. Rather than trying with a capital "T," finesse your way to success.

You are sitting at your computer attempting to work on a project that requires concentration. Instead of whipping out the usual flogger and going to town on your poor self, try a few different strategies. Mix and match them for best results.

- Take a mini meditation or prayer break.

- Get up and move around—if you are really sluggish, make it aerobic.

- Take a brief trip to your favorite humor Web site—don't call it slacking or avoidant behavior. You need a few laughs to wake yourself up.

- Use one of those fidget activities we talked about in the medication chapter.

- Stand on your head . . . maybe the extra blood going to your brain will help.

- Try some emotional-release maneuvers—go break some thrift-store dishes or throw ice cubes in the bathtub. Create a little harmless excitement for yourself.

- Take those breaks, relax, have some fun and keep going back to the task. You will get it completed if you persist.

2. Check In with Yourself

Take Your Cognitive Temperature. Don't go running off to the drugstore in search of a specialized thermometer you can insert in your brain . . . we made this one up. Rather, we are suggesting that you devise your own "temperature" scale for your mental functioning. Is your brain "white hot"—ready to rock and roll with the most challenging of creative work? How about "stone cold dead"?—you can barely put one foot in front of the other on your way to bed. "Lukewarm" could mean it's time for routine tasks you have already mastered. Get the picture?

If you have any flexibility in your day or workplace, we suggest that you assess your brain's capacity on an hourly basis and fit your chosen task to your brain's actual functional level. You may need to use an alarm watch or cell phone to remember to do this. If you have little choice about what to do when, at least you may avoid beating yourself up when the work is more of a struggle than you would like. It is not your lack of trying that is the problem, but an ornery brain.

Are You Less Frazzled Yet? If not, go back to #1. You might now be saying, "Why? I already tried that and it didn't seem to work!" Let's return briefly to some of the imagery in the mental hygiene chapter for an example. There may be a lot of stuff to be cleared out, so it may take more than once for a technique to work all the way to completely clear it. Or you may think of a time when you needed to flush a toilet more than once to get to the desired result. Sometimes we just need to repeat an action to get the job done.

3. Try Doing Some Very Routine, Repetitive Task

The simpler the task, the better. If you can get some momentum going on the really easy things, you may be able to shift to something a bit more challenging once you have made some progress. And it sure helps to get the volume down on The Judge's criticisms when you can point to some success in moving forward on the "to do" list.

4. Check In with Yourself

How is your mental state (what's your "cognitive temperature")? Are you calm, agitated, curious, bored? How about your body? Are you tense? You may need to stretch or move around a bit before continuing.

Are you ready to do what you set out to do when you became overwhelmed? If not, go back to #3.

You may find that it takes several repetitions of checking back, doing the simplest tasks, and taking short breaks to get things moving. Before we introduce some more helpful tools for avoiding "stuckness," we are going to urge you to include an ADD coach as a key member of your professional helping team. He or she knows ADD from A to Z and is the expert at guiding ADDults through the pitfalls that generally litter our path from intention to action. Go to ADDcoaching.com for more information about ADD coaching and to begin your search for a coach who is a good fit for you. While we are offering a number of tools from our coaching kit in this chapter, reading a self-help book is not enough when you are trying to put more order and forward movement in your life.

First Aid for Decision Making

(What you can do when you are ready to start getting into action but don't know *what* to start on.)

Everything seems equal in importance, and the ability to prioritize seems to have evaporated. In all likelihood, what is happening is that you are still boggled by all the to-do's floating around in your head—and the notion that you have to do them all *right now*. You are not so overwhelmed that you can't function at all, but you are not in a great place to make decisions. You would be a better employee than a manager in this state of mind.

- Save the knotty problems for your coaching session.

- Make some kind of decision and stick to it. If you become aware that you have veered away from what you intended to do (become distracted), say "oops" and move back into your original task.

- In this state of mind, don't waste time and energy trying to make the "best decision." Write a few possibilities down, put them in a hat and pick one at random.

- If there are only two possibilities to choose from, flip a coin.

- The goal is to get moving, not to move in some perfect and efficient fashion.

- Keep the decision demon at bay by having no more than three things on the desktop. This means that you pluck

411

three items from your "to do" list at any given time and write them down. Don't go to your massive "to do" list for more items until you have dealt with the three on your desktop.

- Your coach can help you get started on more complicated decisions. He or she can provide the perspective needed to help you move away from "majoring in minors" while the must-dos go undone.

More on ADD Coaching

An ADD coach is the person who can help you learn how to:

get out of that state of overwhelm more quickly

decrease the amount of overwhelm in your life

take forward steps toward your goals

identify and remove obstacles to the actions you desire to make

gather tools to help you "work with your quirks"

Notice that we included a lot of self-care items.

> **Build a foundation that supports you—eating,
> sleeping, meditation, exercise and play
> (if you don't, that inner five-year-old will get you)**

Self-care is always the first step in any plan for change. You can't think clearly when you are sleep-deprived or have low blood sugar. You would be surprised (don't laugh) at the number of our clients who attempt to manage their complicated lives while running on empty in terms of the basics. Often, the early months of coaching are spent laying the self-care foundation to support a life that really works.

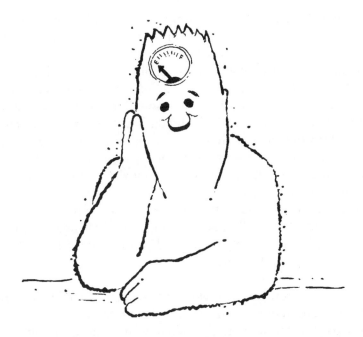

In the first part of this chapter, we have been discussing what to do when you find yourself in a state of overwhelm. We have used different words for this state—*boggle*, *stuckness* and *shutdown*. Perhaps you have never thought in terms of "stuckness" being a problem with overstimulation, but it is. Generally, it happens because there is too much going on in our heads and we are having trouble identifying the pieces and sorting them out. So we can't choose or initiate an action step. In the next section, preventive medicine, we offer strategies for reducing the amount of time you spend in overwhelm, leaving more for taking those forward action steps.

Preventive Medicine (for Staying Out of Overwhelm While Moving Forward)

The Rock-Bottom Plan
Once you have decided to make a major or minor life change, the next step is to design a rock-bottom plan for living. This plan is a simple fallback lifestyle for the times there are lots of to-do's in

your life. Actually, it's an important tool in your box of life strategies even if you are just focused on surviving your everyday life.

Change, of course, always brings some upheaval with it. And life with ADD is rarely smooth sailing. Somehow we have been conned into believing that we "should" be always on top of things and always at our best. If you have been to those seminars and workshops on how to succeed, it can be very intimidating when you compare the how-to instructions to your actual life. They don't say much about dirty laundry and bad brain days, for example. It is then natural to conclude that everybody else bounds out of bed at the crack of dawn, eager to greet a day chock-full of successfully met challenges and productivity. This is simply not true. Even people without ADD have their ups and downs.

Imagine that you have just won an all-expenses-paid trip to the dream location of your choice. The only hitch is that you have to leave tomorrow morning. What would you clear off your schedule today in order to board the plane to paradise on time? Of course, we can hear some of you saying "I would have to drop everything and spend the rest of the day and all night packing . . . and I'm still not sure I could make it." That's the subject of another conversation, but we are all too familiar with ADDult packing challenges.

All right, we'll try another scenario. Your mother is having surgery. You will need to be available to care for her for several days after the operation. What changes do you make to your routine in this case? Carryout food? Paper plates? Do you cancel your usual volunteer activities? What about going to the kids' soccer games? Do you ignore the laundry and dishes piling up as you deal with your mom's needs? Do you let some things slide at work so you can leave a little early?

You can probably do this for your mom, but what about yourself? We know, this one is harder, especially if you aren't having surgery or something that dramatic happening in your life. You are just having a "bad brain day," sort of like a bad hair day only worse. Even with the best of treatment for your ADD, those functional dips do happen.

The key to riding out those less than stellar days is a pre-planned strategy for a modified routine—the rock-bottom plan. Before your next bad brain day, sit down with pencil and paper and design a schedule that eliminates all nonessentials. Keep your list in a handy place so you can just read the directions when you need them—when you are on overload is not the time to be thinking or planning.

We bet that you have had quite a number of these days and that you are not completely unfamiliar with the numbers of the local carryout joints. The difference between what you have done in the past and what we are suggesting you do now is that you may never have taken a guilt-free meltdown day. Instead, you ordered the pizza or slunk off to bed, all the while calling yourself a lazy slacker.

Make no mistake about it, every time you talk to yourself in this way, you set yourself back. The antidote to taking a step back in this way is to reverse your usual standards for yourself. In the infamous words from Despair.com, you are "increasing success by lowering expectations." Consider rock bottom to be your lowest functional point. Any behavior over and above this baseline is cause for congratulations. Avoid defeating yourself by expecting a higher level of functioning at any given time.

Use your "rock-bottom plan" as the baseline that you return to whenever you need it. When you are making changes in your life, start at rock bottom and add things gradually. You'll be amazed at how much simpler a major change can be when you aren't trying to rehab the kitchen, solve the problem of world hunger and write the great American novel all at the same time! Whenever you find that you had been sailing along, but then added so many activities that you got overwhelmed again, start back at rock bottom.

Put Your Own Oxygen Mask on First

Take this little mantra from the airlines and memorize it. Post it on your computer, your bathroom mirror and on the toilet seat. Write it down a thousand times. Whatever it takes to permanently imprint these words on your brain. One of the biggest obstacles to making positive life changes is trying to take care of everybody else. It is just not possible to keep on giving from an empty pot.

Action Steps—Breaking It Down

One of the most common stoppers for our coaching clients is trying to take action steps that are too big. For example, one of Kate's clients (we'll call her Pat) is interested in becoming a coach. Pat has a natural affinity and talent for coaching and has heard a great deal of supportive feedback in the training classes she is enrolled in. Recently, she took a marketing class and was encouraged to write articles, get speaking engagements and develop a Web site. Pat was more than a little freaked out by this advice, as she is currently a homemaker and mom with almost no experience in the world of business. Those particular action steps seemed too big and scary to Pat.

The remedy was to help Pat come up with a smaller step, a baby step if you will. Rather than write an article for publication, she determined that putting some musings down on paper on a particular topic was doable. The next step will be to show those musings to a safe person who will not judge them—her coach!

Sometimes the obstacle to taking certain steps is fear, and sometimes it is being overwhelmed and unsure of where to start. The solution to overwhelm is to break the action down into small steps, with a timeline for the whole project. The timeline, however, should never be set in stone. Forgive the delay or detour and set a new date for the subsequent steps to completion. When a client is unsure of where to start, they usually lack some information about what is involved in a given action. Putting up a Web site is a big project, with multiple steps. There is a learning curve involved and a lot of information to gather before action is taken. As ADDers, many of us carry a lot of shame about our gaps in knowledge. This can make it hard for us to admit that we need help and information.

Crises are nature's way of forcing change.
—Susan Taylor

How Can I Be Sure I Have What It Takes?

You have done a whole lot of work with yourself, to accept your ADD and to clean out much of the mental gunk you accumulated before you understood how ADD affected your life. You now have enough brain space available to actually think about the life changes you want to make. These changes can be little or big, from cleaning out that messy closet to going to school, changing careers, getting married or getting a divorce. Of course, you are the only one who can determine the magnitude of the change you are contemplating. For some of us, the messy closet may be a bigger deal than completing years of school. The apparent size of any project has more to do with the emotional charge associated with it than the actual amount of work needed to complete it. That said, we know that the ADD brain tends to look at a task and do one of two things: (1) think it will be an absolute breeze, because the brain has not really processed all the steps and potential obstacles to be dealt with, or (2) freeze up because the brain has seen all the work involved in the change and thinks it all has to happen *now*.

Moving Forward at the Speed of Light

Of course, many ADDers are not at all reluctant to take action, and to take it swiftly. Many successful entrepreneurs are fast-moving, decisive guys and gals. Those with ADD who use this style effectively tend to have at least one farmer (see Thom Hartmann's *Attention Deficit Disorder: A Different Perception* for a description of farmers) as a key team member to handle the details and ensure that appropriate information is available before a decision is made. Without that balancing factor, ADDers can get in trouble, either on a work project or with relationships with others.

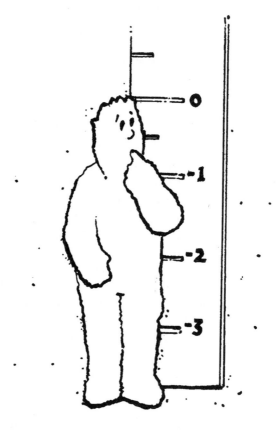

Don't Be Fooled by Appearances—
Even When You Seem to Be Terminally Stuck,
There Is Forward Motion

As you know, computers work on many levels. We can be working on a spreadsheet, for example, while the download function is doing its thing in the background. Our brains can do something similar. When we dream, we are processing and reprocessing the events of our day in order to integrate our experience. We also have unconscious thought processes that go on in the background of waking consciousness.

Even though we have seen sudden shifts in our clients many times, it is always a wonderful gift when a big change seems to come out of left field. They are stuck in the same patterns for quite a while, with seemingly endless repetitions of the old habits. Then one day there is a big aha! The learning is integrated and new ways of behaving appear, as if by magic. The appearance of "stuckness" was just an illusion, as there was steady work going on in the background the entire time.

An experienced coach, however, is never totally shocked by the big shifts. Part of the job is to catch the smaller changes along the way and point them out to the client.

We know from our own lives that the ADD experience is often "as if" one foot is nailed to the floor while we go around in circles with the other. Certainly, we do seem to meet those same life lessons over and over again. But have you ever considered that you may be learning something new each time around? What can seem like movement without progress may actually be just gradual progress.

One of the best ways to visualize this is as a spiral. Sure, we're coming around to a very familiar situation again, but haven't we moved up a level, maybe ever so slightly? What looks like "returning full circle" if we only notice the length and width of our path, becomes a spiral that keeps moving upward with each cycle when we see its height. Like ascending a spiral staircase, we may find that we have been going upward at the same time we were winding around the center.

It is by tiny steps that we ascend the stars.

—Jack Leedstrom

Allow Yourself to Take Baby Steps

One of the biggest obstacles to moving forward is to sabotage yourself by giving up because you are not seeing results as rapidly as you expect. Here comes another coaching commercial: Get a coach who can help you to notice and acknowledge the more subtle positive steps you are taking. He or she has a long-range perspective gained from working with many people who have also traveled a bumpy road. These are folks just like you who have successfully overcome the challenges.

You won't need to sign up for a lifetime of coaching. A good coach will teach you the skills needed to coach yourself.

Say Oops and Then Move On
In Kate's all-time favorite movie, *The Producers* (1967), the opening scene features Zero Mostel as a cheesy, second-rate producer, reduced to wooing little old ladies to get financial backing. He is playing a racy little game with one of his elderly paramours when Gene Wilder walks in on them. Gene, playing an anxious accountant prone to panic attacks, freezes and starts hyperventilating. Zero, in a soothing voice (but with an underlying subtext of menace), talks Gene out of the room. He says, "Oops, just say oops, back out and close the door . . ."

Learning to "just say oops" is not an easy task, but it is essential for successfully moving forward. Years of comments about our *not living up to our potential* leave their marks on our hearts. As adults, we take over where our parents and teachers left off, berating ourselves for every misstep. The way out of the failure cycle is to reset our expectations and give ourselves the permission to be less than perfect. To forgive ourselves. To just say oops. This process often takes a long time. In the beginning, the coach does the forgiving, the client eventually learning the difficult lesson of self-forgiveness. Then, with more realistic expectations, the client is poised to get into action and move forward.

Dark Humor and What We REALLY Think
When you get really fed up with those chipper folks who try to force-feed you that "just do it" nonsense, we suggest that you take a little trip to Despair.com. This Web site offers an abundance of demotivators—motivational products and posters for pessimists, underachievers and the chronically unsuccessful.

Darker humor is a soothing salve for those moments when you wonder if you will ever stop going around in circles.

In the words of thinkrightnow.com, if your mind were a computer, your beliefs would be the operating system. The reason those inspirational posters are so annoying to many of us is that we basically think they are a "crock of s—t." Our true beliefs are reflected in "despairational" slogans like these:

Success—a tiny oasis in a sea of chaos

Failure—is not what you do, it's what you are

Mistakes—the one thing you can count on

Losing—take heart, you can only lose if you were in the game to begin with

Stupidity—thinking that there is any conceivable reason to get out of bed in the morning

Goals—those ridiculous statements you write on Post-its and paper your walls with

Procrastination—what you do to give people the impression that you actually intend to do anything at all

Laziness—if you wait long enough, the items on your "to do" list will become obsolete

Planning—a wildly optimistic vision of what you would like to happen

Success—if at first you don't succeed, start another project

We laugh at this stuff, because, on one level, we think it is ridiculous. On another, however, we know that we actually buy into the ideas behind the joke. How many of us have a core belief that we really are failures, for example. Or that we are not in the game at all, not really a contender.

You Gotta Start Somewhere
(The Couch Potato Shuffle)

Somebody somewhere told us about a doctor who hands out unusual prescriptions to his patients in dire need of exercise. Naturally, these are folks who are also fatally allergic to the very concept of getting up off the couch for any reason. Not because they are lazy, mind you, but because they are terrified of going through repeated episodes of extreme physical and mental misery, leading to yet another dismal failure to follow through.

This enlightened physician tells them that all they have to do is stand in front of the TV and walk in place for five minutes. Anybody can do that, right? (As long as you are ambulatory, anyway.) Sounds ridiculous, doesn't it? The patients are stunned, and then they laugh, and then they go home and do what he says. Wonder of wonders, they often find themselves going for an actual walk after doing that couch potato shuffle—even outdoors!

This is surprising only if you believe that lack of motivation is (a) some incurable disease, or (b) an intractable character flaw. If you have read this book up to this point, we would be surprised if you still bought into "b." As for "a," "low-motivation-itis" is a stubborn virus, but it can be conquered, though not through a head-on confrontational approach. Break up the tasks leading to your goals into microscopic particles, too tiny to scare you. Have a ball making up your versions of the couch potato shuffle.

Paperwork and Other Busywork
(Working with Resistance)

One of the most common problems ADDers struggle with is difficulty in completing paperwork. Many of us do very well with the other aspects of our jobs, but are terrified our supervisor will find out about the mounds of backlogged paperwork we just can't seem to complete. Or our supervisor is all too aware of the problem and is losing patience as the stuff keeps piling up.

Well, of course the paperwork is the last to-do on the list. It is boring, tedious and often downright silly. An awful lot of the documentation we are required to do on the job is the result of overregulation and a "cover your butt" mentality. Our minds naturally are more attracted to more immediate and compelling concerns. The mental hygiene problem in this case is that we make ourselves wrong for the way we are. We decide that there is something wrong with us because we don't just loooove spending hours and hours filling out forms.

We don't have to love it, we don't even have to like it. If your job requires the paperwork and there is no getting around it, it is a matter of setting up a system to get the darn stuff off your desk. Your coach can help with this. The best system in the world, however, will not work if you are struggling with your resistance to doing the job at all. Your resistance has a number of components (we are not going to go into Freud and that kind of resistance):

- Anger at having to do something you really hate to do

- Anger because nobody knows how hard this is for you

- Fear that once you start you will never get to the end of it . . . you will spend eternity in paperwork hell

- Anger because you think the paperwork is really stupid

- Basically, it's "I don't wanna and you can't make me"

And on top of all that, our inner critic is making harsh judgments. Some self-talk snippets include:

- You are such a baby . . . whining about having to do something you don't like

- Just suck it up and do it

- Boy, that "you can't make me" attitude is really mature

- Your attitude is terrible

- It's your own fault—you procrastinated and now you have to pay the consequences

- You deserve to do time in paperwork hell

Do you still wonder why that big pile of paperwork has now become much, much more than a pile of tasks you would rather not do? It has now become a huge psychological mountain you can't imagine scaling. Before you even begin the climb, there is a jungle of thorny vines at the base to hack your way through.

There is, however, a way to get through the thorny section and ascend the mountain.

The first step is to acknowledge that what you are facing is indeed a mountain. It does no good whatsoever to tell yourself that it "shouldn't" be a mountain, because other people do it so easily . . . blah blah.

Honor and respect the journey you are taking to conquer this mountain, because it is not trivial. It is a "hero's journey" to fight your way through all the crap that is holding you back. Once you have learned to use your sword and shield to make your way through the jungle of poisonous thinking in one instance, you will be able to make it through the next obstacle course, and the next . . . until you are home free.

So, how do you hack your way through the jungle and get to the top of that mountain?

424

Know That It *Is* a Mountain

Some of you are now saying, "It feels like a mountain, but that's just plain silly."

No, it's not. It is a mountain because:

- You look at the piles and you are overwhelmed by their size.

- Your mind does not automatically chunk the job down to smaller work bites.

- You see it as a whole big hateful pile of work that you have to do all at once.

- Your inner adolescent rebels.

- When the few pieces of paper have grown into large piles, you have been looking at those same papers for some time.

- While you have been looking at the papers/piles you have been beating yourself up for procrastinating.

- You have tried and failed to tackle those piles many times.

Each time you made up your mind to do the paperwork and then could not make yourself follow through, it reinforced the idea that this job was just too much for you.

You have been calling yourself stupid, lazy and a lot of other unkind names for a long time in relation to that pile of paper.

When you look at the pile now, it represents a lot more than a bunch of work you would prefer not to do.

It is now a big heap of shame, fear, anger and other emotions.

Of course you are stuck! Who wouldn't be, under these circumstances?

Probably you have already experienced some relief as you recognized the painful emotions associated with your paper pile job. Perhaps you shed a tear or two, or spent some time pounding an inanimate object. Congratulations, you have taken a step toward healing the emotional baggage that surrounds your ADD. First you acknowledge that you have the feelings and then you allow them to come out somehow. The hard part is letting yourself have your feelings . . . knowing that you are not just being silly or immature. That you are an earnest soul who has been doing the best you know how.

Treat It Like a Mountain
Realize that you are going to be going uphill.

This is bad news and good news. The bad news is that the grade may be steep and involve some huffing and puffing. On the other hand, aerobic exercise can feel pretty good once you get in the groove. The sitting around doing nothing but worrying how high the mountain is can be a lot more work, stress and strain. So maybe the bad news is really good news. The good news is that you are going up.

Experienced mountaineers may just charge up that mountain if the challenge is not too great and they are in terrific shape.

If, however, you are not in top shape you will need to take it in stages.

- Be sure to take enough snacks and nourishment for the journey

- Sit down and rest when you need it

- Give yourself a big pat on the back at the end of each leg of the journey

- If you get out of breath after going a hundred feet, take a rest and tell yourself you did a good job going that far

In the case of paper piles, you may want actual food-type snacks or it might be some other type of reward. Music is very nourishing to the soul, but sometimes we forget to turn it on. Usually, it is because we don't feel that we have earned the right to be happy. If you still believe that you have to earn happy-making treats (and most of us do), think of it as an incentive plan in reverse order. You give yourself the treat during the job in order to lift your spirits enough to do it at all. Often, you need to give yourself the reward before even starting the job.

KK: "I often give new clients a prescription to do away with their 'to do' list for a few days (or as long as it takes to relax). Their only focus during that time is self-care. They can meditate, listen to music, take a bath—anything that feeds them. Usually they start getting naturally activated even while the prescription is in effect. Taking the 'shoulds' away has an amazing effect."

When you are ready to ascend that mountain, make sure you have the proper gear. Is your chair comfortable? Do you have enough light? Is the music on (or off—your preference)? Have you written reminders to yourself? Such as:

Take a break when you need it.

You are already doing a good job—you are facing your fear and beginning to take the action steps needed to get through your paper pile.

You are allowed to have feelings about doing this job—take a tantrum break if you need it.

And do anything you want for yourself in the way of encouragement.

It is hard to let old beliefs go. They are familiar. We are comfortable with them and have spent years building systems and developing habits that depend on them. Like a man who has worn eyeglasses so long that he forgets he has them on, we forget that the world looks to us the way it does because we have become used to seeing it that way through a particular set of lenses. Today, however, we need new lenses. And we need to throw the old ones away.

—Kenichi Ohmae

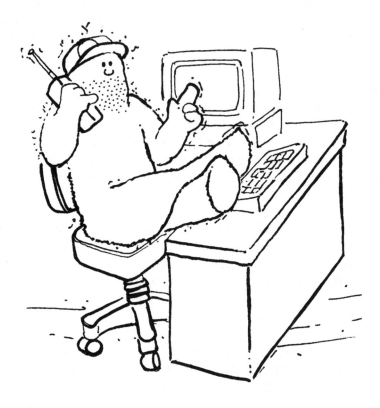

We'd suggest that you pause a moment before continuing to read. Mr. Ohmae's metaphor contains a compelling message, reminding us of a power we often forget—the power to change our feelings by changing our thinking. On those days when you are frustrated, feeling that you will never adequately maintain the forward momentum, take the metaphoric lenses out of your eyeglasses and replace them with a new set, as Mr. Ohmae suggests. Seeing the situation differently expands your thinking so you can consider your situation from a different perspective. And with changed thinking, you will experience changed feelings, fear being a big one that often ties us up in knots.

Fear of Taking Action

Peeling back the layers of the fear that can confront us as we begin moving forward on a significant change in life, we run into some common themes:

> If I take this step it will eventually lead to doing or being something I don't feel ready for.

> If I take this step I will fail . . . again.

> If I take this step (even if I am successful) I will drop the ball later on and fail to follow through.

> If I take this step I will have to make all these other scary changes (doing something my husband/wife doesn't approve of means I will have to get a divorce).

The key to addressing these fears is to remind yourself that you can take a break in the forward action any time you need to. Give yourself time to adjust to each step on the road to your goal and you will be more likely to stay the course.

Beware of Playing the Catch-Up Game

One of the big obstacles to forward motion is the strange notion that we are behind and somehow have to catch up with everyone else. The comparison game, of course, is always a losing proposition. Without exception, if you look around you will find people who seem to be doing better than you are. Why do we want to engage in a surefire losing proposition anyway?

The backlog of all those half-done, not-good-enough efforts from the past can drag your current projects down so heavily that they come to a standstill, relegated to the slush pile once more. This happens because the new project has too many expectations attached to it. We are trying too hard to prove that we are really okay. No matter how spectacular our work in progress is, it can't make up for all the things we didn't do, or did poorly in the past. Take another look at the section called "Toxic Mental Debris: The Vicious Cycle of Shame, Perfectionism and Procrastination" at the end of the mental hygiene chapter for more on this one.

Follow-Through and Accountability

We bet that the mere mention of those words sends shivers up your spine. You envision a sadistic slave master who is giving you the lash as, once more, you confess that the dog ate your homework. When you have been "guilted" for most of your life, eventually guilt loses its power as a motivator. It wasn't a great strategy to begin with, but once upon a time it may have set you in motion, after a rather miserable fashion. Now, you still get to feel rotten, but your butt refuses to unstick itself from the chair when you are made to feel guilty. Sometimes it is you who is doing the guilt tripping and sometimes it is somebody "out there." Either way, guilt is worse than useless—it is a demotivator that contributes to backward motion.

Still, we can't avoid those follow-through actions if we want to make progress toward goals. The key to success in developing follow-through skills is to keep practicing them, without making yourself wrong when the actions don't quite match your intentions in the beginning. We don't recommend that you try to go it alone. It is all too easy to slide into old patterns of beating yourself up in the privacy of your thoughts. A good ADD coach can help you by continually reminding you of your goals and intentions, while at the same time asking the right questions to discover the things that are stopping you from taking action. Your "failures" to follow through are then simply viewed as clues that will lead the way to solutions.

Using Play to Boost Productivity

The reason we have such an aversion to work is that there is not enough play in it. Really. The people who told you that you are an adult now and it's time to put the toys away and get to work were just plain wrong. Think about some of the most dysfunctional working environments in existence. Not only are they unbearably grim, but they tend to put the brakes on actual output. Why do you suppose there are so many reports in the news about going postal? And then we have the IRS, which hounds the poor wage-slave but can't keep its own house in order.

We have worked for "the man" in employee situations and we also have logged many years in self-employment. Our most productive work environments included a liberal dose of fun. Without it, those creative juices just evaporate. You don't have to be a painter, dancer or writer to be creative, by the way. Anything we do can be improved when we flex those muscles that produce novel solutions. You may need to use stealth if your workplace is very repressive. If anything except following orders is forbidden, find ways to doodle in the margins of your binder, so to speak. Or better still, look for a more congenial way to earn your paycheck.

A User-Friendly Life?

It is time to wrap this chapter up. Perhaps you wondered exactly where it was we were going with all this talk about the things that get in the way of forward motion. There is a point to all this—honest! When we wrote the first edition of the "lazy crazy" book, the final chapter was called "From Obstacle to Opportunity," and it was filled with stories about ADDults who were living joyful lives that were a good fit for their unique selves. It was written fourteen years ago, when we were blissfully unaware of just how much housecleaning it would take before our own dreams would be realized. We have both been through a divorce since then, and a number of other difficult transitions that sometimes made it seem as if there would never be any real forward progress in our lives. We are intimately acquainted with the thoughts and beliefs that can get in the way. We also know, without a doubt, that it is possible to make your way to success from some very stuck and seemingly hopeless places. We know this because we are advanced students in the School of Hard Knocks. It doesn't do any good to present a Pollyannaish view of all the wonderful ADD characteristics.

We can't tell you exactly where you are going. That depends on your dreams and your personal value system. As coaches, we would ask you the questions to help you uncover the "what" and the "why" of your personal vision. With that picture firmly in mind, we would help you to navigate your chosen path, teaching you the tools that you can use to move yourself in the direction you desire. This chapter, of course, is just a snapshot of the stoppers and work-arounds that would be discussed in a coaching relationship. That's why we strongly urge you to work with a coach. We can deal with generalities in a book but not the specifics of your situation.

Success is achieved when you figure out what you were born to do and fashion a lifestyle that enables you to do it.

If we were to make a statement that applies to all of us it would be this: We want to design and live a user-friendly life. One that uses the gifts (strengths) we have and doesn't require us to spend a whole lot of time doing things that are a struggle. Your job, your relationships, leisure-time lifestyle . . . all of it needs to come up for review and revision.

If you take the "dis" out of disabilities, you will find abilities.

Lest you think that the whole purpose of ADD recovery and self-help is to banish all those embarrassing differences, consider this phrase from the fellowship of Alcoholics Anonymous: *God doesn't make junk.*

We firmly believe that there are positive uses for every seemingly strange talent, trait and "symptom." It is often a matter of first accepting ourselves and then rearranging how our differences are used to come up with a formula that works. Read our second book, *The ADDed Dimension,* for more perspective on the positive side of the ADD experience.

We challenge you to work hard at your recovery. We challenge you to set aside your defenses and squarely face the reality of your ADD. We challenge you to use your self-knowledge to work on the weaknesses that have a negative impact on your recovery. Most of all, we challenge you to celebrate your unique gifts and talents.

Never lose sight of the many gifts you possess! We truly believe that ADD is more than just a disability . . .

It is also an ADDed Dimension!

Epilogue

Imagine a world without ADD.

We invite you to glimpse such a futuristic world created by the imaginative mind of our colleague, Darlene Contadino of Cincinnati, Ohio.

Thank you for your insights, Darlene, and for your permission to include your essay in our work.

We think it is a compelling conclusion for this book . . .

Galaxy 298	Planet Press	May 10, 2390

Scientists Debating Wisdom of TNT Gene Removal

Dr. Smarty is credited with the original discovery in 2275 of the elusive TNT gene that caused impulsivity, distractibility and poor reinforceability. The discovery of this gene and the subsequent development of a surgical procedure to remove it from patients constituted a major scientific breakthrough.

With this discovery scientists made great strides in eliminating most maladaptive behaviors. But in a recent Gene Removal Conference, scientists from around the galaxy gathered to debate the wisdom of the decades-old TNT gene removal project.

The original discovery was welcomed by people everywhere. Society did not know what to do with people who were born with this gene. Many of these people failed to contribute to the goals of the community, refusing to attend the Intergalactic Training Academy and never fulfilling their responsibilities in society. Half the people in our prisons exhibited these maladaptive behaviors as did some who were addicted to illegal drugs and alcohol.

Therefore it was reasoned that if the gene that caused these dysfunctional behaviors could be eliminated, these people would be relieved of their suffering and society as a whole would greatly benefit. So the Gene Removal Project was undertaken in 2290 to eliminate this troublesome gene from the Galaxy's populations.

Initially this appeared to be a wise decision. Fewer schoolchildren displayed behavior and learning problems. No longer inattentive, they readily acquired great knowledge. Eliminating the insatiability of these children caused a significant reduction in the rates of juvenile delinquency because these individuals were no longer driven to seek out adventures.

But as a fourth generation of children whose TNT genes were surgically removed reach maturity, some rather disturbing facts can no longer be ignored. It was largely unnoticed in the early stages of the Gene Removal Project that scientific research and discovery have gradually slowed and come to a virtual standstill. Without the insatiable curiosity to drive the scientific process, increasing numbers of scientists have become content with the status quo. Only now are people in our society becoming aware of the glaring absence of new scientific and medical discoveries since the project began.

There has been a parallel decrease in the numbers of new developments in business and industry. It is now hypothesized that when impulsivity was erased, people were no longer capable of taking risks. Virtually no new management systems have been introduced since the project began. The technology used today has evolved little from that used many years ago.

There appears to be yet another troubling by-product of the TNT Gene Removal Project. Many members of our society at large report a general discontent with their lives and the communities in which they live. Paralleling the elimination of impulsivity, spontaneity seems to have disappeared from their lives. There is no more adventure. The lives of many people in our society are well planned but mundane—it has been many years since anyone has climbed a mountain or explored a cave.

The worlds of literature, art and music also appear to have suffered. Since the elimination of distractibility, people have not been compelled to write imaginative poetry, paint the colors of a sunset or compose beautiful songs.

It is impossible to ignore the benefits enjoyed by our society in the years since the removal of the TNT gene. Without the troubling maladaptive behaviors caused by this gene, life has become significantly more orderly. But the behavior of many of our citizens is beginning to resemble that of computer robots.

The recently held meeting was to study the data compiled in the years since the project began. The questions raised at the Gene Removal Conference can be summarized as follows:

"Has Science created efficient machines, lacking in creativity and initiative? Has Society killed personality in the name of order?"

The scientists in attendance were in unanimous agreement that the answer to these questions is "Yes." It was noted in the records of the proceedings that the Gene Removal Project may have had some unexpected negative results and that future scientists might at some point choose to revisit the decision.

This journalist is concerned that a third more important issue was not raised:

"How can we put the gene back?"

Unfortunately even the brightest of our scientists appear satis-fied to inquire no further than simply to review and comment on existing data, so things are unlikely to change in the foresee-able future.

After all, there is no one with the passion and imagination to ask the questions . . .

Web-Based Resources

Nonprofit Organizations

add.org—National ADDA. The first national organization for adults with ADD. Annual conference, teleclasses, articles, personal stories, interviews with ADD professionals, book reviews and links to other ADD-related sites.

addresources.org—Free articles, National ADHD Service Provider Directory, telecourses, links to a hundred related sites and a list of Washington State support groups. A lending library is available to members.

chadd.org—CHADD (Children and Adults with Attention-Deficit/Hyperactivity Disorder) is a nonprofit organization that offers information to parents, educators, professionals, the media and the general public.

Coaching and Coach Training

addcoach.com—Home of the Optimal Functioning Institute. Offers comprehensive ADD coach training, books and resources.

addcoachacademy.com—The ADD Coach Academy (ADDCA) Coach Training Program offers long-distance training to new and experienced coaches.

addcoaching.com—Web site for information on awesome coaching from Kate Kelly, Peggy Ramundo or one of their associates. ADD coach training program.

flylady.net—A personal online coach to help you regain control of house and home.

americoach.org—American Coaching Association. Founded with the goal of making individualized coaching available to everyone who may desire it.

powersystemscoach.com—A collaborative team approach to ADD coaching. Home of the powersystems planner.

Women with ADD

ADDvance.com—Internationally recognized authors Patricia O. Quinn, M.D., and Kathleen Nadeau, Ph.D., answer questions for parents, adults, teens and professionals. Online resources for women and girls with ADD.

ncgiadd.org—Web site for National Center for Gender Issues and ADHD. NCGI was founded by Patricia Quinn, M.D., and Kathleen Nadeau, Ph.D., to promote awareness, advocacy and research on AD/HD in women and girls.

SariSolden.com—Web site hosted by the author of *Women with Attention Deficit Disorder.* Features include articles, discussion board and resources.

General

ADD.about.com—A family-oriented site with an abundance of information ranging from recommendations on books and tapes to articles on alternative treatments and how to help your child organize for school in the morning.

addforums.com—Online Web community for adults, teens and parents.

adhdnews.com—Offers periodic newsletters with information on the research and treatment of ADHD, online support, announcements and resources.

additudemag.com—A subscription-based magazine. Information and inspiration for adults and kids with ADD.

drhallowell.com—A Web site hosted by the Hallowell Center, featuring articles, links, referral assistance and a message board.

thomhartmann.com/home-add.shtml—a Web site for parents and professionals hosted by a well-known ADHD author. Features include articles, discussion board and resources.

Online ADD Store . . . and More

addconsults.com—A virtual online ADHD clinic. Browse the store for ADD-friendly products. Talk one-on-one with experts. Get help finding an ADD-savvy professional. Online conferences, workshops and directories are also available.

Motivation and Demotivation

Despair.com—If you are in need of a good chuckle, this is the place to go. They describe themselves as a motivational Web site for pessimists, underachievers and the chronically unsuccessful.

Suggested Reading

Books you may find helpful:

Adamec, Christine. *Moms with ADD*. Dallas: Taylor Trade Publishing, 2000.

Amen, Daniel. *Healing the Hardware of the Soul*. New York: Free Press, 2002.

———. *Windows into the ADD Mind*. Newport Beach, Calif.: Mindworks Press, 1997.

Andrews, Joan, and Denise Davis. *ADD Kaleidoscope*. Duarte, Calif.: Hope Press, 1997.

Brown, Lisa Blakemore. *Reweaving the Autistic Tapestry*. London: Jessica Kingsley Publishing, 2001.

Brown, Thomas. *Attention Deficit Disorders and Comorbidities in Children, Adolescents and Adults*. Arlington, Va.: American Psychiatric Association, 2000.

———. *Attention Deficit Disorder: The Unfocused Mind in Children and Adults*. New Haven: Yale University Press, 2005.

Carson, Richard. *Taming Your Gremlin*. New York: Harper Collins, 2003.

Friends in Recovery. *The Twelve Steps: A Guide for Adults with Attention Deficit Disorder.* Centralia, Wash.: RPI Publishing, 1996.

Glovinsky, Cindy. *Making Peace with the Things in Your Life.* New York: St. Martin's Press, 2002.

Goleman, Daniel. *Emotional Intelligence.* New York: Bantam, 1997.

Hallowell, Edward. *Worry.* New York: Ballantine, 1998.

Hallowell, Edward, and John Ratey. *Delivered from Distraction.* New York: Ballantine, 2005.

Halverstadt, Jonathan. *ADD and Romance.* Dallas: Taylor Trade Publishing, 1998.

Hartmann, Thom. *Attention Deficit Disorder: A Different Perception.* Grass Valley, Calif.: Underwood, 1997.

————. *Beyond ADD: Hunting for Reasons in the Past or Present.* Grass Valley, Calif.: Underwood, 1996.

Hartmann, Thom, and Richard Brandler. *Healing ADD.* Novato, Calif.: Underwood-Miller, 1998.

Hill, Robert W., and Eduardo Castro. *Getting Rid of Ritalin: How Neurofeedback Can Successfully Treat ADD Without Drugs.* Charlottesville, Va.: Hampton Roads Publishing Company, 2002.

Jamison, Kay Redfield. *An Unquiet Mind: A Memoir of Moods and Madness.* New York: Vintage, 1997.

Kelly, Kate, and Peggy Ramundo. *The ADDed Dimension.* New York: Scribner, 1997.

Kennedy, Diane. *The ADHD Autism Connection.* Colorado Springs: WaterBrook Press, 2002.

Kohlberg, Judith, and Kathleen Nadeau. *ADD Friendly Ways to Organize Your Life.* New York: Brunner-Routledge, 2002.

Latham, Pat, and Peter Latham. *Attention Deficit Disorder and the Law.* Washington, D.C.: R.K.L. Communications, 1997.

Ledingham, D. Stephen. *The Scoutmaster's Guide to Attention Deficit Disorder.* Cincinnati: PositivePeoplePress, 1994.

Mate, Gabor. *Scattered.* New York: Plume Books, 2000.

Matlin, Terry. *Survival Tips for Women with AD/HD.* Plantation, Fla.: Specialty Press, 2005.

Miller, David, and Kenneth Blum. *Overload: Attention Deficit Disorder and the Addictive Brain.* New York: Andrews McMeel Publishing, 1996.

Nadeau, Kathleen, ed., *A Comprehensive Guide to ADD in Adults.* New York: Taylor & Francis Group, 1995.

Nadeau, Kathleen G., and Patricia O. Quinn, eds. *Gender Issues and AD/HD: Research, Diagnosis and Treatment.* New York: Taylor and Francis Group, 1995.

————. *Understanding Women with AD/HD.* Altamonte Springs, Fla.: Advantage Books, 2002.

Novotni, Michele, and Randy Petersen. *What Does Everybody Else Know That I Don't?* Plantation, Fla.: Specialty Press, 1999.

Quinn, Patricia O., Nancy A. Ratey, and Theresa L. Martland. *Coaching College Kids with AD/HD.* Altamonte Springs, Fla.: Advantage Books, 2000.

Ratey, John. *A User's Guide to the Brain*. New York: Vintage USA, 2002.

Ratey, John, and Catherine Johnson. *Shadow Syndromes: Recognizing and Coping with the Hidden Psychological Disorders That Can Influence Your Behavior and Silently Determine the Course of Your Life*. New York: Bantam, 1998.

Richardson, Wendy. *The Link Between ADD and Addiction*. Colorado Springs: Navpress, 1997.

———. *When Too Much Is Not Enough*. Colorado Springs: Pinon Press, 2005.

Ross, Julia. *The Mood Cure*. New York: Penguin, 2003.

Solden, Sari. With foreword by Edward Hallowell. *Journeys Through ADDulthood*. New York: Walker & Company, 2004.

———. *Women with Attention Deficit Disorder*. Grass Valley, Calif.: Underwood, 1995.

Weiss, Lynn. *ADD and Creativity*. Dallas: Taylor Trade Press, 1997.

Of course, new books about ADD will just keep popping up. For an up-to-date reading list, please visit us at addcoaching.com.

INDEX

445

Prozac, 377
psychologists, 99–100
psychotherapy, 106–7

QEEG, 101
quiet zones, 213
Quinn, Patricia O., 230, 242–43, 346

random access memory (RAM), 63–64
Ratey, John, 101, 378–79
reaction time, 56–58, 66
reading skills, 163
recovery:
    acceptance and, 113–16
    balance and, 117–19
    balance inventory and, 124
    complexity of, 341–42
    definition of, 104
    depression and, 111–13
    goal of, 124, 432–33
    grief process in, 106–10
    hitting rock bottom and, 118, 413–15
    self-evaluation and, 128–33
    "should-do's" and "must-do's," 134–38
    social benefits of, 121
    twelve-step programs and, 121–24
    see also treatment
reframing, 390, 396, 428–29
registration, memory and, 62–63
rehearsal, memory and, 62–63
relationships, 62–63
    dating, 194–200
    descriptions of, 153–54,

165–68, 194–98, 200–207, 208–11
    feedback and, 163–64
    in groups, 153–65
    impaired social skills and, 68–70
    one-on-one, 165–72
    survival tips for, 159–65, 168–72, 176–87, 198–200, 211–16
    at workplace, 173–93
    see also communication; family relationships; speech
relaxation, in meditation, 329, 332
relaxation, techniques for, 309
religion, 140–41
remedial writing classes, 182
reminder lists, 292
rest and relaxation zones, 212–13
retrieval, of memory, 65–66
return address stamps, 275
"revolutionary bed ejector," 137
Richardson, Wendy, 360
risk taking:
    in adolescence, 73–75, 235
    in adulthood, 48
    childhood accidents and, 48
    as defense mechanism, 73–75
    sexual, 234–36
Ritalin, 47, 55, 86, 110, 351, 352, 355, 359, 369–70
rock-bottom plan, 413–15
role-playing, sexual, 252
rote memorization, 63, 65, 312–13
Rotz, Roland, 383

watches, waterproof and alarm,
293–94
"we," "me" and, 199
week-at-a-glance planners,
290–91
weekly schedules, 126
Wellbutrin, 245, 249, 376
What Drives Me the Craziest list,
267–68
When Too Much Is Not Enough
(Richardson), 360
"who cares" attitude, 78–80, 82
Wilder, Gene, 420
will, paralysis of, 56
see also mental fatigue
withdrawal, as defense mechanism, 82–83
Witness, The, 390–93, 395
women:
ADD and, 230–44
hormones and, 231–32
as household managers, 236–38
language of men vs., 145
learned helplessness and,
87–88
as parents of ADD children,
238–39
self-blame in, 239
self-esteem in, 233–34
sexual risk taking in, 234–36
*Women with Attention Deficit Dis-
order* (Solden), 236
work, 118
choice and change of, 139,

187–90
difficulties in, 37–38
inner circle at, 178–79
medication and, 185
noise, doors and telephones
at, 183–85
office equipment and, 181–82
office management and,
272–74
productivity and, 402–4
rules and, 176–79
self-employment, 191–92
selling your ideas at, 177–78
social relationships and,
173–93
stress and, 185, 403–4
technology and communica-
tion at, 179–82
temporary, 192
written communication at,
182
workaholism, 18, 119
"work details," 224, 229
working (immediate) memory,
63–64, 301
Wright, Sarah, 383
written communication, 182,
323

yellow pages, personal, 282
you-messages, 170

Zametkin, Alan, 231
Zoloft, 246

About the Authors

Kate Kelly, M.S.N., A.C.T., is one of the pioneers in the field of adult ADD. She is coauthor of *You Mean I'm Not Lazy, Stupid or Crazy?!* and *The ADDed Dimension.* Her background includes experience as a nurse/therapist, college educator and coordinator for psychobiological research. Currently, Kate is an ADD life coach, and founder of the ADDed Dimension Coaching Group. She is a nationally recognized speaker and workshop leader. Even more important than her professional credentials is the fact that Kate is an ADD adult herself. She feels that she learned much more from experiencing life with a hidden disability than she ever did in school. Kate lives in Cincinnati with her partner, Paul, and their two kitties, Luna and Helios.

Peggy Ramundo, B.S., A.C.T., is an educator by background who has been working in the field of ADD for eighteen years. Nationally known for her work with ADD children, adolescents and adults, she is currently in private practice as an ADD coach. Peggy is the coauthor of two books for adults with ADD, *You Mean I'm Not Lazy, Stupid or Crazy?!* and *The ADDed Dimension.* She cofounded the Attention Deficit Disorder Council of Greater Cincinnati, and was lead instructor for the Optimal Functioning Institute (for ADD coach training). Peggy is currently a senior staff member of the ADDed Dimension Coaching Group, as well as a seasoned speaker and workshop leader. In her spare time (what?), she is an avid collector of all things antique, and has a passion for animals. Peggy is also the proud parent of two adult ADD children.